The NEW Me

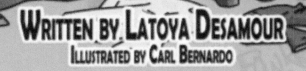

WRITTEN BY LATOYA DESAMOUR
ILLUSTRATED BY CARL BERNARDO

Ordering Information:
Quantity sales. Special discounts are available on quantity purchases
by corporations, associations, and others. For details, contact
the publisher at the web address below.
Printed in the United States of America.

www.LatoyaDesamour.com

ISBN 978-1979184663

Library of Congress Number: 2017916768
First Edition

Acknowledgements: Thank you to Janet Caruthers for being my mentor.
Your assistance with developing extended resources is invaluable to student success.
To my husband Clef, thank you for always believing in and supporting my passions.

For D6
-L.D.

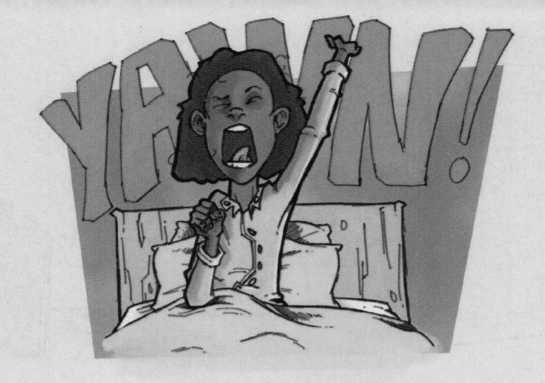

WAKE UP IN THE MORNING,
IT'S TIME TO GO.

WILL THIS DAY BE AWESOME,
OR ONLY SO-SO?

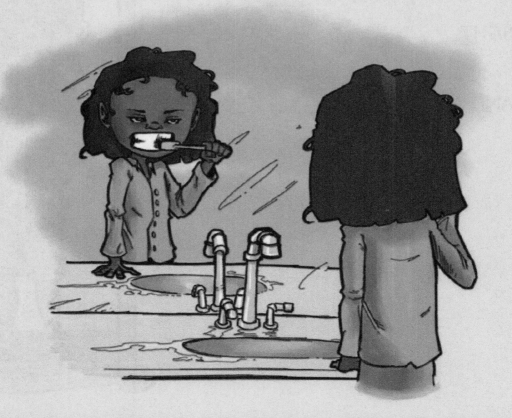

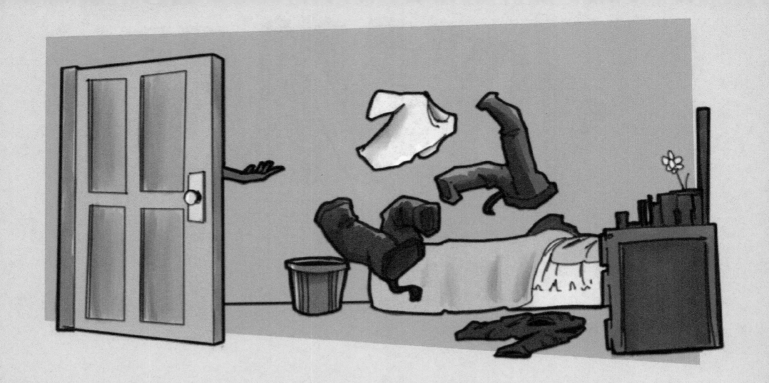

For nine years straight, I have done what I was told.
But today is the day I'd break my mold.

Starting out fine with a FUNKY HAIRDO

Some bright PINK SOCKS

AND A TEMPORARY TATTOO.

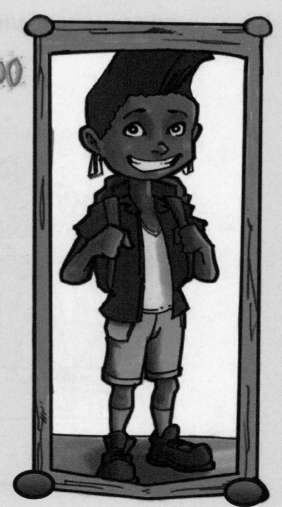

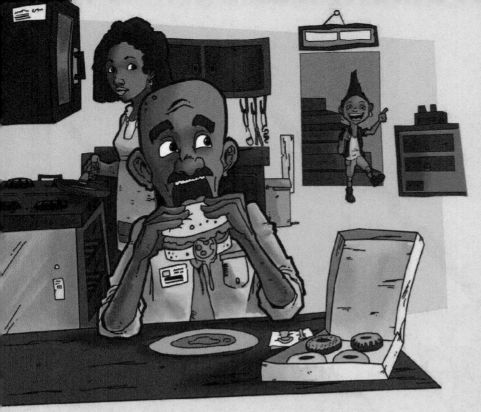

"No toast for me; I'm living ON THE EDGE,"

I told my mom as I grabbed a donut instead.

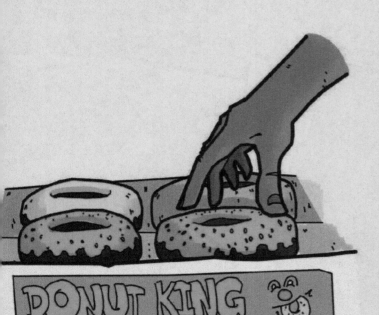

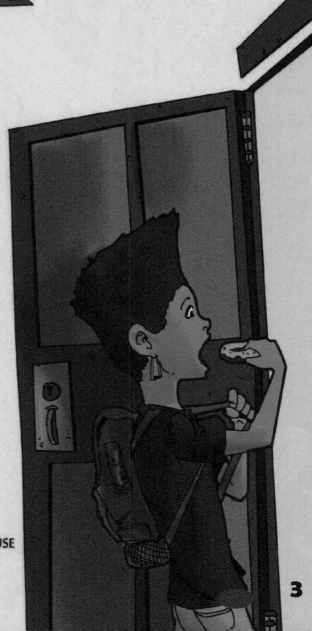

"I'm free; I'm nine; and I'll do as I please,"

I said to my dad who looked quite displeased.

But they uttered not a word as I walked out of the house

In my yellow tank top and open black blouse.

3

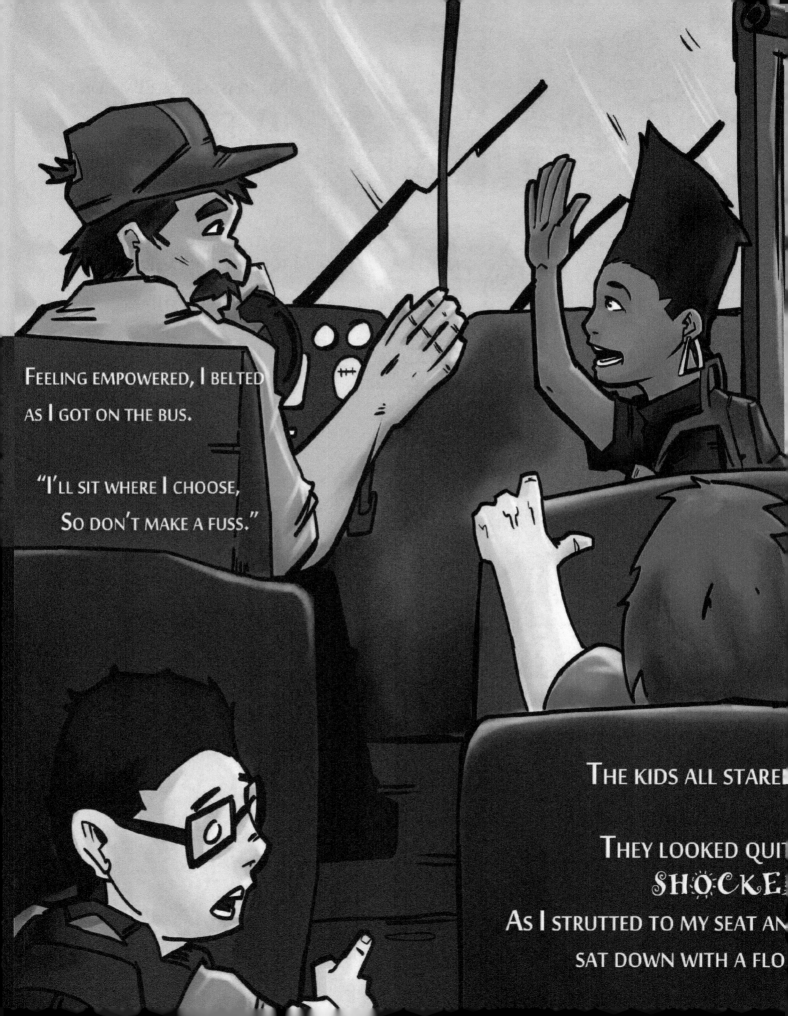

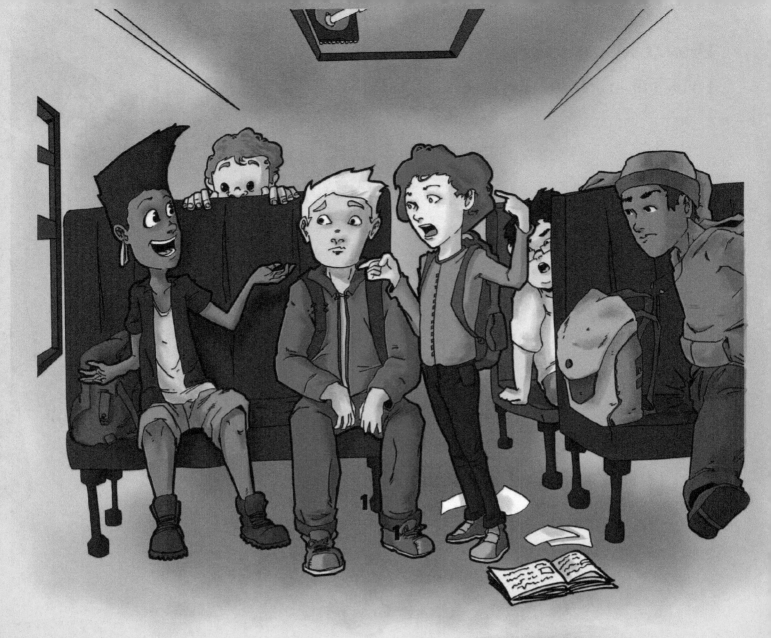

RIDING TO SCHOOL,
I FELT THIS DAY WOULD BE FINE

EVERYONE WOULD LIKE THE NEW ME,

A BURST OF SUNSHINE.

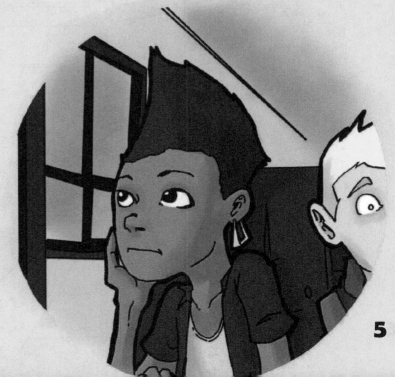

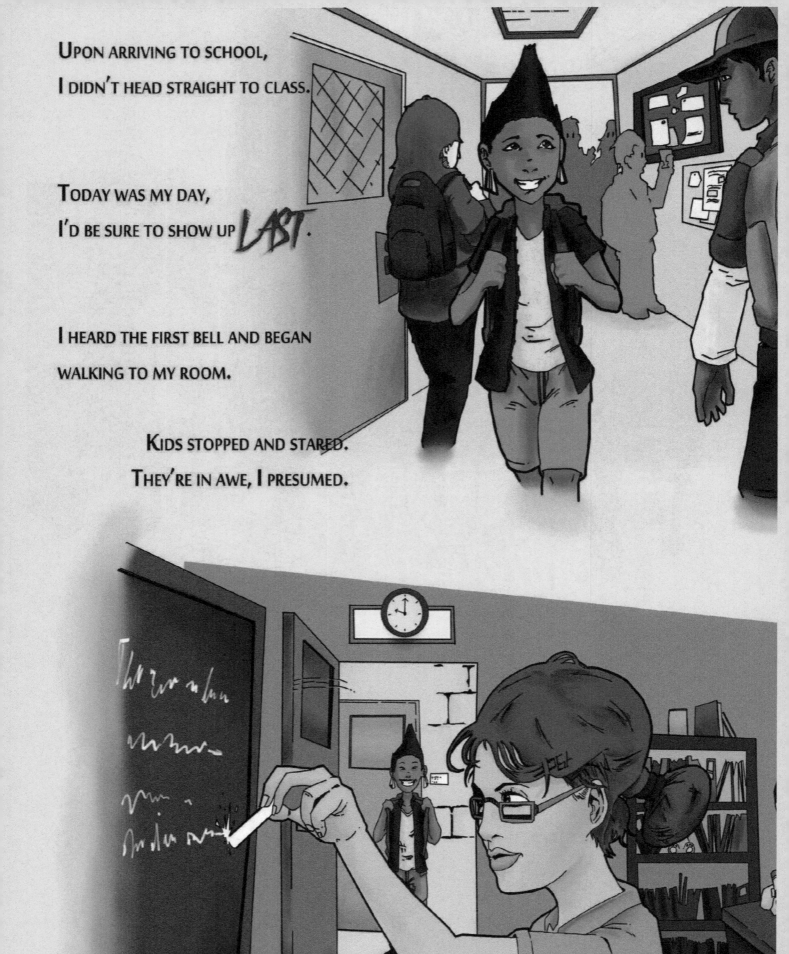

Upon arriving to school,
I didn't head straight to class.

Today was my day,
I'd be sure to show up *LAST*.

I heard the first bell and began
walking to my room.

Kids stopped and stared.
They're in awe, I presumed.

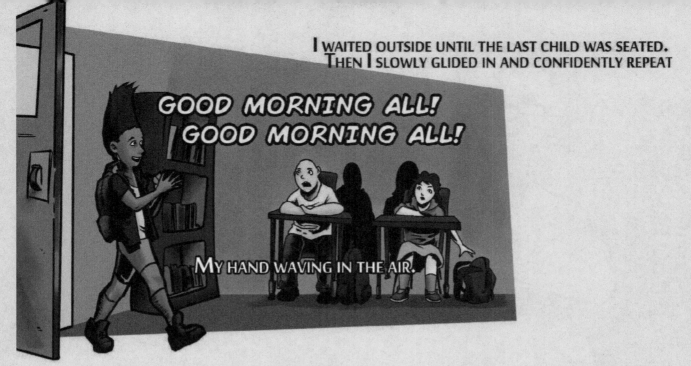

"Good morning, Hannah.

WHAT ON EARTH HAPPENED TO YOUR HAIR?"

My teacher exclaimed, curious as ever.

I declared, "Why Ms. Burns, it's the new me.

Is it not clever?"

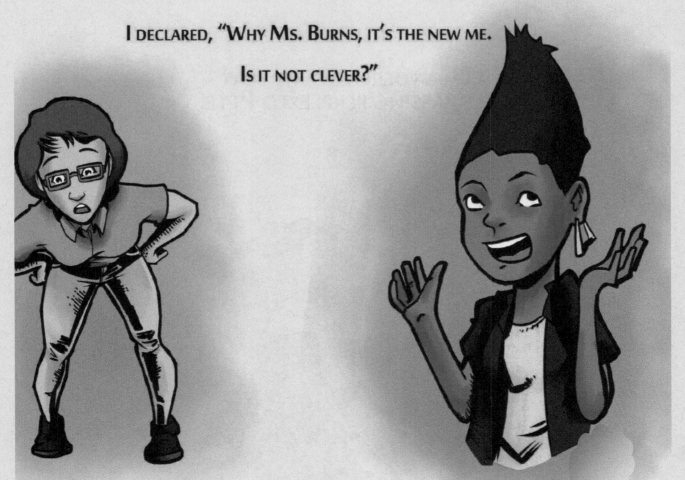

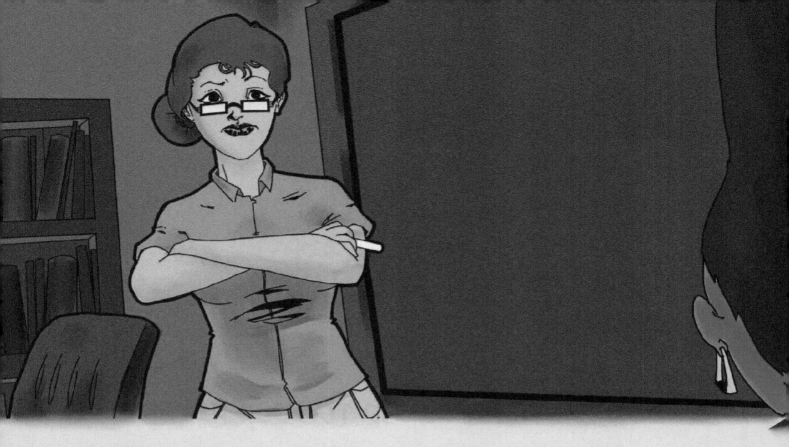

THE EXPRESSION ON HER FACE SEEMED TO DISAGREE.

SO I WANDERED TO MY SEAT
WHILE PASSING PERPLEXED PETE.

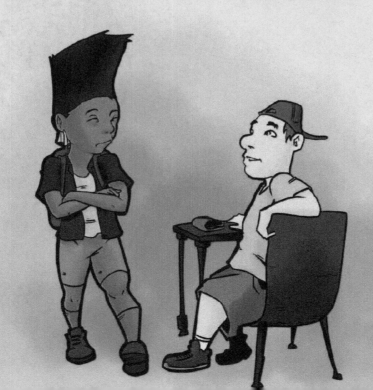

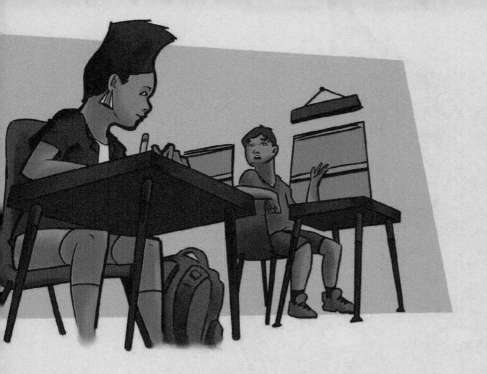

While sitting in my chair,
    I kept myself busy

By twirling my pencil
    Which made me half DIZZY.

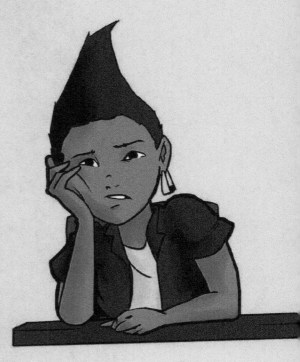

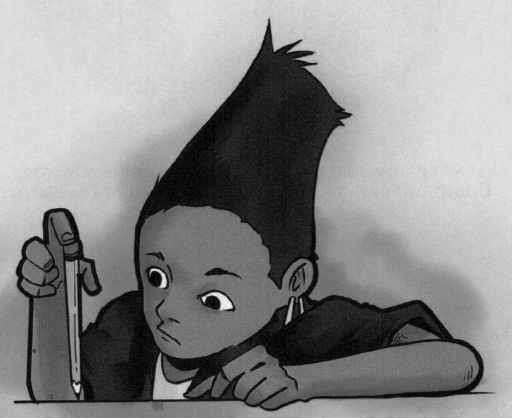

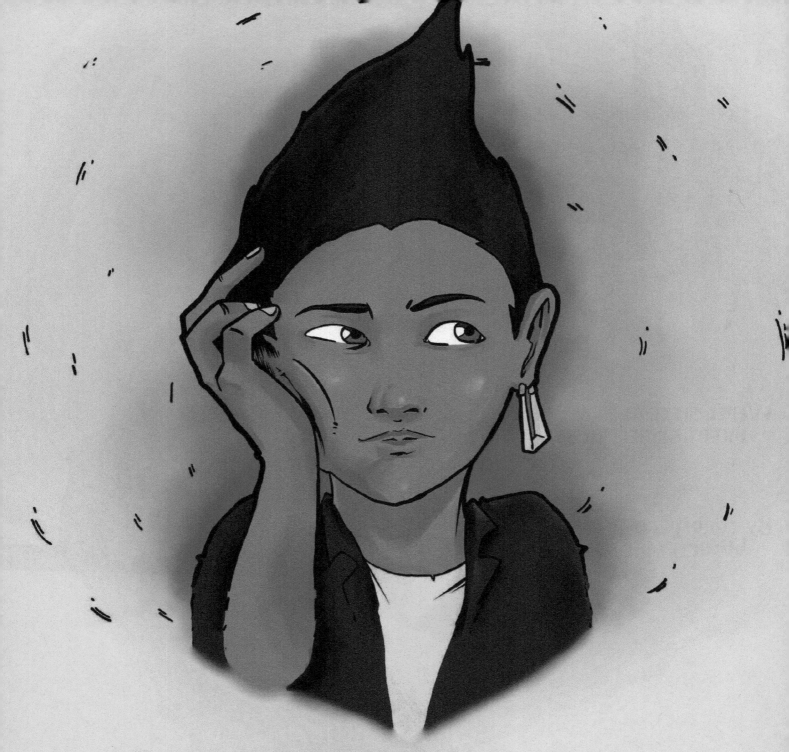

I'M NOT PAYING ATTENTION, AND I'M NOT DOING ANY WORK.
COULD THIS DAY GET ANY BETTER? I THOUGHT AS I SMIRKED.

THIS TUESDAY WAS MY DAY.
MY DAY OF TRANSFORMATION.

THE OLD, SIMPLE ME WAS ON A MUCH NEEDED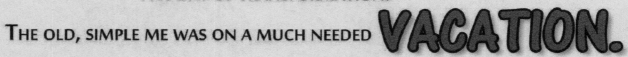

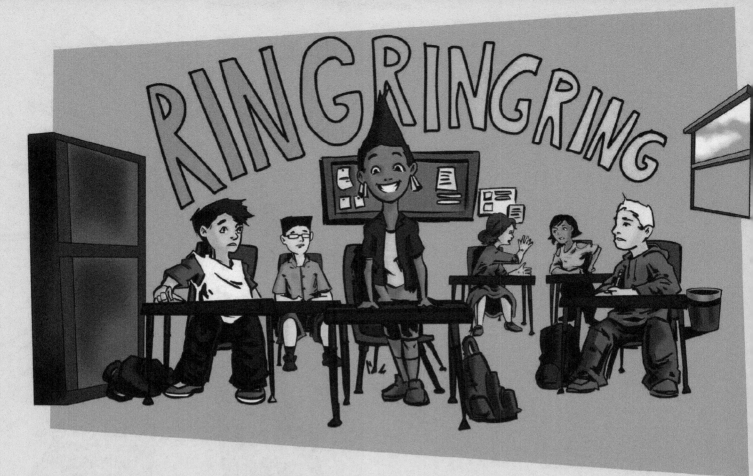

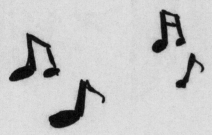

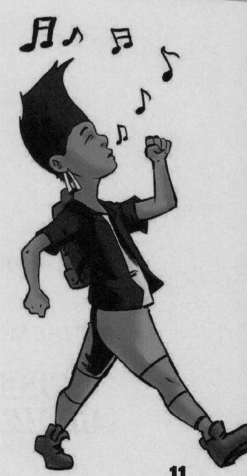

ALAS, THE BELL **RANG** AND I WAS OFF TO EAT.

TODAY I'LL SIT WITH THE **COOL PEOPLE**,

NOT MY USUAL PEEPS.

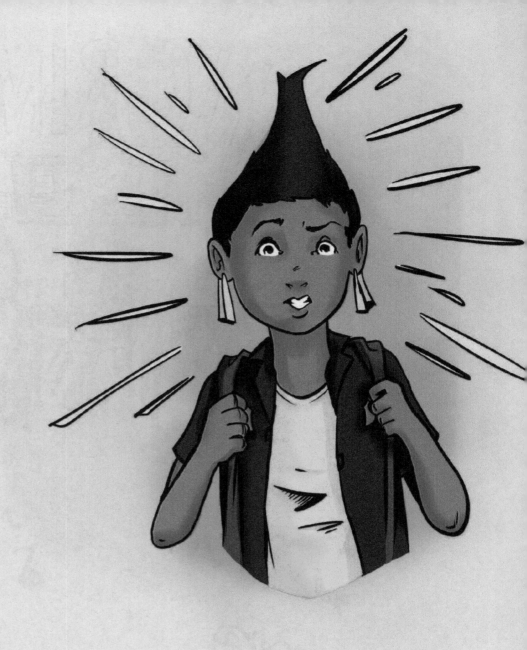

I'LL BE HIP.

   I'LL BE HOT.

I'LL BE THE MOST AWESOME GIRL THEY'LL SEE,

ONCE THOSE POPULAR KIDS FINALLY GET A FRESH LOOK AT THE NEW ME.

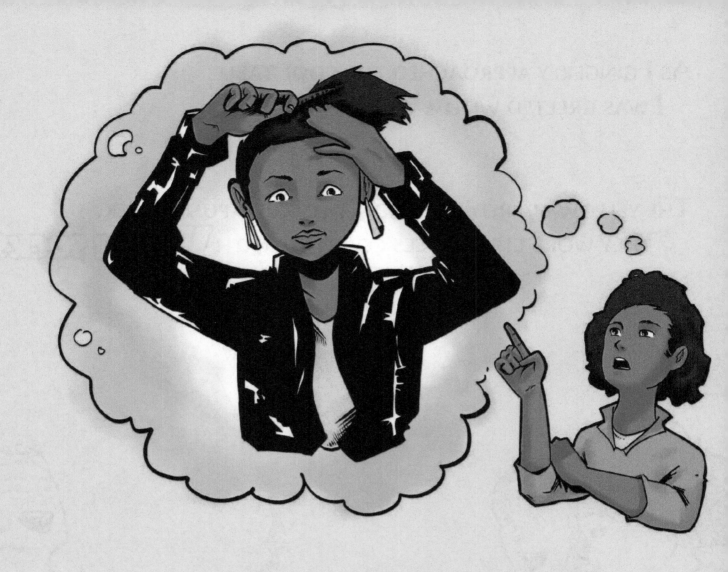

I KNOW BEING DIFFERENT IS THE ONLY WAY TO GO.
THE OLD PERFECT HABITS, I HAD TO **OUTGROW**.

I'M TIRED OF BEING PERFECT.
AND I'M TIRED OF BEING SMART.

AFTER TODAY, I'D GET A WHOLE NEW START.

As I gingerly approached the cool table,
I was greeted with a SHOCK.

The yellow-haired kids didn't look so punk-rock.
They wore classic tees complete with **WHITE SOCKS**!

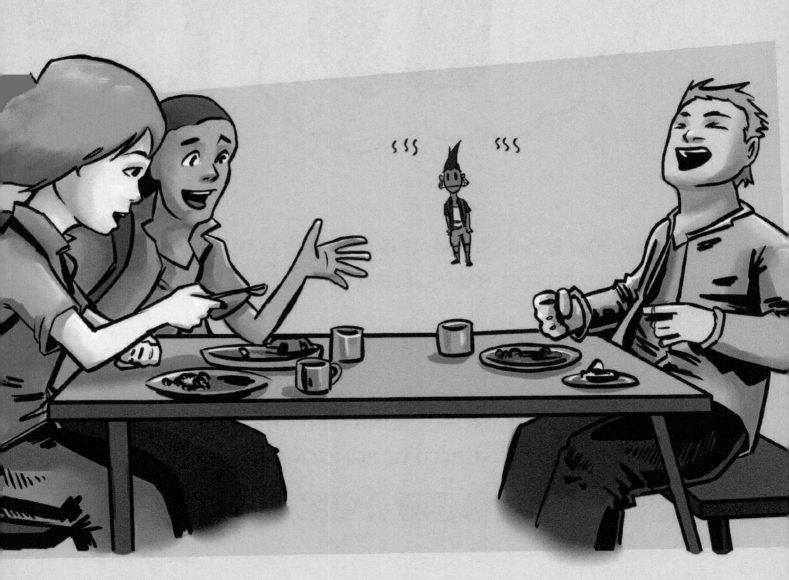

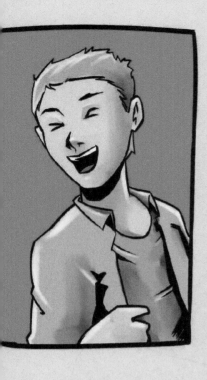
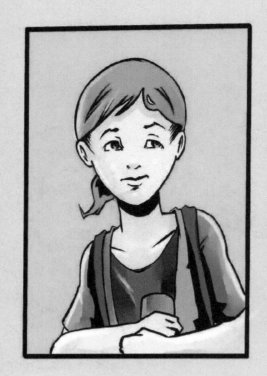
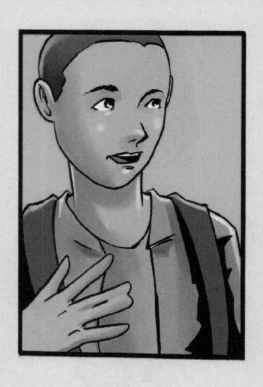

"WHAT'S GOING ON HERE?"

I ASKED THEM TO SHARE.

"WE JUST WANTED TO FIT IN, TO WEAR WHAT YOU WEAR,"

THEY ALL MURMURED SHEEPISHLY AS I CONTINUED TO STARE.

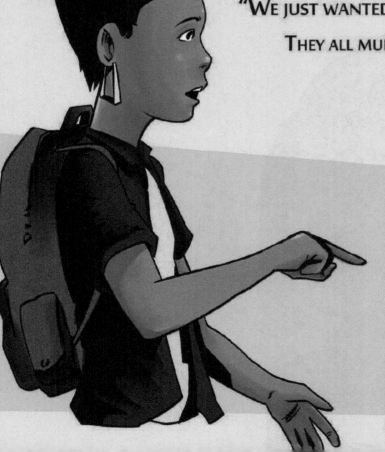
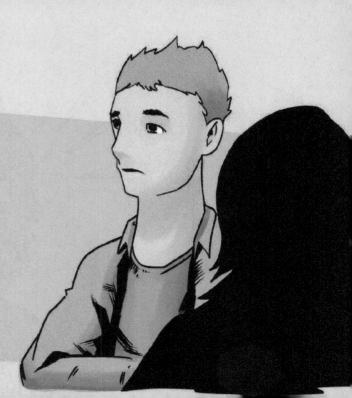

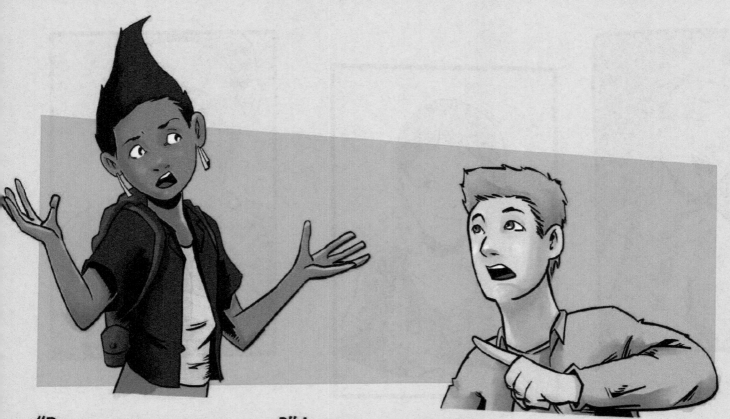

"But whatever do you mean?" I asked with curiosity.

"I'm as plain as can be. Why would anyone want to look like me?"

As they searched for an explanation, a crowd began to gather. Everyone was CONFUSED. They wanted to know what was the matter.

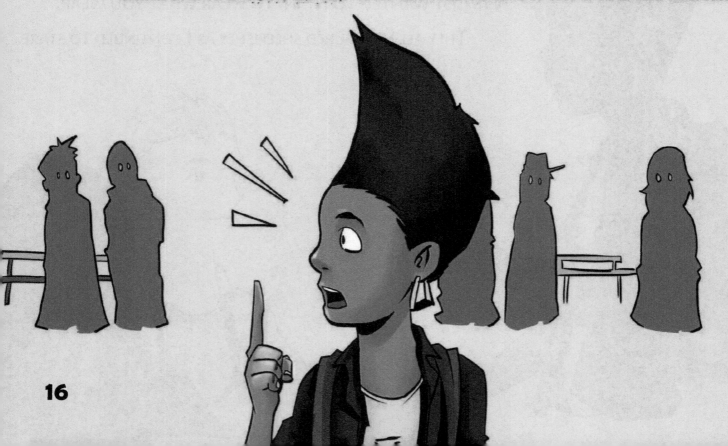

MR. SYKES CAME OVER TO EXAMINE THE CHATTER.

"WHAT WE HAVE HERE IS A CLASSIC CASE OF IDENTITY SWAP.

PEOPLE AREN'T HAPPY WITH THEMSELVES, SO THEY'D RATHER BE SOMEONE THEY'RE NOT."

"BUT WHO YOU ARE IS GOOD, SO CELEBRATE.
FOR YOUR DISTINCT QUALITIES ARE SUITED FOR YOU,
THEY'RE NOT FOR SOMEONE ELSE TO IMITATE.

SO BE YOURSELF AND ALWAYS KNOW
THAT BEING YOU IS AS GOOD AS GOLD."

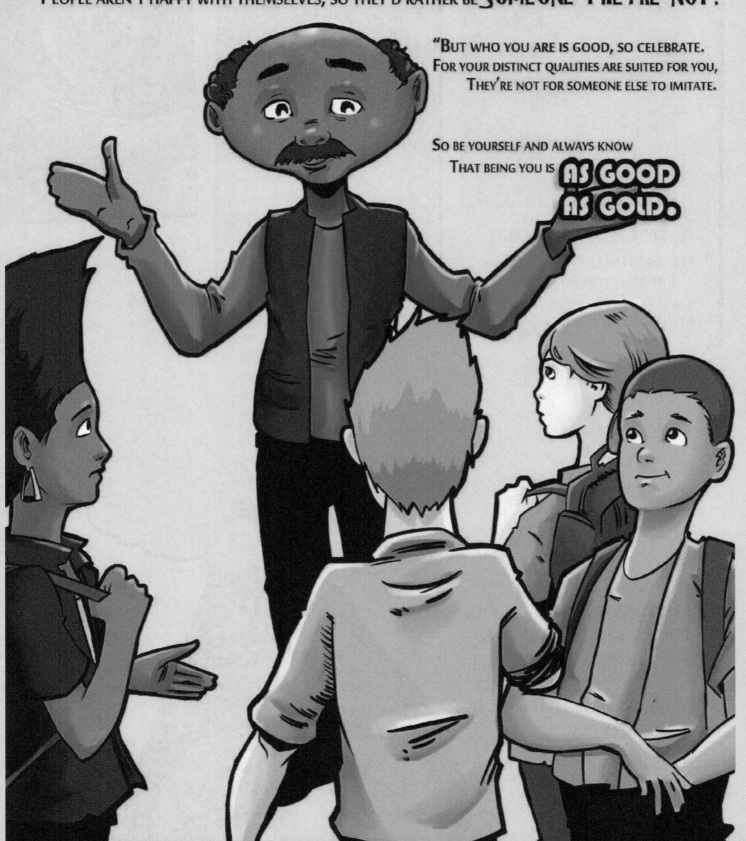

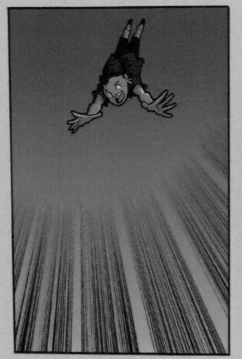

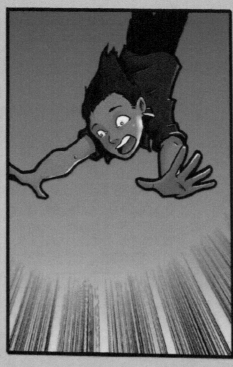

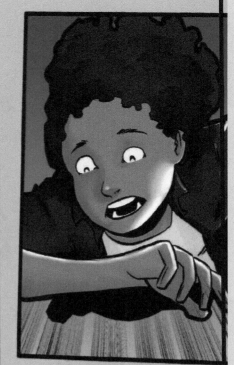

As I looked around and pondered those words,
I realized something great.

I was special being just me,
I DIDN'T HAVE TO IMITATE.

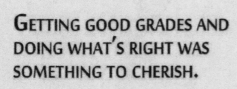

Getting good grades and doing what's right was something to cherish.

I didn't have to let the old me simply perish!

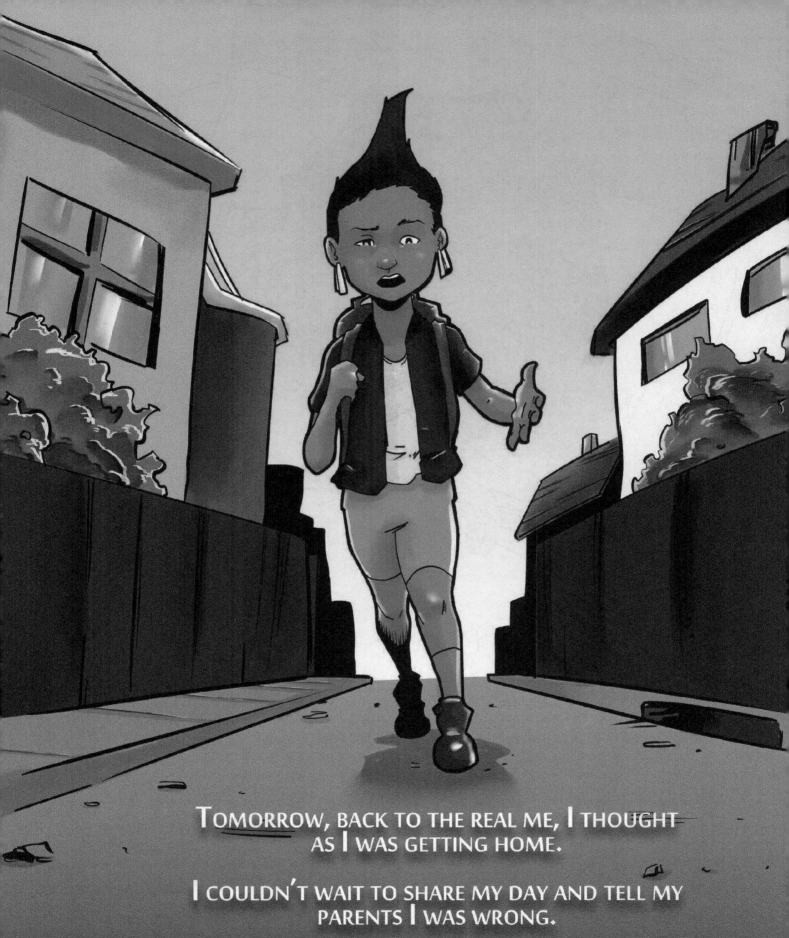

TOMORROW, BACK TO THE REAL ME, I THOUGHT
AS I WAS GETTING HOME.

I COULDN'T WAIT TO SHARE MY DAY AND TELL MY
PARENTS I WAS WRONG.

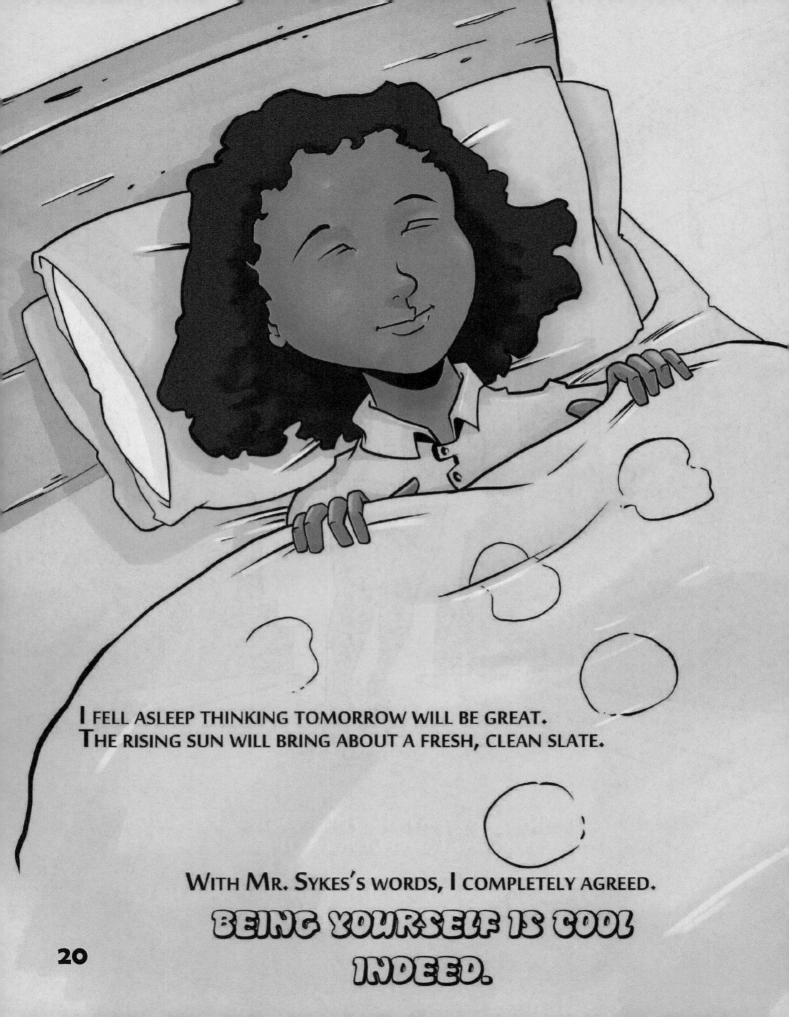

I FELL ASLEEP THINKING TOMORROW WILL BE GREAT.
THE RISING SUN WILL BRING ABOUT A FRESH, CLEAN SLATE.

WITH MR. SYKES'S WORDS, I COMPLETELY AGREED.
BEING YOURSELF IS COOL INDEED.

GLOSSARY

awe: feeling of respect or amazement

belted: to shout or speak loudly

clean slate: to start over

chatter: to communicate by talking

cherish: to love or protect

confidently: having a strong belief; sure

declared: to make known or state clearly

distinct: different in nature or quality

empowered: having power or authority

exclaimed: to cry out or speak suddenly as in surprise, strong emotion, or protest

gingerly: with great care or caution

habits: things you do all the time

identity: who you are inside

indeed: true

imitate: to copy someone or something

murmured: to utter words in a low tone; to make a low, rumbling sound

perish: to pass away or disappear

perplexed: confused; puzzled

pondered: to think deeply about something

presumed: to think something is true without knowing it's true

sheepishly: embarrassed or bashful, as by having done something wrong or foolish

strutted: to walk proudly as if expecting to impress observers

swap: To switch; trade

transformation: a complete change in someone's or something's appearance

Reading Comprehension Questions

1. Why did Hannah dress differently?

2. What did Hannah mean when she said, "I'd break my mold"?

3. In the morning, what did Hannah do that showed she was "living on the edge"?

4. Why were the kids on the bus shocked?

5. Why was Hannah strutting on the bus? What does that tell you about how she feels about herself?

6. What did Hannah mean by she would be a "burst of sunshine"?

7. Why do you think Hannah wanted to be the last one in class?

8. Describe Mrs. Burn's reaction to Hannah.

9. In class, how is Hannah acting differently than usual?

10. How were the kids at the cool table dressed?

11. On page 13, Hannah says she should outgrow her "perfect habits." List at least 5 perfect habits that Hannah PROBABLY had?

12. What explanation did the cool kids give about why they were dressed differently?

13. The story says that "Mr. Sykes came over to examine the chatter." Another way to say that would be, "Mr. Sykes came over to _____."

14. Summarize what Mr. Sykes told the children.

15. Hannah couldn't wait to get home to tell her parents she was wrong. What was she wrong about?

16. At the end, what does Hannah mean by, "The rising sun will bring about a fresh clean slate"?

17. How did Hannah's feelings change from the beginning of the story to the end?

Conversation Questions

1. What is the main character's conflict?

2. Does Hannah struggle with embracing who she is in the beginning of the story? Explain your thinking.

3. Why is being yourself important?

4. What are some negative consequences that come from giving in to peer pressure?

5. Do you think a person can be bullied or harmed on the internet?

About The Author

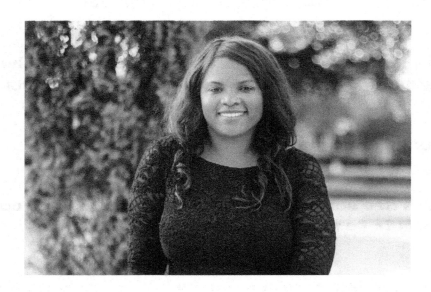

Latoya Desamour is an author and elementary teacher who has taught for over 13 years in Tampa. She was born and raised in Jacksonville, Florida and left home to attend the University of South Florida in Tampa. She graduated with a B.S. in Elementary Education and a Master's Degree in Educational Leadership. She is married to an extremely supportive husband and together, they have 4 wonderful children.

About The Illustrator

Visit https://www.artofcarl.com/ for more information.

CPSIA information can be obtained
at www.ICGtesting.com
Printed in the USA
LVOW05*0914161117
556448LV00004B/8/P

Nursing Home Care

NOTICE

NURSING HOME CARE

John E. Morley, MB, BCh
Dammert Professor of Medicine
Director, Division of Geriatric Medicine
Department of Medicine
Saint Louis University School of Medicine
St. Louis, Missouri, USA

Joseph G. Ouslander, MD
Professor and Senior Associate Dean
 for Geriatric Programs
Charles E. Schmidt College of Medicine
Professor (Courtesy), Christine E. Lynn
 College of Nursing
Florida Atlantic University
Boca Raton, Florida, USA

Debbie Tolson, PhD, MSc, BSc (Hons), RGN, FRCN
Alzheimer Scotland Professor of Dementia/Director
Alzheimer Scotland Centre for Policy and Practice
School of Health, Nursing and Midwifery
University of West of Scotland
Hamilton, Scotland, United Kingdom

Bruno Vellas, MD, PhD
Professor of Internal Medicine and Geriatrics
Gerontopole, University of Toulouse
INSERM U 1027
Toulouse, France

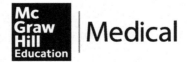

New York   Chicago   San Francisco   Athens   London   Madrid
Mexico City   Milan   New Delhi   Singapore   Sydney   Toronto

Nursing Home Care

1 2 3 4 5 6 7 8 9 0   QDB/QDB   18 17 16 15 14 13

ISBN 978-0-07-180765-4
MHID 0-07-180765-9

This book was set in Warnock Pro by Thomson Digital.
The editors were Jim Shanahan and Karen G. Edmonson.
The production supervisor was Richard Ruzycka.
Project management was provided by Ritu Joon, Thomson Digital.
The cover designer was Thomas DiPierro.
Quad/Graphics was printer and binder.

This book is printed on acid-free paper.

Library of Congress Cataloging-in-Publication Data

Nursing home care / John E. Morley ... [et al.].
   p. ; cm.
 Includes bibliographical references.
 ISBN-13: 978-0-07-180765-4 (hardcover : alk. paper)
 ISBN-10: 0-07-180765-9 (hardcover : alk. paper)
 I. Morley, John E.
 [DNLM: 1. Homes for the Aged—organization & administration. 2. Nursing Homes—organization & administration. WT 27.1]
 RA999.A35
 362.16068—dc23
                                    2013016064

McGraw-Hill Education books are available at special quantity discounts to use as premiums and sales promotions or for use in corporate training programs. To contact a representative, please visit the Contact Us pages at www.mhprofessional.com.

CONTENTS

Color insert appears between pages 208 and 209.

FOREWORD

Nursing Home Care: An Equal Challenge for All IAGG Regions

Nursing home care has developed significantly in many countries and is probably one of the most challenging aspects of gerontology and geriatrics. Changes in the structure of the family and in life expectancy increase the chance of many older adults becoming severely dependent due to disabilities, including dementia, and increase the probability of them spending their final months of life in a nursing home. It remains a challenge since it can be a turning point in life, despite the great improvement in nursing home facilities and the care achieved in the last few years. However, heterogeneity can be considered a hallmark in nursing home assistance, since great variability may be observed within the same country as well as among different countries. The demographic/epidemiological transition of most countries in the world is facing great limitations for continuing care in hospitals; thus, innovative forms of care are necessary. Technology will create facilities as is the case of telemedicine. However, care is a person-to-person relationship with no substitute. It goes beyond a technical approach since its major demand is solidarity. All forms of community care are to be explored, mainly home assistance, notwithstanding nursing home care and hospice care that will remain a huge demand in the future.

The aims of this textbook are:

- to improve knowledge on quality of care nursing home to nursing home, and country to country;
- to share experiences in the multiple aspects of nursing home care and management;
- to share the knowledge from new evidence-based medicine, evidence-based nursing and social care, and clinical research. For a long time, clinical research has been excluded from the nursing home setting. It is only by translating evidence from clinical, nursing, social, and psychological research that we will be able to improve our practice and share our experiences;
- to create a community of health and social care professionals, practice leaders, and managers to improve our works.

In the past, the IAGG has taken several interdisciplinary initiatives under the leadership of J.E. Morley (Saint Louis University) in collaboration with the World Health Organization's world program on aging. This includes international workshops, publications of Task Forces in the field, and continuing education courses. This book is the result of these initiatives aiming to generate a new worldwide generation of nursing homes and residential homes providing the same standard of care and living conditions in all countries around the world and for all the older adults who need it.

IAGG is happy, in association with this text, to offer a certification of nursing home competence. This can be accessed at http://www.garn-network.org.

VELLAS Bruno, IAGG President
GUIMARAES Renato Maia, IAGG Past President
CHA Heung Bong, IAGG President Elect

The Future of Long-Term Care

Populations around the world are rapidly aging, and this will impact significantly on almost every area of life. Today, one in every nine people in the world is 60 years of age or older. This is expected to increase to one in five people by 2050.[1] Population aging is not just an issue for the rich world. The majority of older people already live in low- and middle-income countries, and this is where some of the fastest aging is occurring.

If societies do not adapt, this demographic transition will present many challenges. These include a shrinking workforce alongside increasing demand for health and social care and social security.[2] However, since older people are a significant resource for their families, communities, and society as a whole, population aging also offers many opportunities particularly if older people can retain their health.[3]

WHO has recently defined four key strategies for countries seeking to respond to this demographic transition. These are the prevention of chronic diseases common in older age; the strengthening of health and social care systems for older people; the promotion of enabling, age-friendly environments; and the re-conceptualization of aging itself.[4]

Effective adaptation to population aging requires all of these strategies to be put in place. Many older individuals retain good health and function until quite advanced years. While there is evidence that this subset of older populations want a more active role in society than in previous generations,[5] many of these individuals face discrimination and marginalization. This is a wasted human resource and there is a strong economic argument to address these barriers.

But one of the hallmarks of aging is diversity, and there will also be many individuals of the same age who struggle with poor health, often with complex geriatric syndromes and comorbidities. This is a burden that is often shared by their families who may lose a previously productive member, and may face severe health care costs or see younger members diverted from employment or education to provide social care.

These older individuals have complex care needs. They need access to integrated and affordable systems designed to foster the best trajectories of health and function. These should encompass prevention, rehabilitation, clinical care, nursing services, social care, and palliative care, and need to be accessible from many settings ranging from their home through to supportive living arrangements and institutional care.

If we are to develop these comprehensive care systems for older people, we must take account of dramatically changing population dynamics. In the past, much of long-term care, particularly in low- and middle-income countries, has been provided by family members, generally women. But the proportion of younger family members available to provide care is dramatically shrinking. There is an increased likelihood that older people will live alone rather than as part of the extended families, which makes this type of support more practical and, these days, younger women may have other aspirations. Furthermore, unless adequately supported and trained, family members are in no position to provide the complex care that older people actually need.

Long-term care systems of the future must therefore include both informal and formal care, and carers across these systems will need to be better provided with support and training. The artificial distinction between home and institution should be reconsidered. Flexible arrangements that span both settings may become more common and funding systems must be designed to ensure that there are no artificial distinctions between settings that lead to "cost shifting" to the detriment of care.

But financing and workforce issues should not be the main driver of these systems. Instead, we need to design systems that best meet the real needs of older individuals. The focus should be on optimizing functional trajectory and doing this in a way that fosters well-being and ongoing social participation. This will require a better understanding of health trajectories in older age, and better collection of data.

Optimizing functional trajectory requires services that span the care spectrum from prevention to palliative care. Health promotion can start in the community (e.g., community-based programs supporting physical activity), or be institution based (e.g., Thai Chi groups to foster good balance and prevent falls). Clinical disease prevention (e.g., control of hypertension to prevent cardiovascular disease) can prevent the onset of new disease, and chronic disease management (through nursing care) can help maintain health; thus, integration with primary care services is critical. Early identification of functional decline can lead to interventions to reverse it, or at least minimize progression. As functional capacities become impaired, service provision to support function will be important, and this needs to span both home environments and institutional settings. Both these settings need to take account of technological advances in assistive living. Finally, adequate palliative care is needed to ensure all older people are able to die with dignity and free of pain.

Governments around the world face constrained resources, yet demand for these services is going to inevitably increase. One estimate from Australia suggests that around 10% of the total expected increase in health care costs over the next 20 years will come from increased demand for care for dementia alone. In Europe, projections for the next five decades suggest that costs for long-term care services as a percentage of GDP will more than double. Optimists among us will hope that these pressures will lead to innovative responses that are not just affordable, but also effective and meet the health and social needs of older people.

This book is a clear step on the path to this innovative future. Many long-term care models are presented, with examples of best practice being provided from countries around the world. With an emphasis on alternative approaches to institutional-based models, this book contains a substantial section on programs that promote aging at home and comprehensive service provision in noninstitutional settings. Denmark, Japan, and Canada have all developed strategies to increase care delivery in home environments and can serve as examples for other nations striving to implement quality programs. But nursing home care will continue to play a key role in meeting the health care needs of older people, and strategies by which to improve care in this setting can translate into benefits across care continuums. This book highlights recent evidence from nursing home care and suggests innovative new approaches. It is unlikely that a single best practice model exists and this book provides an overview of existing models that can be adapted to specific needs of regions or countries.

I think the book is also important for another reason. Long-term care has for too long been marginalized professionally and academically. I hope that the rigor and ambition of these chapters help foster the inexorable shift to a more central position in the thinking of decision makers around the world.

John R. Beard, MBBS, PhD, Director
Andrea Foebel, PhD
Department of Ageing and Life Courses
World Health Organization

References

1. UNDESA. *World Economic and Social Survey 2007: Development in an Ageing World.* New York: United Nations Department of Social and Economic Affairs; 2007.
2. Sikken B, Davis N, Hayashi C, Olkkonen H. *The Future of Pensions and Healthcare in a Rapidly Ageing World.* Geneva, Switzerland: World Economic Forum; 2009.
3. Beard JR, Biggs S, Bloom DE, et al. *Global Population Ageing: Peril or Promise?* Geneva: World Economic Forum; 2012.
4. WHO. *Good Health Adds Life to Years: Global brief for World Health Day 2012.* Geneva: World Health Organization; 2012.
5. Age Wave, *Sun America. Age Wave/SunAmerica Retirement Re-Set Study.* Los Angeles: Sun America; 2011.

INTRODUCTION

"I was one of those people who thought going to a nursing home would be terrible – now that I am here I am having a great time!"

—Anonymous nursing home resident

The publication of the IAGG-WHO 2011 Taskforce, quality improvement and research development agenda for nursing homes, provided the impetus for this book. The Taskforce recommendations brought into sharp focus the need for resources and opportunities for nursing home practitioners to develop knowledge and skills and to gain recognition for their expertise. This unique practical text book serves as a rich evidence-based resource to provide practitioners with the information and practical know-how to advance nursing home care with and for older people. Additionally it serves as the course textbook for the online IAGG Certificate in Nursing Home Practice. Each chapter includes a summary list of key learning points for quick reference, and multiple choice questions. In addition, a number of extra online components are provided and a full slide kit for teaching purposes is also available. Completion of additional online learning activities is required to achieve IAGG certification. Details and course registration can be accessed at http://www.garn-network.org.

The book reflects IAGG's conviction that nursing home practice is an interdisciplinary endeavor that requires a sound theoretical, scientific, and values base in addition to practice know-how. Diversity in nursing home provision around the world manifests in different delivery models and variations in the contributions and role functions of specific disciplines. Mindful of the influences of different cultures and context the premise of this book is that there is a shared and common knowledge base to guide nursing home practice and approaches to caring that are universal. We believe that in the quest for excellence all staff should appreciate the essence of this knowledge, ideally most should be skilful with demonstrable competencies relevant to their role; some will need advanced practice skills, and some will be expert practitioners with leadership roles. Terminology is explored and explained as we recognize that internationally nursing homes and nursing home practice are not uniform, and it is important that this is acknowledged.

The balance between health and social care aspects of nursing home provision for older people shades contemporary debates about what constitutes quality. In this unique interdisciplinary textbook our mission has been to explicate, in a way that will be helpful to the international community of nursing home practitioners, the state of the art and science of nursing home practice. We acknowledge that this has been a complex and ambitious undertaking that has challenged us as practitioners and scholars, at times, requiring us to set aside our cultural and professional heritage to expose the essentials of nursing home practice.

A consistent assertion of this book is that to advance nursing home practice requires international and inter-professional learning, research, and leadership with policy impact. It is also essential that we listen, embrace, and respond to the views of older nursing home residents and their family and friends.

The book has been prepared in four parts, each with its own distinctive feel. We have devoted half of this book to the management of common age-related conditions and diseases as these often co-exist with amplified impact on the well-being, independence, and quality of life of nursing home residents. Understanding the relationship between geriatric syndromes and other co-morbidities is crucial to decisions about the appropriate pathway of care for an individual resident. For some readers we anticipate that this second part of the book may become a well-thumbed practice handbook. We do however encourage all to take the time to start at the beginning with Part 1 to build understanding of the origins of the nursing home movement, alternative approaches including aging in place, and importantly appreciate what older people are saying about nursing home life and culture change. We look in depth at nursing home admissions, the characteristics and care needs of older nursing home residents, and associated costs. Nursing home design is explored and illustrated with selected international examples of contemporary nursing homes highlighting the need to pay attention to the sense of place and the sense of home as much as clinical needs. Readers will be left with no doubt that a prerequisite to delivering high-quality care is the ability to create a good living and working environment within the nursing home in addition to attending to the clinical and wider care needs of an individual. Aligned with the IAGG Nursing Home Global Improvement and Research Agenda (presented in Chapter 1) the essentials of culture change are explored. Compelling arguments are presented for involving nursing home residents and their visiting families and friends in culture change projects.

Part 2 focuses on the fundamentals of working as part of a nursing home team providing day-to-day care and the leadership essentials to drive the quality improvement agenda. International examples of nursing homes are showcased to illustrate the range of facilities and different models that exist. Care principles that are internationally considered to underpin practice that is person centered, dignified, and respectful are examined from a practical perspective. We reflect on the impact of truth-telling practices within nursing homes, dwelling on the issue of trust and a person's sense of security and well-being. Strategies to make the admission experience as positive and reassuring as possible are considered alongside assessment tools including the minimum data set and other tools.

We discuss our collective professional and moral responsibilities to protect vulnerable older nursing home residents from physical, psychological, sexual, and financial abuse and poor practices including inappropriate prescribing and restraints. Practical tips are included for managing and preventing accidents including trips, slips, and falls. Learning points from recent major USA and UK incidents related to fire prevention and management and disaster preparedness in nursing homes are shared. Part 2 concludes with a debate about the state of the art of contemporary nursing home research and education, reviewing progress and achievements and exposing our weaknesses and development priorities.

The benefits of comprehensive assessment of geriatric conditions are well known and all older nursing home residents present with complex problems and multiple conditions. Part 3 of the book addresses the most common conditions experienced by older nursing home residents. The clinical implications and management considerations for each condition are explored, alongside consideration of emotional impacts and strategies to enhance resident's well-being. Screening and assessment methods are discussed along with selected care pathways and other toolkits for practice and local policy development.

Part 4 addresses clinical and nursing aspects of disease management. This section will be particularly useful to physicians and advanced practice nurses, but also will guide day-to-day nursing approaches to common diseases in the nursing home. The key points are presented in tabular form or in figures, to allow rapid access to the basic knowledge.

This book would not have been possible without the support of the European Union and the IAGG-WHO commitment to enhancing care for older persons in nursing homes. We are grateful to John R. Beard and Andrea Foebel for writing the Preface.

Specific thanks go to Valerie Tanner for her editorial and administrative skills that she deployed to keep manuscript preparation on track and on time. We thank James Shanahan and Karen Edmundson from McGraw-Hill for their enthusiastic efforts at bringing this book to fruition.

We thank Yves Rolland for his contributions to the Education and Research Chapter; Marilyn Rantz for the photo of a nursing home in Columbia, Missouri; Ligia Dominguez for her pictures of nursing homes in Italy; Mel Richter for the photos of a nursing home after a tornado in Joplin, Missouri; Stephen Feman, Scott Fosko, Nicole Burkemper, and Jeff Lorraine for supplying photographs of eye and skin lesions; and Petrina Sweeney and Kenneth Shay for oral health photographs. We also thank Karen Barney for supplying pictures of assistive devices and Jenny Lee for her picture of the 3 generations of walkers.

Nursing Home Care

Part 1

INTRODUCTION TO NURSING HOME LIFE AND ALTERNATIVES

Chapter 1

LONG-TERM CARE NEEDS IN AN AGING WORLD

Population aging is a worldwide phenomenon and the graying of the population will have a profound impact on societies and on healthcare and social systems. Since the 1950s, the proportion of older people has steadily risen from 8% in 1950 to a projected 22% in 2050. In 2008, 313 million (62%) of the older population lived in developing countries; more than half of this population lives in China and India. By 2040, there will be more than 500 million older persons in these countries alone. From 2010 to 2060 the numbers of people 80 years of age and older is predicted to triple in Europe from 4% to 12% of the total European population (Figure 1–1).

Between 2006 and 2050 the number of Americans aged 85 years and older will grow from 5.3 million to nearly 21 million (Figure 1–2). Although population aging is a wonderful achievement, many older adults experience a combination of age-related changes, challenges, and comorbidities that limit their ability to live independently and increase their need for specialized housing and skilled care. Although it is recognized that for most elderly aging in place in their own home is ideal, this is not always feasible. For this reason, there is an increasing need to develop long-term care solutions. There is no universal or ideal long-term care solution as all options inevitably require adjustments to home, home life, or place of residence in ways that can profoundly impact on individuals, family, and communities. Determination of the best long-term care arrangements for a person involves multiple considerations, including their healthcare and social needs, individual choice, locality, availability of programs, and fiscal resources. In some regions, the nursing home is the major component of long-term care services, but it is important to recognize that there are many other alternative community models evolving. The International Association of Gerontology and Geriatrics (IAGG) recognizes and values diversity in quality long-term care provisions appropriate to regional resources and culture, and recognizes that there are multiple interpretations of what constitutes quality. An important part of the long-term care development journey is to understand current best nursing home practices so they can be shared and to learn lessons that can be applied in other community-based innovations. This chapter sets out alternatives to nursing home care and the IAGG 2011 nursing home-improvement agenda.

TERMINOLOGY

When making comparisons about nursing home practices around the world, it is important to note that there is no universal definition as to what is meant by the term *nursing home*. Consequently, it is important to understand the contextual and cultural differences of the term when comparing studies and making inferences for local practice. Chapter 2 examines the concepts of *nursing* and *home* more closely, but here we highlight some international differences between the facilities that are described as nursing homes.

We use the following definitions:

- *Nursing home:* An institution providing nursing care 24 hours a day, assistance with activities of daily living and mobility, psychosocial and personal care, paramedical care, such as physiotherapy and occupational therapy, as well as bed and board. May or may not have physicians seeing residents in the facility.
- *Residential home (assisted living):* An institution providing living conditions adjusted to the needs of residents, usually requiring no more nursing care than can be given by a visiting nurse. In general, admission results from an inability to manage at home. Assistance can be provided for some basic activities of daily living, including assistance with dressing. Meals might be provided in either a communal or private room. Most care is provided by nursing aides and personnel with little or no training.

These terms or derivatives are applicable across many regions of the world, although there are some anomalies. In the United States, residential homes are described as assisted living facilities. In the United Kingdom, the term *nursing home* is no longer used; instead, there are 2 types of care homes: (a) care homes that provide personal care (help with washing, bathing, and medications), board, and lodging, which are akin to European residential homes, and care homes that provide skilled nursing care supervised by a registered nurse 24 hours per day and are often nurse led. There is also a range of other housing and retirement community solutions designed to assist older people to age in place, as is discussed in Chapter 2. It is similar in France, with EHPAD (the institution for dependent old adults) and the EHPA institution for nondependent older adults, which regulate the residential homes.

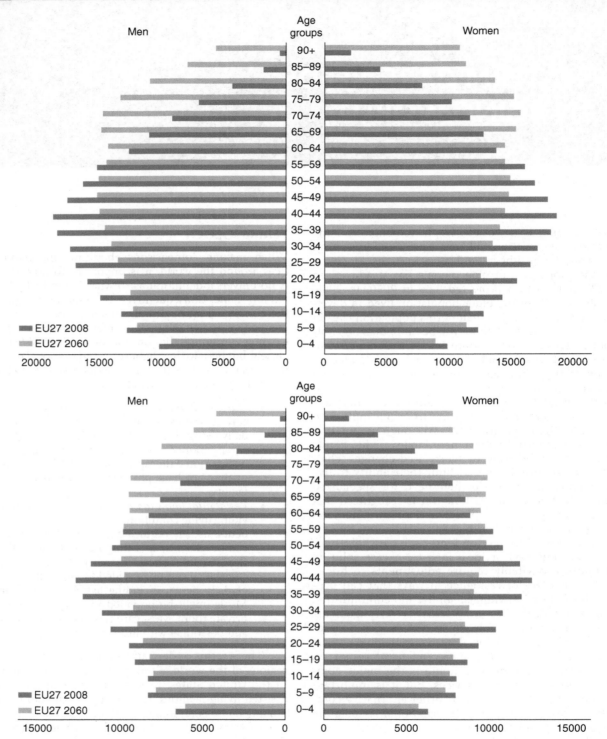

Figure 1–1. Changes in the European Union population structure from 2008 to 2060. EU represents countries in the European Union. (http://ec.europa.eu/economy_finance/publications/publication14992_en.pdf)

Number of older Americans, 1960–2040 (in millions)

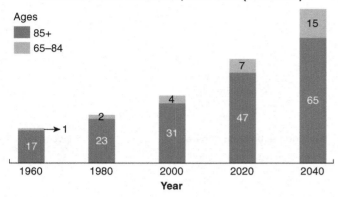

Figure 1–2. The increase in old-old in the United States.

Thus when reading this book and thinking about the implications for local practice it is important to remember that the term *nursing home* is not used consistently, and the roles and functions of physicians and nurses vary by country, and to some extent by provider. Furthermore, there are variations in the ways that nursing home practitioners are prepared and regulated, and it is important to appreciate these contextual and administrative differences.

SOCIAL DETERMINANTS OF INDEPENDENCE IN LATER LIFE

There is no doubt that living with a partner and having family or neighbor support are critical determinants of later-life well-being (Table 1–1). Although with increased longevity it is reasonable to assume that today's older population has access to support from multiple generations, such support is not always realized. In many regions, increased geographical mobility and migration has put physical distance between generations. Social isolation brings multiple challenges for the older person and caring at a distance brings with it stresses and strains for family members. In China, the stresses of young people moving from rural areas to the cities is compounded by the 1-child policy, which is leading to a decrease in the number of available caregivers. Although communication technologies enable distant family members to keep in touch, there

Table 1–1.	SOCIAL DETERMINANTS OF INDEPENDENCE IN OLD AGE
Self-care capacity	
Living with supportive others	
Supportive neighbors/informal caregivers	
Family solidarity with caregiving capacity	
Social care services	
Domiciliary visits	
Financial Resource	

Also see Table 1–4.

is no substitute for proximity and having someone close to hand, who can provide direct care and help out when problems arise. Caregiving is often undertaken by a spouse, who may himself or herself be older, or an adult child, most often a daughter. However, it is important to remember that some older people have life-long caring responsibilities, such as those who have adult children with learning difficulties.

Although much of healthcare policy espouses care in the community as something provided through formal services, the majority of social care is provided through informal unpaid family and friends. A recent cohort study undertaken in Japan, demonstrated that insufficient informal care levels were strongly associated with the discontinuation of living at home and institutionalization. Poverty is also a major consideration, and in some regions, elder abandonment is reported. Although the history books would suggest destitution is a thing of the past for some older persons, without material or social means it still feels a reality and their options are limited to homelessness or hostel-style accommodation (see Chapter 2). Post retirement low pensionable income is a common phenomenon. Aging brings the economics of later-life independence into sharp focus, be it the cost burden to the individual who must self-fund domestic or nursing help, or the family member who may need to choose between paid employment or unpaid caring responsibilities, or municipalities and governments with responsibilities toward the increasing numbers of older people. A universal challenge is the development of payment and copayment methods to support the rising costs of all forms of long-term care. Where copayment is required, the emotive issue of needing to sell your home to pay for long-term care fuels debate about the economic imperative and highlights the need to evolve long-term care insurance. Although many health inequalities persist into old age, it is important to remember that many people do age in relatively good health and continue to live active and independent lives.

HOME VISITING

The availability of home visits by nurses, other healthcare workers, and social workers to older people living in their own homes or within social housing is a major factor influencing the opportunity of the elderly to remain in their own home. Around the world a variety of approaches are taken to home visiting—some are preventative and focus on health maintenance, others provide personal care and skilled nursing care. The frequency of home visits varies from brief visits several times in the same day, to as-needed visits and to annual checkups.

In Japan, preventative home visits are provided to nondisabled home-dwelling older people who are functionally independent; the intent is to prevent functional decline. The ethos of the Japanese approach is echoed in healthcare policy in other countries. In Wales (UK), for example, there is a policy-level commitment to older people to help them to stay safe, healthy, and independent for as long as possible, and to manage effectively within the community health conditions that arise,

Table 1–2.	ELEMENTS OF MEDICATION ASSESSMENT FOR COMMUNITY (HOME) NURSES TO CONFIRM ABILITY OF PERSON TO TAKE HIS OR HER OWN MEDICINES

- Reads label and name of drug and understands its purpose
- Understands dosage, when to take drug, and what to do if a dose is missed
- Understands relationship to food and taking of drug
- Accurately demonstrates drug preparation (where necessary) and drug administration
- Recognizes how drug should be stored

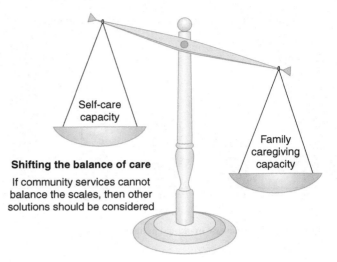

Shifting the balance of care

If community services cannot balance the scales, then other solutions should be considered

Figure 1–3. Shifting the balance of care.

thereby avoiding crisis or inappropriate hospitalization or premature admission to a nursing home.

Medication management is a major risk to frail or cognitively impaired persons and community nurses can play an important role in promoting medication safety in the home. A simple nurse-administered Safe Medication Assessment Tool (SMAT) can be used to gauge medication risk. SMAT approaches are based on the patient's self-reported drug consumption, adherence, knowledge about the drugs, and observation of them taking their medication. These approaches can identify patients who are at risk of unsafe self-medication. A recent SMAT study of 160 older patients in Sweden found that 70% could not describe the medicines they were taking or the correct dose. Thirty-five percent required help from another to take the medications out of the bottle or package, but the prescriber had not appreciated their difficulties. Many factors influence an older person's ability to safely administer prescribed and over-the-counter medications, and periodic review using instruments such as SMAT is an important part of chronic disease medication management in the community (Table 1–2).

Some older people rely on daily home visits to help them to get in and out of bed, for personal hygiene and more technical tasks such as urinary catheter care. These essential visits tend to be relatively brief in duration and are rarely provided during the night. In some countries, such as Scotland, state-funded intensive home support is provided for people with dementia for up to 12 hours per week. However, the impact of such strategies of shifting the balance of care to the community for people with complex health needs remains unclear.

As an individual's dependency increases or their health declines, the burden of care can exceed the combined resources of the family and community services, precipitating the need for alternative solutions (Figure 1–3). The next section discusses a number of options to support both aging in place and alternatives to nursing home care.

AGING IN PLACE

More than 90% of older persons have no need for nursing home placement and successfully live in the community with help from family and friends and the same healthcare systems available to younger persons. Persons who have multiple disabilities, are demented, or are frail and lack a strong community support system often will need to go to a nursing home. Older persons would prefer to stay at home or at least not be institutionalized. This has led to the "aging in place" movement. "Aging in place" denotes not needing to leave one's house or apartment to obtain the required health and social services support services and remain safe in one's home environment. It is the emerging creative social effort to maintain the "person–place whole" in a meaningful way that will overcome the problems faced by an older adult. The principles underpinning aging in place align with the United Nations Principles for Older Persons, which designates 5 principles for any social policy for older people: independence, participation, care, self-fulfillment, and dignity.

In the United Kingdom, the government policy to try to keep persons at home began in 1954 when the Ministry of Health stressed the importance of "the task of enabling old people to go on living in their own homes as long as possible." Although this concept is laudable, it has been criticized for giving families no choice but to provide non-reimbursed care in the home, and for failing to recognize that for an older person to live in impoverished conditions does not equate to the older person being happy. Aging in place also requires adequate supportive services to be available to allow for healthy aging and a negotiation with the older individual to allow the "invasion of their home by strangers."

It is interesting to look at the success of aging-in-place initiatives in countries such as Hong Kong that have high average life expectancies at birth; for example, life expectancies in Hong Kong in 2009 were 79.7 years for men and 85.9 years for women. In Hong Kong, the institutionalization rate of 10% of those age 65 years and older is higher than the rate of other industrialized cities such as London (2.3%). This goes against the finding that older people prefer to receive care at home rather than being institutionalized and highlights the real and complex challenges in

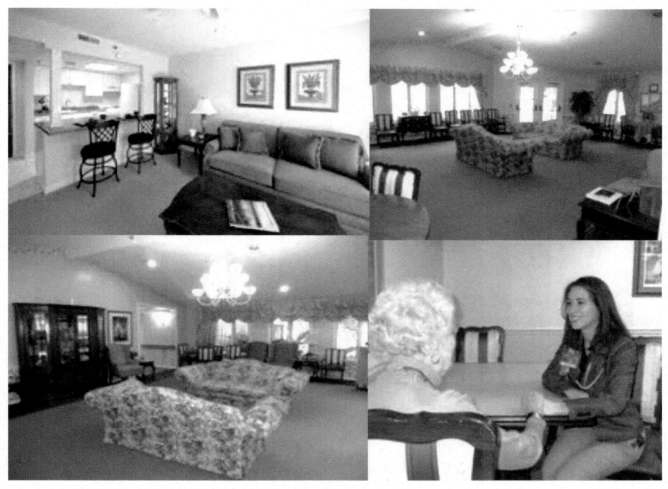

Figure 1–4. Example of an assisted living facility in the United States with a physician doing a "home visit."

achieving the aging-in-place imperative. Between aging in place and being admitted to a nursing home are a range of supported-living options, which in the United States are known as assisted living facilities, while elsewhere they may be known as residential homes.

The Danish government has placed a special emphasis on "aging in place" and has stopped the building of new nursing homes (*Plijchejm*) since 1984. Nursing homes have been replaced by "elderly housings" (*Eldreboliger*). Elderly housings represent dwellings designed to be handicapped accessible so as to allow an older person to live independently. In Denmark, 5.5% of persons 65 years and older live in these houses. In Sweden, comprehensive services are provided by municipalities through the Home Help program and county councils provide primary healthcare.

In the United States, a number of "senior communities" (continued care retirement communities) have developed in which a person can buy a property associated with a centralized community center, nursing home, and assisted living that will allow them to "age in place." The "village" model is a group of older persons who come together and establish a community where they help one another remain

in their own home and remain independent as long as is possible.

Assisted living centers are apartment complexes that provide help with controlling medicines, meals, housekeeping, some assistance with dressing, and safety supervision (Figure 1–4). Most will have a nurse present for some period of time during the day. Physical and occupational therapy are available in the building. Transport may be provided to physicians or physicians may make "house calls." For persons recently discharged from hospitals or homebound persons who are falling, Medicare will provide home visits by nurses, physical therapists, occupational therapists, and social workers as needed. A small number of physicians do make home visits.

A number of demonstration "smart houses" have been built to allow older persons to be electronically monitored. An advanced example of this is Tiger Place, which is associated with the University of Missouri in Columbia. Tiger Place uses electronic monitoring to detect falls and to analyze gait problems of older persons living alone (Figure 1–5). The computerized data alerts staff to changes in the resident's normal behavior that may signal something is wrong or unusual. In this way, the nursing team can

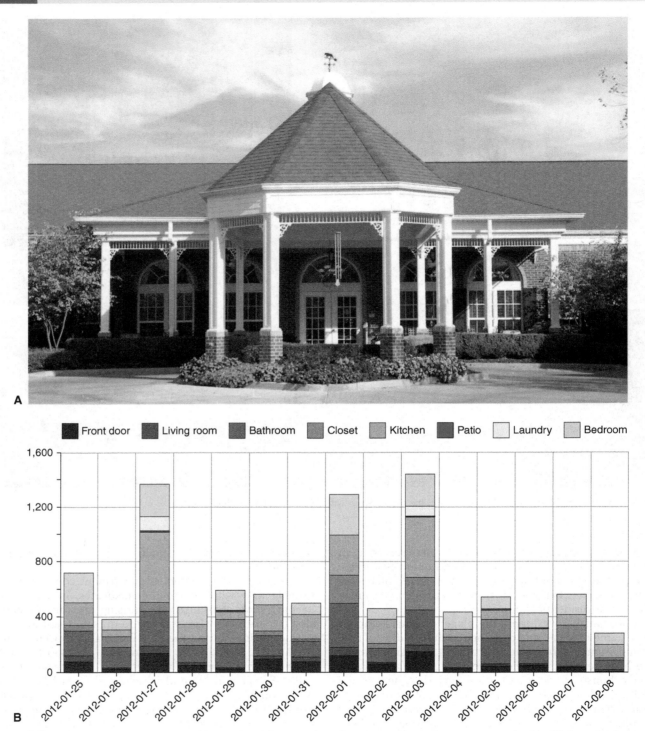

Figure 1–5. (**A**) Tiger Place is a computerized living center where people can be monitored so as to improve personal safety. (**B**) Example of computer print out of resident's daily activity pattern. (Photo by Dr. Marilyn Rantz, Univ. Missouri School of Nursing, Columbia, Missouri.)

work in partnership with the resident to plan appropriate interventions or provide immediate assistance as required.

The Program of All-inclusive Care for the Elderly (PACE) is a comprehensive community-based program for persons who would normally need nursing home care (Figure 1–6). This program developed out of "On-Lok" (a peaceful happy abode), an alternative to nursing home

care for the Chinese community in San Francisco that started in 1979. At present there are 61 PACE programs in 30 U.S. states. PACE programs provide coordinated community-based healthcare and transportation. PACE is based on a central facility that also provides day care and home visits when necessary. The PACE program has been demonstrated to provide a number of positive outcomes

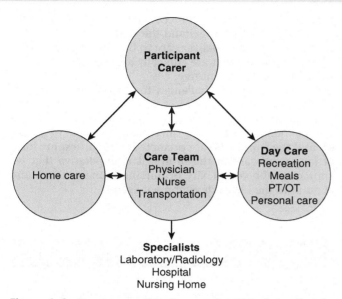

Participant
Carer

Home care

Care Team
Physician
Nurse
Transportation

Day Care
Recreation
Meals
PT/OT
Personal care

Specialists
Laboratory/Radiology
Hospital
Nursing Home

Figure 1–6. Components of the Program for All-Inclusive Care for Elderly (PACE). This is a coordinated care program where primary providers interact with participant and caregiver to limit inappropriate access to expensive care. OT, occupational therapy; PT, physical therapy.

(Table 1–3). Best outcomes are seen in the old-old who live alone, use ambulatory aids, and require help with instrumental activities of daily living.

In Holland, a variety of innovative projects for seniors living in the community have been developed. These include gardening projects for person with dementia and free exercise club memberships for frail older persons. The EASYcare study is a nurse-driven geriatric assessment program for patients who are identified by the general practitioner as having mobility problems, weight loss, dysphoria, or cognitive problems. In consultation with a geriatrician, the nurse develops a management intervention.

In Japan, many older persons have prolonged stays in hospitals. To be more cost-effective, in 2000 the Japanese government introduced a nationwide long-term care insurance system for the Koki (old and rare, i.e., persons older than 70 years of age). Among the innovative programs introduced were the field medicine projects in the Kochi

prefecture. All persons age 65 years and older receive a yearly health-related questionnaire assessment and those age 75 years and older have yearly geriatric examinations. Interventions include an explanatory meeting on results with the participant and family member. Other interventions include exercise classes, cognitive rehabilitation classes, home blood pressure monitoring, home visits by community nurses, and lectures. This intervention has led to an increase in activities of daily living (ADL) independence and a reduction in medical expenses.

In Montreal, Canada, a nurse case manager has been used to ensure continuity of care, to direct the nursing needs of the patient, to provide an engaged partnership with the older person, to provide care to prevent illness and functional decline, to facilitate coordination of the healthcare team, and to make invisible institutional boundaries.

In France and Spain, healthcare is paid for by the national social security system with the cost of dependency (help for ADL) partially paid by the regional authorities. The family has to pay for lodging and meals.

The Cochrane Database of Systematic Reviews found strong evidence that day hospital attendance leads to better outcomes, decreased mortality, and a reduction in ADL deterioration. Similarly, home care geriatric assessment, management, and preventive programs appear to improve outcomes of those who are "aging in place." Community volunteers have been shown to be capable to doing some of these tasks. Hospital at-home programs can prevent unnecessary hospitalization at the end of life and decrease hospitalization in debilitated patients who are not yet at end of life.

"Aging in place" for many older persons is feasible and can be cost-effective. It requires a coordinated, government-supported system to make it feasible for the average older person. There are numerous services that need to be in place to allow this to be successful (Table 1–4).

Table 1–3. POSITIVE OUTCOMES OF THE PROGRAM FOR ALL-INCLUSIVE CARE FOR THE ELDERLY (PACE)
• Cost-effective
• Participants twice as likely to die at home as nonparticipants
• Reduced hospitalizations and nursing home admissions
• Longer survival times
• Better health
• Better quality of life
• Better functional status
• Greater satisfaction

Table 1–4. PROGRAMS NECESSARY TO ALLOW SUCCESSFUL "AGING IN PLACE"
• Meals on Wheels
• Community nurse visits
• Transportation
• Housing adapted to needs
• Adequate home heating/cooling system
• "Friend at hand" or "befriending" service providing volunteers as companions and helpers
• Assistance with bathing and hygiene
• Home-therapy services
• Telecare
• Physician home visits
• Respite care for family
• Day care and/or social centers for seniors
• Care coordination
• Ideally, assistive technology in the home to simplify tasks and monitor safety

In examining whether a person is better "aging in place" or moving to a nursing home, one needs to follow the United Nations Principles for Older People set out in 1999. **Independence** requires the older person to remain at home as long as it can be done safely. The author JEM uses the Rule of Bungee Jumping for his patients. Bungee Jumping is clearly unsafe, but legal. Thus, a person can remain at home as long as it is no more risky than Bungee Jumping. Persons should be provided with choices and alternatives. "Aging in place" needs to continue to provide older persons the opportunity to **participate** in activities with younger persons and not to become isolated. In many countries **care** delivery needs to be no longer focused on hospitals or institutions but moved into the community. Older persons need to have access to community events be they spiritual, cultural or recreation to allow them to maintain **self-fulfillment**. All persons who interact with older persons "aging in place" need to recognize the importance of maintaining the older person's **dignity** and make sure the older person is treated fairly. In the end, to enable older persons to happily "age in place" society needs to be prepared to shoulder the costs and to work in partnership with individuals and family caregivers.

INTERNATIONAL NURSING HOME DEVELOPMENT AND RESEARCH AGENDA IAGG-WHO

In 2010, the IAGG working with the World Health Organization (WHO), assembled an international Nursing Home Taskforce that met in Toulouse, France. The impetus for the work was the known variation in standards of nursing home care around the world and a desire to promote evidence-informed improvements, mindful of the rights and preferences of older people. Specifically, the Taskforce was charged with identifying the clinical, quality, and research concerns and development priorities. This was achieved following a review of evidence, the holding of an international workshop where key issues were presented and debated, and preparation of a consensus paper, which was published in 2011. Readers can view the presentations at the IAGG website (www.iagg.info-who/workshops). The recommendations extended across the 4 improvement domains shown in Table 1–5 that need to be addressed to achieve sustained improvements.

A total of 15 specific recommendations were identified, as listed in Table 1–6. Nursing home providers, administrators, and policy makers have a collective responsibility to address the quality, cultural, and training issues raised by the Taskforce. Practitioners are responsible for ensuring that they understand the evidence base for their own practice and to deliver care to the best of their ability using approaches that are clinically appropriate, dignified, respectful, and restraint free.

There are many challenges to the provision of high-quality nursing care, not least of which are those associated with cost and historic underinvestment. If we are to provide quality care for the increasing numbers of people around the world who are predicted to require some form of long-term care in the future, it is imperative that we appreciate the complexity of nursing home practice and commit to the IAGG development agenda.

Table 1–5. THE 4 IAGG NURSING HOME IMPROVEMENT DOMAINS
1. Reputational Enhancement and Leadership
2. Clinical Essentials and Care Quality Indicators
3. Practitioner Education
4. Research

Table 1–6. IAGG RECOMMENDATIONS
Reputational Enhancement and Leadership
1. Effective leadership structures are established that, where possible, include an expert physician (medical director), an expert registered nurse (nursing director), and a skilled administrator.
2. An international alliance is formed to develop nursing home leadership capacity and capabilities.
3. International exemplars of excellence in nursing home practice are showcased to raise awareness of the demonstrable benefits for older people and the high standards achieved through expert practice.
4. Positive working conditions for nursing home practitioners are created with attractive career development opportunities, recognition, and similar rewards enjoyed by healthcare workers in comparable roles within the acute care services.
Clinical Essentials and Care Quality Indicators
5. Nursing home quality indicators are developed that are sensitive to clinical and care needs and the right of older people to care that is dignified and respectful.
6. The use of physical and chemical restraints should be reduced to those that are absolutely indispensable.
7. "Meaningful activities" are offered to residents to provide physical and mental exercise and opportunities to participate within the nursing home and in community life, enhancing personal autonomy, social relationships (including intergenerational relationships), and social support.
8. Evidence-informed pain assessment and management programs are introduced into all nursing homes.
9. Evidence-informed end-of-life and palliative care programs are introduced into all nursing homes.
10. National drug approval agencies consider requiring drug trials that are age appropriate and inclusive of nursing home residents before they are approved.
Practitioner Education
11. The International Association of Gerontology and Geriatrics develops international certification courses for nursing (care) home health professionals.
12. Pilot the use of "Community of Practice Models" as a practice improvement method for nursing homes, using both face-to-face interdisciplinary training and virtual team support.

(continued)

Table 1–6.   IAGG RECOMMENDATIONS (CONTINUED)

Research

13. A universal ethical approach to obtaining informed consent and monitoring the appropriateness of research is developed.

14. Nursing home research capacity in developing nations is developed.

15. An investment is made in research priorities that address major public health problems and inequalities that affect older people receiving long-term care. Research priorities for which a high need is recognized include the following:

   a. A worldwide survey of different models of care, nursing home structure, and issues in improving quality of care.

   b. A worldwide survey of older persons and their families to determine their preferences for long-term care.

   c. A cross-national, prospective epidemiological study measuring function and quality of life in nursing homes.

   d. Culturally appropriate standardized assessment instruments are developed, including those involving social participatory methods.

   e. A function-focused approach to the prevalence of geriatric syndromes, their impact on function, and development of strategies to improve care for these syndromes needs to be developed.

   f. Research that evaluates the impact of different models of care against trajectories of physical and cognitive function.

KEY POINTS

1. Population aging around the world means there is an ever-increasing need to develop long-term care solutions.

2. Most older people would prefer to remain in their own homes, if they can do so safely and with appropriate support.

3. The majority of older people are active, independent, and can live their lives within the family home or social housing without need for long-term care.

4. To achieve aging in place there needs to be a balance between the individual's self-care capacity and the family capacity to supplement care needs, accessing where necessary community care.

5. The social and health determinants of a person's need for long-term care are complex and change with time.

6. A proportion of older people with complex needs will require some form of long-term care. For those with the highest level of need, this is likely to be provided within nursing homes.

7. The IAGG Global Nursing Home Improvement Agenda makes 15 important recommendations, which if delivered, will assist reform, raise the status of nursing home practice, and, most importantly, promote the high quality of nursing home practice care that our eldest and frailest deserve.

SUGGESTED READINGS

Ball J, Haight BK. Creating a multisensory environment for dementia: the goals of a Snoezelen room. *J Gerontol Nurs.* 2005;31:4-10.

Cairns D, Tolson D, Brown J, Darbyshire C. The need for future alternatives: an investigation of the experiences and future of older parents caring for offspring with learning disabilities over a prolonged period of time. *Br J Learn Disabil.* 2013;41(1):73-82. Available at http://onlinelibrary.wiley.com/doi/10.1111/j.1468-3156.2012.00729.x/pdf.

Forster A, Young J, Lambley R, Langhorne P. Medical day hospital care for the elderly versus alternative forms of care. *Cochrane Database Syst Rev.* 2008;(4):CD001730.

Gusdal AK, Beckman C, Wahlstrom, Tornkvist L. District nurse's use for an assessment tool in their daily work with elderly patient's medication management. *Scand J Public Health.* 2011;39:354-360.

Guttman R. Case management of the frail elderly in the community. *Clin Nurse Spec.* 1999;13(4):174-178.

Hirth V, Baskins J, Dever-Bumba M. Program of all-inclusive care (PACE): past, present, and future. *J Am Med Dir Assoc.* 2009;10(3):155-160.

Katz PR. An international perspective on long term care: focus on nursing homes. *J Am Med Dir Assoc.* 2011;12:487-492.e1.

Kris AE. Understanding older adults: US and global perspectives. In Lange JW (ed). *The Nurse's Role in Promoting Optimal Health of Older Adults; Thriving in the Wisdom of Years.* Philadelphia: F.A. Davis; 2012:41-53.

Kuzuya M, Hasegawa J, Hirakawa Y, et al. Impact of informal care levels on discontinuation of living at home in community-dwelling dependent elderly using various community-based services. *Arch Gerontol Geriatr.* 2011;52(2):127-132.

Kwon S, Kim K. Architectural types of residential unit in nursing homes. *J Asian Archit Build Eng.* 2005;112:105-108.

Matsubayashi K, Okumiya K. Field medicine: a new paradigm of geriatric medicine. *Geriatr Gerontol Int.* 2012;12:5-15.

Melis RJ, van Eijken MI, Borm GF, et al. The design of the Dutch EASYcare study: a randomised controlled trial on the effectiveness of a problem-based community intervention model for frail elderly people (NCT00105378). *BMC Health Serv Res.* 2005;5:65.

Minner D, Hoffstetter P, Casey L, Jones D. Snoezelen activity: the Good Shepherd Nursing Home experience. *J Nurs Care Qual.* 2004;19(4):343-348.

Ribbe MW, Ljunggren G, Steel K, et al. Nursing homes in 10 nations: a comparison between countries and settings. *Age Ageing.* 1997;26(suppl 2):3-12.

Rolland Y, Abellan van Kan G, Hermabessiere S, et al. Descriptive study of nursing home residents from the REHPA network. *J Nutr Health Aging.* 2009;13:679-683.

Shepperd S, Wee B, Straus SE. Hospital at home: home-based end of life care. *Cochrane Database Syst Rev.* 2011;(7):CD009231.

Tolson D, Rolland Y, Andrieu S, et al. IAGG WHO/SGFF (World Health Organization/Society Français de Gérontologie et de Gériatrie). International Association of Gerontology and Geriatrics: a global agenda for clinical research and quality of care in nursing homes. *J Am Med Dir Assoc.* 2011;12(3):185-189.

van Exel J, de Graaf G, Brouwer W. Care for a break? An investigation of informal caregivers attitudes toward respite using Q methodology. *Health Policy.* 2007;83:332-342.

MULTIPLE CHOICE QUESTIONS

1.1 Which of the following is *not* necessary to allow successful aging in place?

   a. Supportive relatives/friends
   b. Financial resource
   c. Minimal self-care capacity
   d. Social care services
   e. Physician home visits

1.2 What percentage of older persons living at home are unaware of the medications they are taking or the correct dose?

    a. 10%
    b. 30%
    c. 50%
    d. 70%
    e. 90%

1.3 Which of these countries has the highest institutionalization rate for older persons?

    a. Hong Kong
    b. South Korea
    c. United States
    d. United Kingdom
    e. Sweden

1.4 "Smart houses" utilize electronic monitoring of falls, gait, toileting, and food usage to allow older persons to age in place with minimal invasion of their home by healthcare workers. This is

    a. True
    b. False

1.5 The Program for All Inclusive Care for the Elderly (PACE) has been shown to have all of the following outcomes except:

    a. Cost-effective
    b. Participants less likely to die at home
    c. Reduction in hospitalizations
    d. Greater satisfaction
    e. Reduction in nursing home admissions

1.6 What prompted the IAGG to convene an International Nursing Home Taskforce?

    a. Population aging
    b. High cost of long-term care
    c. Variations in the quality of nursing home practice
    d. Confusion about terminology
    e. Inappropriate use of restraints in nursing homes

Chapter 2

THE NURSING HOME MOVEMENT

The concept of nursing homes began when Emperor Constantine (324-337 AD) moved the capital of the Byzantium Empire to Constantinople (Istanbul). His wife Helena developed a series of homes to take care of the infirm elderly persons, which were called "gerocomeia" (Figure 2–1). Of note is that physicians were required to provide care in the nursing home when these individuals became ill. The Knights Hospitaler of St. John is credited with developing the first hospice care facility in Rhodes (1309-1522). From these beginnings care for the infirm and the elderly was predominately provided by the Catholic Church and associated with monasteries.

In England, after the split with the Catholic Church, the care for the poor, sick, and aged became the responsibility of the parishes under the English Poor Law of 1601. These led to the building of poor houses that eventually evolved into nursing homes. In the United States, in the early 1850s, both Catholic nuns and the Jewish community began to develop nursing homes. In 1965, the passage of Medicare and Medicaid by Congress led to a flood of nursing homes being developed, as government money was made available for the care of the elderly and disabled. In much of the developing world, care of the aged remains the province of religious orders. In recent times in China, there is pressure on the government to develop nursing homes, although most rich, ill, older persons are looked after in hospitals until they die (Figure 2–2).

A number of organizations that champion the care of older persons in nursing homes have developed. A particularly effective group, the American Medical Directors Association (AMDA), was founded by William Dobbs, MD, James Pattee, MD, and Herman Gruber in Hilton Head, South Carolina in 1978. AMDA has become the premier information source on patients in long-term care, focusing on the role of physicians in the long-term care continuum. It provides certification for medical directors of nursing homes, and there is now evidence that certified medical directors improve the quality of care in nursing homes. AMDA produces 2 publications focused on nursing home care: one is a scientifically focused journal, *JAMDA: The Journal of the American Medical Directors Association,* and the other is a news magazine, *Caring for the Ages.* AMDA has developed several clinical practice guidelines and provides many other resources for its members. Opportunity for participation in the work of the association for all disciplines involved in nursing home care exists and the society has developed an international outreach program.

The National Association of Directors of Nursing Administration in Long Term Care (NADONA/LTC) was formed in 1986 in St. Louis, Missouri, to support and educate nurses working in long-term care. They provide certification for directors of nursing, a yearly conference, and a variety of other educational endeavors. Their journal, *The Director,* was first published in 1993.

The Gerontological Advanced Practice Nurse Association (GAPNA) was founded in the United States in 1981, and has special interest groups focused on nursing homes, assisted living, hospice, home care, and transitions. *Geriatric Nursing* is the society's journal.

The American Health Care Association is an advocacy group for long-term care providers. Its magazine is *The Provider.* Leading Age is a second national advocacy organization for long-term care providers, largely not-for-profit, in the United States. In 1989, the European Association for Directors and Providers of Long Term Care Services for the Elderly was founded in Luxembourg.

In addition to the societies named above, there are a number of influential projects that are also concerned with developing nursing home practice, most often on a national or regional basis. One such example is the innovative UK (England) My Home Life project (http://myhomelife movement.org/), which is funded by a consortium of charities. It is a collaborative program aimed at improving the quality of life of those who are living, dying, visiting, and working in care homes for older people. This project seeks the older person's view in all of its activities, which focus on the sharing of best practices and the development of resources to help practitioners and providers to improve experiences of care.

In the United States, the Advancing Excellence in America's Nursing Homes (www.nhqualitycampaign.org) was created in 2006. This organization works directly with more than half of the nursing homes in the United States by establishing an infrastructure for excellence, strengthening the workforce, and improving clinical and organizational outcomes. The goals of the organization are to:

- Reduce staff turnover
- Encourage consistent assignment of staff
- Independence from physical restraints
- Appropriate prevention and treatment of pressure ulcers
- Appropriate care to prevent and minimize pain

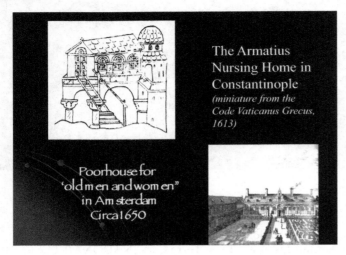

The Armatius Nursing Home in Constantinople *(miniature from the Code Vaticanus Grecus, 1613)*

Poorhouse for 'old men and women" in Amsterdam Circa 1650

Figure 2–1. Examples of early nursing homes. (Reprinted with permission from Morley JE. Geriatric future history. *J Nutr Health Aging.* 2006;10:431.)

- Do advance care planning according to the preferences of the residents
- Assess resident and family satisfaction
- Include staff satisfaction in quality improvement activities

In the United States, the medicalization of nursing homes occurred with the Hill-Burton Act (Hospital Survey and Construction Act) of 1954. This allowed hospitals to build long-term care facilities as part of the hospital. In 1965, passage of Medicare/Medicaid paid for rehabilitation in nursing homes and also for room and board for indigent elderly. Driven by the Institute of Medicare's report suggesting a major need for improving quality of nursing home care, Congress in the Office of Budget Reconciliation Act of 1987 (OBRA '87) passed new legislative requirements for nursing homes. The 4 keys to this legislation were:

- The requirement for a standard assessment (to become the minimum dataset)
- Reduction of restraints, psychotropic medications and Foley catheters
- A need for comprehensive care planning

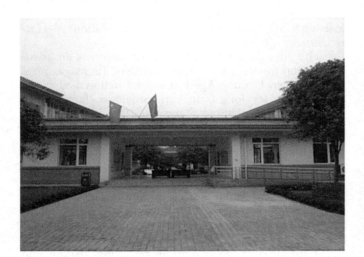

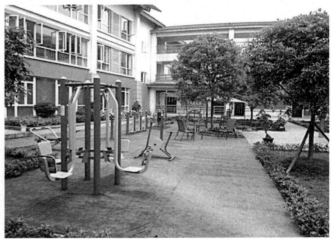

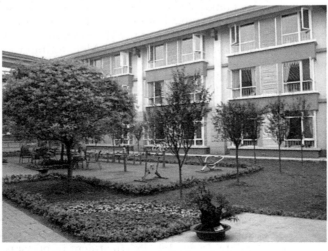

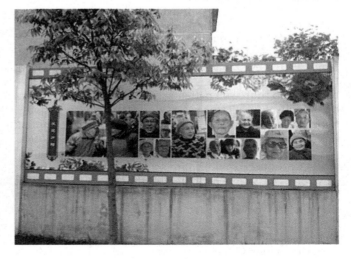

Figure 2–2. Nursing homes in Dujiangyan, China.

- The development of quality indicators
- The introduction of a medical director

This medicalization of American nursing homes has been a two-edged sword, markedly decreasing length of hospitalization and improving medical care in nursing homes, but at the same time deemphasizing the home aspects of long-term care. So, for a time, the standard approach to nursing home care in the United States was based on the hospital and medical model of care delivery. Consequently, nursing homes were built based on clinical design briefs modeling the hospital environment thus creating a sterile interior that was the antithesis of a home. Later in this chapter we explore contemporary views on best practices in nursing home design.

Development of nursing homes in the United Kingdom has seen long-term care beds move out of National Health Service Hospitals, with the remnants of poor law infirmaries, into a predominately (73%) independent sector care home market. In 2010, there were some 20,000 nursing home places caring for approximately 400,000 older residents. In the United Kingdom, a care home is defined as "a residential setting where older people live usually in single rooms with access to onsite care services, with or without nursing services." Only homes that are registered to provide nursing care have an obligation to ensure that care is supervised or administered by professional nurses. Care homes operate a social model of care, with healthcare from the state-funded National Health Service. Medical care is accessed through referral to National Health Service primary care and the family physician visits the person as they would anyone living in the community. For residents who are in care homes without onsite nursing, referral for community nursing services can also be requested. Care regulators focus on social dimensions or care based on nationally agreed minimum standards that come under their jurisdiction, but they do not regulate standards of healthcare. A report by the British Society of Geriatrics was highly critical of the predominant social model of care at the expense of access to expert clinical and nursing services. Medical directors are rare within UK care homes and it is not unusual for a single facility to have 10 to 20 different general practitioner providing care to their residents. These physicians, however, do not have influence on how the home is run.

DIVERSITY OF NURSING HOMES AND LONG-TERM CARE AROUND THE WORLD

Figure 2–3 shows the variability in the percentage of persons 65 years of age and older who are nursing home residents around the world. This varies from 0.2% in South Korea to 10% in Hong Kong.

In the United States, the majority of nursing home residents spend less than 6 months in the nursing home, either receiving rehabilitation with discharge to home or dying (Figure 2–4); 23.5% of short-term stayers who were admitted from a hospital are rehospitalized within 30 days. Only a small number of residents (9%) survive beyond 3 years. In contrast, in the United Kingdom, 27%

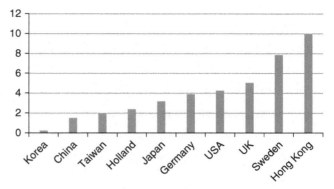

Figure 2–3. Percent of persons 65 years or older residing in nursing homes in selected countries.

of residents survive for more than 3 years, with the longest stayers living for more than 20 years. Similarly, in Australia 23% survive in nursing homes for 5 years or more. In most countries, just under half of the residents spend more than 2 years in the nursing home. As can be seen from Figure 2–5, most persons in nursing homes have a number of problems with activities of daily living associated with living at home.

In most of the world, half of nursing home residents are 85 years of age or older, the exceptions being Japan and Italy where there are more younger nursing home residents. In most countries, 70% or more of nursing home residents have dementia. The exception is the United States where fewer than 50% have dementia, a result of the emphasis on posthospital rehabilitation being carried out in nursing homes. Approximately half of the patients are incontinent of urine, and a smaller percentage are also incontinent of bowel. In France, 19.6% have aggressive behavior, 10.8% disruptive vocalization, and 10.9% are wanderers. The use of physical restraints varies from under 5% in countries such as the United States, Denmark, and Japan, to 20% or more in Hong Kong and Finland. Antipsychotic use is highest in Austria (45%) and lowest in Hong Kong (12%).

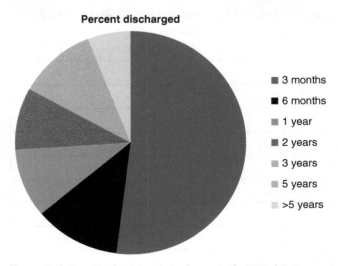

Figure 2–4. Length of stay in nursing homes in the United States.

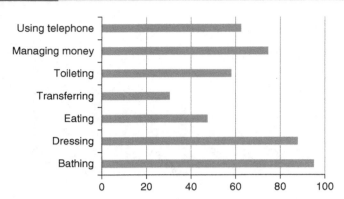

Figure 2–5. The percentage of nursing home residents in the United States needing help with activities of daily living.

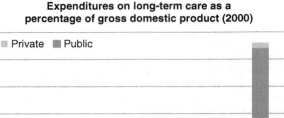
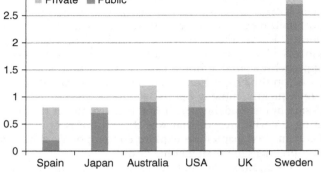

Figure 2–6. Public and private spending on institutional care as a percentage of the GDP in various industrialized countries. (Source OECD.)

Table 2–1 provides selected characteristics of residents in United States and European nursing homes based on the Minimum Data Set (MDS) 2.0. (Inter-Resident Assessment Instrument; Inter-RAI).

Most developed countries spend 0.5% to 1.6% of their gross domestic product on nursing home care. Norway and Sweden spend substantially more and Spain spends less.

The vast majority of nursing home care is publically funded (Figure 2–6). Most funding for long-term care is used for institutional care (Figure 2–7).

NURSING HOME DESIGN

Originally, nursing homes were either designed to be similar to hospitals or adapted available housing environments. In the 1970s, M. Powell Lawton designed the Weiss Pavilion at the Philadelphia Geriatric Center to be helpful to the residents as opposed to focusing on nursing

staff efficiency. Today, it is recognized that the physical environment interacts with individual and interpersonal factors, as well as the organizational environment, to modulate the behaviors of residents in nursing homes. Figure 2–8 provides examples of modern nursing homes in Europe.

Sizes of nursing homes vary. In the United States, approximately half have between 50 and 100 beds, with 7% having more than 200 beds. Recent studies suggest that smaller units with from 9 to 30 residents may be ideal for quality of care and life. Smaller units appear to lead to greater mobility and friendship formation; less agitation, aggression, and depression; and better maintenance of cognition. This has led to an enthusiasm for the Green Houses, which are homes for 9 to 12 older persons with private bedrooms and bathrooms, a communal room, and an open kitchen leading to the dining room. Even in larger nursing homes, private bedrooms are replacing rooms for 2 or more residents (Figure 2–9).

Table 2–1.	SELECTED CHARACTERISTICS OF RESIDENTS IN U.S. AND EUROPEAN NURSING HOMES BASED ON MDS 2.0	
	Characteristic	
	U.S. %	**Europe %**
9 or more meds	68	24
Antipsychotics	19	25
Depression	30	32
Pain	5	36
Falls	13	18
Incontinence	–	73
Weight loss (5%)	9	–
Pressure ulcers	14	10
Behavioral problems	16	27

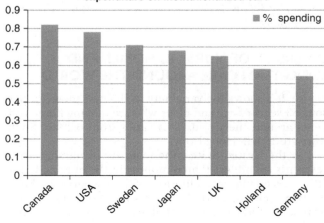

Figure 2–7. Share of total long-term care spent on institutional care. (Source OECD.)

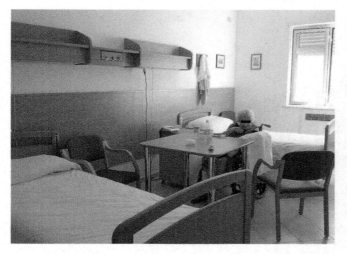
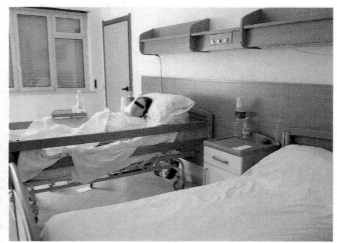
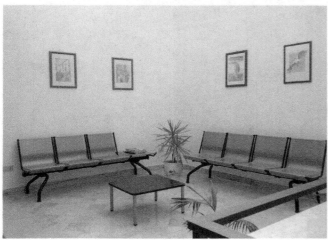
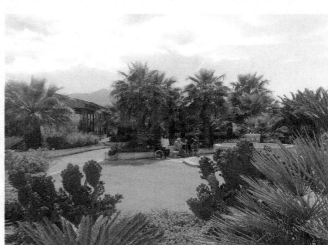

Figure 2–8. Nursing homes in Sicily. (Reprinted with permission from Ligia Dominguez.)

Many larger nursing homes have divided themselves into smaller units, designated Special Care Units, for the care of demented residents. These units often have access to an enclosed garden area with a circular "wander" pathway (Figure 2–10). Outdoor areas appear to be associated with better sleep.

The basic design of residential units is either bedrooms around a long corridor or bedrooms leading into a central community area. With the corridor design, the community area can either be at the end or the middle of the corridor. Bedroom size varies in different countries with the United States having the largest, Korea the smallest, and Japan and the United Kingdom having intermediate sizes. Most homes in the United States, United Kingdom, and Japan have 1 to 2 beds per bedroom, whereas Korea averages 4.9 beds per bedroom. Evidence supports the idea that private bedrooms are associated with greater resident, family, and staff satisfaction, and a reduction in nosocomial infections. Sleep quality is better; there is a decrease in both rummaging behavior and in resident conflicts with private rooms.

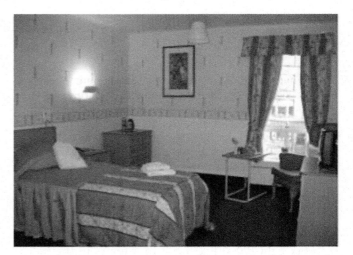

Figure 2–9. Private bedroom with homely furnishing in the United Kingdom.

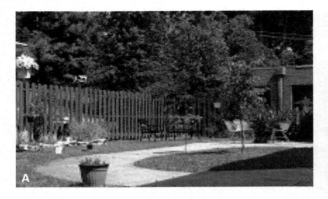

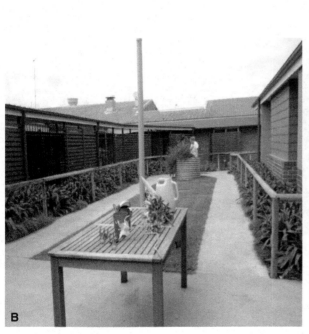

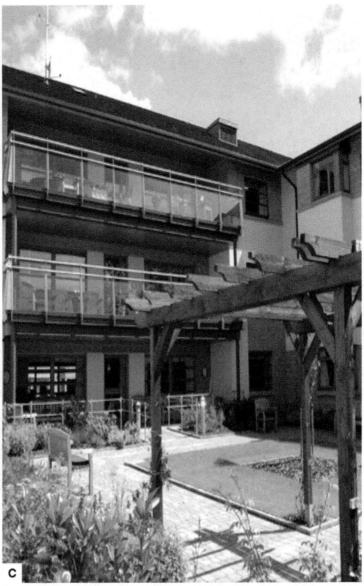

Figure 2–10. (**A**) Wander garden in USA Nursing Home. (**B**) Wander garden in Australian nursing home with fencing looking onto access path taken by staff to create sense of proximity to a street. (**C**) A UK nursing home with garden courtyard.

"Wayfinding" is an important component of design. Besides signage, especially personalized pictures outside rooms, decorating doors differently, and shorter distance to rooms giving direct visibility all allow residents to find their rooms more easily. Signage needs to be at a lower level than for younger persons as unstable persons tend to look lower to the ground. Windows to the outside also improve wayfinding. Many U.S. nursing homes now have "memory tables" outside the room, which contain pictures and meaningful mementos.

Lighting plays a key role in design. Natural light produced by skylights can have positive effects. In addition, high-lux light (2000 lux) for 2 to 4 hours in the morning may reset the advance in circadian rhythm seen with Alzheimer disease and improve sleep. Some studies show that residents have trouble tolerating the light.

Overall, the evidence on the efficaciousness of bright light is variable.

Not having strong contrasts on the flooring may well reduce falls. Accessibility to rooms for wheelchairs and avoidance of stairs or steps are an important component of design. Lack of doors on toilets in the bedrooms often improves access, decreasing incontinence and falls. Addition of grab bars along corridors and in toilets also has a role in reducing falls. Although there is a strong movement to deinstitutionalize nursing homes, the evidence that these changes improve outcomes is lacking. Nursing stations need to be central to minimize distances staff need to travel and should allow easy visual supervision of residents by the smallest number of staff. The inclusion of overhead hoists for ease of getting persons out of bed may be a useful design addition.

Table 2–2.	ATTRIBUTES OF A WELL-DESIGNED NURSING HOME

- Homelike environment with single bedrooms
- Adequate attention to needs for those with physical and visual disabilities
- Enhanced lighting
- Privacy and personalization of residents' rooms
- Environment that modulates the effects of loud sounds
- Soft furnishing to reduce reverberation of sound
- Easy-to-clean environment for incontinence
- Enhanced wayfinding
- High level of ventilation
- Thermal and humidity control
- Free of tripping hazards or distracting floor designs
- Bright open public spaces
- Safe access to outside spaces
- Window height suitable for wheelchair users

Table 2–3.	ORGANIZATIONAL BENEFITS OF EFFECTIVE NURSING HOME DESIGN

- Improves residents' quality of life
- Results in greater staff efficiency
- Is attractive to purchasers and relatives
- Incorporates cost-effective use of space
- Can improve occupancy rates

In designing nursing homes, emphasis needs to be put on the residential features rather than on the medical design. The focus needs to be on the general well-being of the residents rather than on high technological considerations. Table 2–2 summarizes the factors to be taken into account in nursing home design. The design features shown in Table 2–2 promote optimal and enabling conditions for people with age-related changes and frailty. For example, attention to the acoustic environment is important for residents with hearing impairment. Studies estimate that as many as 90% of dependent older people have age-related hearing loss. Older people tend to eat more when they feel relaxed and are socializing, so the meal time environment is important. Avoidance of sedentary behavior has many health benefits so it is important that mobilization is encouraged, that individuals can find their way, and that floor hazards are minimal. Compliant flooring, such as Smart Cell and SofTile floors (www.hiphealth.cu/media/research_cemfia_stephenrabinovitz) can reduce the impact of force on a hip after a fall by 47% (Figure 2–11).

All cement or wooden floors should be covered with carpets to reduce hip fractures.

In commercial terms, effective nursing home design brings with it important benefits for the organization, as shown in Table 2–3.

DESIGNING NURSING HOMES FOR PEOPLE WITH DEMENTIA

The basic accommodation needs of people with dementia are the same as for other residents. However, people with dementia particularly benefit from an environment that provides:

- Small-scale living units
- Familiar features and a homely style
- Scope for involvement in ordinary domestic activities
- Good signage and "cueing" features, for example, by providing well-lit, inviting entrances to day rooms
- Additional space for meaningful daytime activities

Following the principles of dementia-friendly design optimizes opportunity for independence and enhances resident's self-esteem. Features that are orientating and readily understandable and the use of objects of interest can provide important cues for sensing or following route. This is important in terms of encouraging physical exercise and is thought reassuring to those who are wandering.

A SENSE OF PLACE

Our final design consideration is that of place making and here we will borrow Pringle's comparison of the nursing home to an airplane. Both of these places are heavily managed in terms of space and how they permit or restrict certain activities through ritual and routine, and how little sense of control the inhabitants have over their environment. For example, in either environment you cannot choose who you sit beside, you cannot spread out your belongings but must confine them to your allocated space. At times your opportunity to mobilize will be restricted, you will have to wait until the bathroom is available no matter how urgent your need is to use it. If you want help from staff, you will need to wait until they are free, and your priority may not be their priority. The quality of the service you receive in either environment will improve with your ability to pay higher premiums! The key difference between airplanes and nursing homes is that flights are of relatively short duration, after which time you leave and return to normality. However, many older residents will live out the rest of their lives in

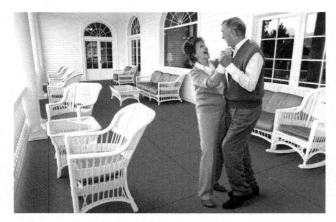

Figure 2–11. Compliant flooring can reduce the impact of falls. (Reprinted with permission from Jeromy Morningstar at Sofsurface.com.)

the nursing home. For air passengers the inconvenience and restrictions of flight are temporary and the tradeoff is that the flight gets us where we want to go. What then is the tradeoff for older persons who, as we saw in Chapter 1, would, if only they could, prefer to be back in their own homes?

The creation of the place that is the nursing home, involves responding to therapeutic demands (care) and the imperatives for safety and social control. This inevitably gives rise to some levels of standardization and uniformity in approach in the form of daily routines and rituals. Harmonizing institutional approaches with more enlightened strategies to enhance a resident's sense of autonomy is a difficult balance. Considerations of quality within the nursing home situation can be thought of in 3 aspects:

1. Quality of care (process or procedure)
2. Quality of life (personal perception)
3. Quality of the place (related to both of the above).

Interpretations of the quality of place go beyond the physical aesthetic to all of the interactions, caring administrations, and the general comings and goings of that place. A further consideration is that for people who do not recall their own recent history, such as people with dementia, place is an abstract concept. Increasingly in nursing literature there is recognition of the importance of thinking about this in terms of "moments of care" and "quality of the moment." Hence nursing home design needs to be considered broadly and encapsulate "place making" for all who may reside within, and for many this is perhaps best thought of as creating momentary positive senses of a good and safe place.

KEY POINTS

1. Nursing homes have inherited a charitable spirit often associated with faiths and support of the elderly infirm.
2. In recent years, a number of groups have emerged around the world to champion provision of high-quality nursing home care.
3. A high proportion of nursing home residents are cognitively impaired and many have multiple long-term conditions.
4. There is diversity in nursing home provision around the world, with some countries focusing exclusively on long-term care and end-of-life care, and others that focus on providing short-term rehabilitative services and respite care.
5. In the 1980s, medicalization of nursing homes, enabled by legislation, heralded a step change in the quality of clinical care provided to nursing home residents in the United States.
6. In the United Kingdom, care homes are based on a social model of care.
7. Contemporary design of nursing homes seeks to create an enabling homely environment for people with physical and cognitive impairments.
8. Place making is an important concept in promoting a homely safe environment.

SUGGESTED READINGS

British Geriatric Society. *2011 Quest for Quality. An Inquiry Into the Quality of Healthcare Support for Older People in Care Homes: A Call for Leadership, Partnership and Improvement.* http://www.bgs.org.uk/campaigns/carehomes/quest_quality_care_homes.pdf. Published by British Geriatric Society. Accessed March 28, 2013.

Calkins MP. Evidence-based long term care design. *NeuroRehabilitation.* 2009;25:145-154.

Cantley C, Wilson RC. *Put Yourself in My Place. Designing and Managing Care Homes for People with Dementia.* Joseph Rountree Foundation. http://www.jrf.org.uk/sites/files/jrf/1861348118. Bristol, UK: The Policy Press; 2002. Accessed March 28, 2013.

Grant LA, Kane RA, Stark AJ. Beyond labels: nursing home care for Alzheimer's disease in and out of special care units. *J Am Geriatr Soc.* 1995;43:569-576.

Hojo C. The VA's transformation of nursing home care: from nursing homes to community living centres. *Generations.* 2010;34(2):43-48.

Katz PR. An international perspective on long term care: focus on nursing homes. *J Am Med Dir Assoc.* 2011;12:487-492.

Kirkevold O, Eek A, Engedal K. Development of residential care services facilitated for persons with dementia in Norway. *Aging Clin Exp Res.* 2012;24:1-5.

Maas ML, Swanson E, Specht J, Buckwalter KC. Alzheimer's special care units. *Nurs Clin North Am.* 1994;29:173-194.

Morley JE. A brief history of geriatrics. *J Gerontol A Biol Sci Med Sci.* 2004;59:1131-1152.

Morley JE. Clinical practice in nursing homes as a key for progress. *J Nutr Health Aging.* 2010;14:586-593.

Morley JE. Geriatric future history. *J Nutr Health Aging.* 2006;10:431.

Nakanishi M, Nakashima T, Sawamura K. Quality of life of residents with dementia in a group-living situation: An approach to creating small, homelike environments in traditional nursing homes in Japan. *Nihon Koshu Eisei Zasshi.* 2012;59:3-10.

Pringle D. Making moments matter. *Can J Nurs Res.* 2003;35:7-13.

Rowland FN, Cowles M, Dickstein C, Katz PR. Impact of medical director certification on nursing home quality of care. *J Am Med Dir Assoc.* 2009;10:431-435.

Sharkey SS, Hudak S, Horn SD, et al. Frontline caregiver daily practices: a comparison study of traditional nursing homes and the Green House project sites. *J Am Geriatr Soc.* 2011;59:126-131.

Tolson D, Morley JE. Medical care in the nursing home. *Med Clin North Am.* 2011;95:595-614.

Tolson D, Nolan M. Gerontological nursing 4: age-related hearing explored. *Br J Nurs.* 2000;9(4):205-208.

MULTIPLE CHOICE QUESTIONS

2.1 The origin of nursing homes was in

a. Paris
b. Constantinople
c. Rhodes
d. Rome
e. Athens

2.2 The major change in nursing home care in the United States was as a result of OBRA. In which year were these nursing home regulations enacted?

a. 1965
b. 1982
c. 1987
d. 1990
e. 1993

2.3 In which country do less than 70% of nursing home residents have dementia?

   a. Japan
   b. United Kingdom
   c. Italy
   d. Sweden
   e. United States

2.4 Which of the following is more common in the U.S. nursing homes than in European nursing homes?

   a. Resident receives 9 or more drugs
   b. Behavioral problems
   c. Use of antipsychotics
   d. Falls
   e. Antipsychotic use

2.5 Which of the following is not an attribute of a well-designed nursing home?

   a. Modulates the effects of loud sounds
   b. Enhanced lighting
   c. Windows at normal height
   d. Easy-to-clean environment
   e. High level of ventilation

Chapter 3

NURSING HOME EXPERIENCE

To understand nursing home life and the many challenges associated with creating a good experience for individuals and families, it is useful to reflect on the meaning of nursing and the meaning of home. In the context of nursing home practice, the term *nursing* can be interpreted in two ways. Nursing can be used to either denote acts of "nursing care," which can be provided by any practitioners, informal caregivers, and family caregivers, or the term can be used to mean the skilled evidence-based practice that is provided by registered and qualified (professional) nurses. The scope of nursing practice delivered within nursing homes varies with region as discussed in Chapter 2, and registered nurses often provide a practice leadership role within nursing home teams. Broadly speaking, professional nursing with older nursing home residents encompasses:

- Curative and rehabilitative dimensions
- Management of long-term conditions
- Care for those who become frail
- Palliative and end-of-life care

The term *nursing* in the context of a "nursing home" suggests that it is a facility where nursing care in its broadest sense is provided (social model). But it can also be a place where residents may benefit from skilled or evidence-based informed nursing provided by registered nurses with advanced skills in working with older people (nursing model). In the medical model, this has been extended to include interaction with physicians and other health professionals (e.g., pharmacists) within the nursing home. In this model, the nursing home also has a medical director or medical coordinator as part of the facility administration.

Home is a word commonly used in many (but not all) societies, and it is important to make a distinction between the place that is home and the building in which people may reside. If we think about home as a place (an aspect of the environment), we begin to realize that building design alone does not turn a building into something that can be experienced by an individual as a home. When people are choosing nursing homes for themselves or loved ones, they often have an intuitive sense of the places in which they would "feel at home" and places where they would not. Developing a sense of belonging and feeling safe is integral to feeling at home. A recent Swedish study suggested that an older person's sense of home depends on the interpersonal relationships and behaviors of all the people who regularly enter a person's life space and interact with him or her, more than the physical space.

MY EXPERIENCE OF NURSING HOMES: VOICE OF THE RESIDENT

There is growing recognition of the importance of listening to what older people say about their experiences of care and respecting their views. Much attention is now placed on personalized approaches to care, and the benefits of knowing the person within long-term care environments are well known. Expectations of older people change with successive generations and are culturally bound, and it is not easy for anyone who is vulnerable and dependent on others to complain. Indeed, gratitude bias, the tendency for older people to be grateful for care and attention regardless of its quality, means that resident satisfaction surveys need to be interpreted with caution. To offset this problem in the United Kingdom, volunteer lay assessors, who are members of the public trained for this role, take part in the Regulator's Inspections of nursing homes and spend time with residents to illicit their feelings. In the United States, ombudsmen (lay volunteers) provide this role on a weekly basis in the nursing home. When complaints are forthcoming, they are often about communication failures and lack of respect or disregard for the resident's right to self-determination.

Many social and nursing care texts espouse the merits of knowing the person through the use of life history (biographical approaches) following humanistic principles. Such approaches are not without their challenges in practice, and it is beyond the scope of this text to explore the arguments fully. Let it suffice to say that to provide personalized care, which is generally considered desirable, requires knowledge of the person who is the recipient of care, including the person's past and present; family and friends; and likes, dislikes, aspirations, and fears. Such personal knowledge permits staff to make emotional connections and anticipate need and plan the best approaches to delivering person-centered care.

The U.K. Alzheimer Society in collaboration with the Royal College of Nursing produced a leaflet "This is Me" to assist practitioners to get to know a person with dementia. The person with dementia and a family caregiver or friend

Table 3–1.   EXTRACT OF "THIS IS ME" GUIDANCE
My name: Full name and the name I prefer to be known by.
Caregiver or the person who knows me best: It may be a spouse, relative, friend, or caregiver.
I would like you to know: Include anything I think is important and will help staff to get to know and care for me (e.g., I have dementia, I have never been in hospital before, I prefer female caregivers, I don't like the dark, I am left handed, I am allergic to …).
My home and family, things that are important to me: Include marital status, children, grandchildren, friends, pets, any possessions, things of comfort. Any religious or cultural considerations.
My hearing and eyesight: Can I hear well, or do I need a hearing aid? How is it best to approach me? Is the use of touch appropriate? Do I wear glasses or need any other vision aids?
My personal care: Normal routines, preferences, and usual level of assistance required in the bath, shower, or other. Do I prefer a male or female caregiver? What are my preferences for continence aids used, soaps, cosmetics, shaving, teeth cleaning, and dentures?

Adapted from Alzheimer's Society. *This is Me Leaflet.* http://alzheimers. org.uk/site/scripts/document_pdf.php?documentID=1290.

complete and update the form in advance of admission so that staff can readily obtain information about the person, communicate appropriately, and begin to personalize care from the outset. The information includes brief details about current and past life, people who are important, activities of daily living abilities, routines, and preferences. An extract of the form is shown in Table 3–1, and it is free to download from the Internet and can be adapted for local use.

The vulnerability that older people feel as a result of their dependence on staff on moving into a care home has been vividly described in many firsthand accounts as has the importance of being able to keep treasured possessions with them (e.g., photographs, ornaments, and other personal items that contribute to a person's sense of identity and belonging). The quotation below and the poem in Table 3–2 both capture the importance of seeing the person and remind us that each older person has a past, a present, and a future.

> *Our main concern was that she would be free from pain; her main concern was that her hair looked nice. Funny that she worried about her hair at that stage in her life. She had her hair done the week she died, insisted she looked nice for her visitors. Said she wanted be remembered as a smart, well-kempt women, even got dressed up for her last photos with her grandchildren.*
>
> (Daughter of former Nursing Home Resident. England, UK).

Table 3–2.   WHAT DO YOU SEE?
What do you see nurses. What do you see? Are you thinking? When you are looking at me? A crabbit old woman, not very wise? Uncertain of habit, faraway eyes, Who dribbles her food, and makes no reply, When you say in a loud voice, "I do wish you'd try." Who seems not to notice, the things that you do, And forever is losing, a stocking or shoe. Who unresisting or not lets you do as you will, When bathing and feeding, the long day to fill. Is that what you are thinking, is that what you see? Then open your eyes nurse, you are not looking at me.
I'll tell you who I am, as I sit here so still. As I use at your bidding, as I eat at your will. I'm a small child of ten, with a father and mother, Brothers and sisters, who love one another. A young girl of sixteen, with wings on her feet, Dreaming that soon now a lover she'll meet. A bride soon at twenty, my heart gives a leap, Remembering the vows, that I promised to keep, At twenty-five now, I have young of my own. Who need me to build a secure happy home.
A woman of thirty, my young now grown fast. Bound to each other, with ties that should last. At forty my young sons now grow and will be gone, But my man stays beside me to see, I don't mourn. At fifty, once more babies play round my knee, Again we know children, my loved ones and me.
Dark days are upon me, my husband is dead. I look at the future I shudder with dread. For my young are all busy, rearing young of their own. And I think of the years, and the Love that I've known. I'm an old woman now, and nature is cruel. It's her jest, to make old age look like a fool. The body it crumbles, grace and vigor depart, There is now a stone, where I once had a heart. But inside this old carcass, a young girl still dwells, And now and again, my battered heart swells, I remember the joys, I remember the pain, And I'm loving and living, life all over again. I think of the years, all too few—gone too fast, And accept the stark fact, that nothing can last. So open your eyes, nurses, open and see, Not a crabbit old woman. Look closer—see me. —Anonymous

Photographs also allow us to connect to a person's earlier life, identity, and sense of person. The bride and groom photograph (Figure 3–1) shows Rita as a 27-year-old bride; her future hopes never included being the "lady in room 9 with dementia."

OUR EXPERIENCE OF NURSING HOMES: VOICES OF FAMILY AND FRIENDS

Knowing the person and taking steps to preserve personhood involves understanding and maintaining relationships with family and friends. Few studies have

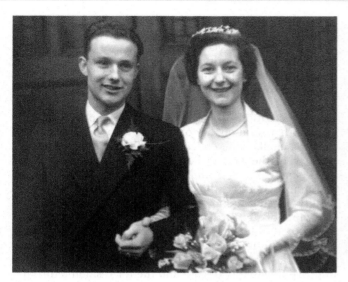 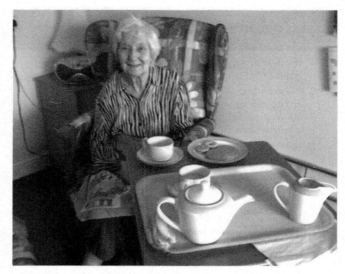

Figure 3–1. Wedding day, age 27 years; afternoon tea, 59 years later in the Dementia Care Unit.

considered the effects on relationships of a spouse or partner moving into a care home. Some commentators liken the experience to an elongated bereavement in that the visiting partner is not free to resume his or her life and move on. A recent study in Hong Kong revealed that many nursing home residents believed that their admission had freed up their partner and alleviated them of the burden of caring. However, the visiting partners reported heightened guilt and distress because the burden of care was reframed by the knowledge that they had failed their loved ones. So it is important that the emotional consequences on the family caregiver are acknowledged and that staff are mindful of the continuing and sometimes acute distress that partners may feel, particularly after admission. The emotionality of visiting loved ones is captured in the following quote from a husband visiting his 83-year-old wife with dementia.

> *The worst moment for me is walking into the day room. Each time I go it's the same. I look along the row of people in chairs, but I don't see my wife; the nurse points her out. I don't recognize her sometimes, and when she cries, it breaks my heart. I give her a kiss hello and hold her hand as you do, but I don't know what to say. What are you supposed to do? It's so hard visiting and so hard if you don't.*
>
> (Mr. Craig. 82 years old, Glasgow).

Relatives are a good source of knowledge about an older person, and finding ways to involve relatives in care has the potential to promote positive experiences. It is, however, important to recognize that family and friends have needs of their own, and a balance is required between involving and overburdening visitors.

In the Netherlands, a study investigating family caregivers' attitudes toward respite services within nursing homes identified two groups of caregivers. The largest group felt misunderstood and abandoned by community services, and the minority group believed that they did not need respite services. It should be noted that the latter group included families that did not access respite because the older person refused this option. Sensitive nursing home practitioners appreciate that family members, particularly those who have shouldered a heavy burden of care, are still recovering from the strain. In addition family members must also adapt to their new role of visitor when formerly they were the main caregivers. Many low-cost interventions can help family caregivers who may be struggling with the emotional burden associated with admission of a loved one to a nursing home (Table 3–3). The one thing that all family visitors want is the reassurance that the person they love is getting good care is settled in the nursing home. It is only natural that we all want the best possible for our older relatives and partners, so visitors are understandably anxious.

Caregiver's Story

> *I looked after Ella all our married life. She was 16 when we married and just as beautiful when she died 70 years later. She hadn't been herself for a couple of years when the doctor said she had dementia and would need nursing. I wanted her to stay at home with me, but in the end, I agreed to try this respite scheme they do. Then she had to go in, you know, and the staff were very kind to her, and they liked my Ella, said she was special and funny. I missed her rotten, but I was more at peace. They called me in when it was her time and let me sit with her. The nurse said I could lie on the bed with her, and I did. She died with my arms around her just like we were at home. They put flowers in her room. She would have liked that, my Ella. Everything I did was for the love of Ella.*
>
> (Ella's husband. Scotland).

Table 3–3.   TWELVE TIPS FOR SUPPORTING FAMILIES IN THE NURSING HOME

1. Greet them respectfully on arrival and ask about their well-being.

2. Reassure them about the well-being of their relative and update them as appropriate on their relative's progress. Offer information about the person's day (e.g., what has the person eaten for lunch); do not wait to be asked.

3. Help them to locate their relative by showing them where their relative is.

4. If the resident is asleep gently, wake him or her and say who is here to visit.

5. Attend to the appearance of the resident. If the resident requires assistance with the toilet, hand washing, or clothing adjustments, provide help promptly to promote dignity and demonstrate respect.

6. If the resident wears spectacles or a hearing device, ensure that he or she has to help him or her converse more easily and hear what visitors have to say.

7. Offer to move the resident to a preferred location for the visit; this may be in the resident's room, a day area, or perhaps outside in the fresh air.

8. Offer a tray of tea or cold drinks to be shared with the resident if possible.

9. Be mindful of the difficulties of visiting an uncommunicative person. When a visitor is not resourceful, suggest how he or she might engage the person's attention such as by looking at old photographs.

10. Ask visitors how they think their relative is settling in and be responsive to concerns even if they seem trivial.

11. Ask visitors if there is anything worrying them and update them on changes to treatment plans.

12. Some visitors find a visitor's diary useful to communicate with other visitors and with healthcare professionals.

WORKING IN A NURSING HOME

The International Association of Gerontology and Geriatrics Taskforce on Nursing Homes recognized that working in a nursing home has in many regions been afforded a low status, giving rise to recruitment and retention challenges and workforce instability. This applies to nursing staff, administrators, and physicians, who often feel disadvantaged in terms of pay, reward packages, and career opportunities. Major challenges for nursing homes are staff turnover and absenteeism. Turnover rates of 25% or more are common in European nursing homes. It will come as no surprise that a stable team is more likely to have capable and stable leadership, be more likely to deliver higher quality care and obtain a reputation for high standards, and be more likely to attract higher caliber staff than a nursing home with a poorer reputation. Workforce and employment issues are thus inextricably linked to care quality.

The explanations for this lie in the growing evidence base that the key to a good life for older people with high support needs are:

- Personalized support and care
- Meaningful daily and community life
- Meaningful relationships
- Personal identity and self-esteem
- Home and personal surroundings
- Personal authority and control

The creation of a place where older people experience both a good quality of life and a good experience of care is a challenging endeavor, and our understanding of underlying theory and best practice is emergent. What we do know is that in addition to maintaining family and community relationships an essential ingredient of high-quality nursing home care are the caring attributes and behaviors of staff. It is well known that when employees deal directly with clients, the satisfaction of the client—in our case, the nursing home user—is directly influenced by staff attitude and affect. Furthermore, strategies to improve the quality of care and life for residents through culture change approaches (see Chapter 4) rely on committed staff with an appropriate value base and practice know how working in an atmosphere where mutual respect and reciprocity thrive. Job satisfaction among nursing home staff is an important determinant of their ability to sustain high-quality care delivery, and this in turn requires organizational valuing of staff and appropriate rewards systems. Numerous studies have shown that workers who receive adequate pay and benefits are more likely to stay within an organization when this is coupled with possibilities of career advancement and a sense of autonomy to improve practices. A salient feature of many culture change projects is the empowerment of frontline nursing home practitioners, and this is thought likely to reduce staff turnover through greater job satisfaction. Strategies to reduce staff turnover are critical to the success of individual nursing homes and for the sector at large because high turnover makes for an unstable workforce. Workforce instability and recruitment and retention of nursing home personnel are universal challenges. A major concern is the current high use of immigrant workers in direct care roles within nursing homes because immigrant employment status, rightly or wrongly, is associated with low-status, low-skilled positions. Immigrant workers also seem to be poorly supported through development opportunities. The United States, for example, has high numbers of nursing staff coming from Mexico, the Philippines, Africa, and Caribbean. Japan and Italy, two countries with the oldest populations, rely heavily on workers from less developed nations. In France, a growing proportion of nursing home staff originate from North Africa, where most older people would expect to remain within the family home. Although there is much to celebrate in cultural diversity, for some older residents, being cared for by staff who do not share their own cultural heritage is not ideal. Thought should be given to including local cultural heritage information within orientation programs for all newly hired staff. This will help staff to find topics of conversation and reminiscence triggers that will help them to relate to residents.

Job satisfaction is inherently linked to perceptions of stress in the workplace, and the increasing pressure for better standards of care in the nursing home can inadvertently compound staff stress. Three features of work-related stress need to be recognized within nursing homes and other long-term care settings:

1. Quantitative overload
2. Qualitative overload
3. Qualitative underload

To put this simply, staff are at risk of both "burnout" and "rustout." Burnout is associated with sustained high demand on staff. In comparison, rustout is associated with staff boredom often associated with unrewarding relationships (e.g., with cognitively impaired residents who are uncommunicative). Although the triggers for underload and overload are different, the consequences within long-term care environments for older people are similar in that practitioners begin to disengage emotionally and detach themselves from their practice and in turn the residents. Thus, burnout and rustout not only directly impact the individual staff member and threatens his or her sense of well-being but also have a negative impact on his or her relationships with colleagues and undermine care quality. An extreme consequence of staff stress is serious abuse of people entrusted to their care (see Chapter 5); more often staff stress leads to more subtle emotional abuse of residents or neglectful acts.

The experience of working in contemporary nursing homes is inevitably influenced by the historical development of the sector as described in Chapter 1. Devaluation of nursing homes and nursing home practice is reported throughout international literature. Furthermore, in some regions, the charitable status of nursing homes and institutional approaches and a general devaluing of the skills and knowledge base required to deliver high-quality long-term care is pervasive. The high proportion of unqualified caregivers working in many nursing homes throughout the world and lack of professional recognition are major sources of concern. A Swedish study revealed that caregivers with no formal competence (untrained) assessed their workload as higher and perceived more work-related stress compared with caregivers with formal competence (trained workers). This indicates that where recruitment of qualified staff is difficult and workforce models rely heavily on untrained assistants, training programs and supervision arrangements must be in place. The absence of such mechanisms for untrained staff who lack essential competencies increases their risks of burnout, which predisposes residents to unsatisfactory experiences of care. In addition, it is important to appreciate that immigrant staff who lack language fluency in their host country may be vulnerable to faster "rustout" than those able to converse more easily and form meaningful relationships with older people.

Although many challenges are associated with working in a nursing home, for practitioners who are committed to working with older people, the rewards are high. In Part 2, we explore in more detail the contributions from a range of disciplines, nursing home leadership, and strategies that have been shown to promote culture change and achievement of an enriched environment of care.

KEY POINTS

1. The term *nursing home* conveys the expectation that it is a place where older people are able to experience the sense of "feeling at home" and where they can expect to receive nursing care in its broadest sense but also to benefit from evidence informed professional nursing.
2. Staff behavior and interpersonal communication are key factors in the development of a sense of home.
3. Personalization of care and approaches that demonstrate respect for individual care choices and preference are associated with good experiences of care.
4. Personalization of care is central to culture change and improvement of quality within nursing homes.
5. To achieve personalization of care, staff need to see each person and feel his or her personality. When the individual has limited ability to convey this, then staff can invite family and friends to help them to build a picture of the person, including their interests, likes and dislikes, and some key facts about his or her life and the people that matter to the person.
6. Family members and intimate partners can find the transition from being the main caregiver to the visitor of a relative within a nursing home distressing. It is important to find a balance between involving them within nursing home life and direct care and enabling them to adjust to a phase in the relationship with their loved one.
7. Working in a nursing home has historically been afforded a low status. As we move forward, it is essential that nursing home careers are seen as positive choices with rewards and incentives to ensure recruitment and retention of high-caliber staff.
8. Research has demonstrated that staff with no formal competences struggle to deliver care at its best. It is essential that all staff receive appropriate preparation and supervision to develop and embed good practice.
9. The emotional labor of working in a nursing home exposes staff to the risk of "burnout" through high demand and "rustout" through lack of stimulation and feedback from uncommunicative residents.

SUGGESTED READINGS

Andrew GJ, Holmes D, Poland B, et al. "Airplanes are flying nursing homes": geographies in the concepts and locales of gerontological nursing practice. *J Clin Nurs.* 2005;14(8b):109-120.

Bishop CE, Squillace MR, Meagher J, et al. Nursing home work practices and nursing assistance job satisfaction. *Gerontologist.* 2009; 49(5):611-622.

Bishop CE, Weinberg DB, Leutz W, et al. Nursing assistants' job commitment: effect of nursing home organizational factors and impact on resident well-being. *Gerontologist.* 2008;48(special issue 1):36-45.

Bowers Helen, Clark A, Crosby G, et al. *Older People's Vision of Long Term Care.* York. England UK: Joseph Rowntree Foundation; 2005.

Engstrom M, Skytt B, Nilsson A. Working life and stress symptoms among care givers in elderly care with formal and no formal competence. *J Nurs Manage.* 2011;19:732-741.

Gillsjo C, Schartz-Barcott D. A concept analysis of home and its meaning in the lives of three older adults. *Int J Older People Nurs.* 2011;6(1):4-12.

Nolan M, Grant G. Rust out and therapeutic reciprocity: concepts to advance the nursing care of older people. *J Adv Nurs.* 1993; 18:1305-1314.

Redfern S, Hannan S, Norman I, Marti F. Work satisfaction, stress, quality of care and morale of older people in a nursing home. *Health Soc Care Community.* 2002;10(6):512-517.

Stone RI, Weiner JA. *Who Will Care for Us? Addressing the Long-Term Care Workforce Crisis.* http://www.futureofaging.org/ publications/pub_result.asp?workforce=1&housing=0&improvem ent=0. Published 2005. Accessed March 24, 2013.

Sloane PD, Williams CS, Zimmerman S. Immigrant status and intention to leave of nursing assistants in US nursing homes. *J Am Geriatr Soc.* 2010;58:731-737.

Tolson D, Rolland Y, Andrieu S, et al. The International Association of Gerontology and Geriatrics/World Health Organization/Society Française de Gérontologie et de Gériatrie Task Forces. A global agenda for clinical research and quality of care in nursing homes. *J Am Med Dir Assoc.* 2011;12(3):185-189.

van Exel J, de Graaf G, Brouwer W. Care for a break? An investigation of informal caregivers attitudes toward respite using Q-methodology. *Health Policy.* 2007;83:332-342.

MULTIPLE CHOICE QUESTIONS

3.1 Which of the following is characteristic of the medical model of nursing homes?

   a. Nursing is provided by registered nurses.
   b. The nursing home has a medical director or a medical coordinator.
   c. Residents are provided with help with activities of daily living.
   d. End-of-life care is provided.

3.2 Which of these is *not* a requirement of personalized care?

   a. Requires knowledge about the life history of the person receiving care
   b. Requires knowledge about the individual's likes and dislikes
   c. Requires a knowledge of the person's friends and family
   d. Requires a knowledge of history at the time the person was young
   e. Requires a knowledge of the person's likes and dislikes

3.3 Which of the following is true of the attitude of nursing home residents and families to admission to nursing homes?

   a. Many new residents believe that their admission freed up their partner and reduced their burden of caring.
   b. Visiting partners do not feel guilt.
   c. There is a high level of stress in the person still living at home.
   d. The emotional consequences of being admitted to a nursing home are minor.
   e. Visiting a partner in the nursing home is not hard.

3.4 Which of the following is associated with staff "burnout?"

   a. Boredom
   b. Unrewarding relationships
   c. High demand
   d. Qualitative underload
   e. Working with uncommunicative persons with dementia

3.5 Which of the following is most compatible with "rustout" of staff?

   a. No formal training
   b. Lack of language fluency
   c. High workload
   d. Qualitative overload
   e. Quantitative overload

Chapter 4

ADVANCING NURSING HOME PRACTICE THROUGH CULTURE CHANGE

Achieving best nursing home practice requires an understanding of the influence of culture on both organizational and staff behaviors. A simple way of thinking about organizational culture is "how things are done around here." "How things are done" is a product of deep-seated assumptions about ways of doing the work of the organization. Thus, the culture within the organization concerns values, dictates receptiveness to change and learning, and embeds ways of doing things that become unquestioned routines. Improvement efforts will only succeed in a positive culture in which staff:

- Experience pride in their work
- Feel committed to improvement
- Sense shared accountability
- Respect one another's expert contributions
- Believe that they have opportunity to own and collectively solve problems
- Perceive that they are a valued members of an effective team

As the above list suggests, perceived values or perceived culture plays an important part within improvement projects. It is also necessary to appreciate that there are other dynamics at play, including market forces and external positioning of the organization to compete, and the bureaucratic controls that regulate and monitor. So when an organization may strive for flexibility but the bureaucratic compliance agenda demands uniformity and prioritization of its mandates, there are inevitable tensions. Hence, a range of internal and external forces impact the organization shape administrative leadership responses and sometimes are thought to be competing with each other. Organizational development experts have described this in terms of the "competing values framework." Table 4–1 presents some questions that will help staff to get insight into the culture of the nursing home where they work and appreciate some of the tensions.

From your answers to the questions in Table 4–1, you should get an idea if the culture is essentially positive or negative. An interesting exercise is to compare how different staff groups within the same nursing home respond to these sets of questions. Studies have repeatedly shown that in negative cultures, there are wide variations between different staff groups and a lack of awareness between the groups of these felt differences.

CHALLENGES TO PROVIDING QUALITY CARE

The Royal College of Nursing U.K. has published three national surveys exploring the quality of nursing home care within England in 2004, 2010, and 2012. The latest 2012 survey was completed by 584 nurses working within care homes in England. Comparing the findings of the three surveys has identified 10 persistent challenges to the provision of high quality care. These challenges summarized in Table 4–2 are not peculiar to the United Kingdom but reflect universal core problems.

APPROACHES TO ADVANCING PRACTICE

Internationally, there have been a range of approaches used to enhance healthcare practice. The popularity of approaches reflects regional and constitutional differences and disciplinary perspectives. There is no doubt that the evidence-based practice movement has been a major force, and this has led to a proliferation of evidence-based guidelines and care standards. There are a plethora of practice development methodologies, organizational development frameworks, and improvement strategies that all seek to advance evidence-informed changed. Interestingly, systematic reviews of the impact of even the most popular developmental methods have failed to show superiority of one approach over another. It would thus seem reasonable to conclude that there is no "golden bullet" that will suit all situations and that nursing home leaders must be discerning in their choice of methods. In terms of changing nursing home culture, transformative approaches are required, and two movements warrant attention: practice development and culture change. The International Practice Development Colloquium offers the following definition:

> Practice development is a continuous process of developing person-centred cultures. It is enabled by facilitators who authentically engage with individuals and teams to blend personal qualities and creative imagination with practice skills and practice wisdom. The learning that occurs brings about transformations of individual and team practices. This is sustained by embedding both processes and outcomes in corporate strategy.
>
> Manley K, McCormack B, Wilson V, eds. *International Development in Nursing and Healthcare.* Oxford, UK: Blackwell Publishing; 2008:9.

Table 4–1.   UNDERSTANDING NURSING HOME CULTURE
1. Based on your experience, what do you understand to be the main strategic driver for the organization?
2. Do the written mission statement and declared values of the organization reflect your day-to-day working experiences?
3. How would you characterize the management style of the organization based on how you are treated as a member of staff?
4. If you have an idea for improving an aspect of care, how easy is it for you to take the idea forward?
5. Overall, what would you say the nursing home is like, and how is success defined, rewarded, and celebrated?
6. What is the organizational glue that holds together the nursing home and the staff team?

Practice development involves a collection of participatory interventions based on transforming behavior and culture. Originally associated with nursing practice in the United Kingdom, practice development is now popular across the northern and southern hemispheres. The principles of practice development are based on partnerships that include service users in the quest to achieve person-centered and clinically effective healthcare in an enriched environment of care. Progress occurs as cycles of development and growth that encompass planning, designing, reflection, implementation, and evaluation. Similar to many methods that drive for sustained change, the relationship between the evidence, the context, and facilitation are critical, and organizational commitment is a prerequisite to success. Practice development approaches have been successfully used to transform caring cultures in a diverse range of settings, including hospitals and nursing homes across Europe, Australasia, and North America. There are some similarities between practice development and culture change methods; both seek transformational change. The culture change journey and core values touch many aspects of nursing home operation, including systems, decision making, accountability, environmental changes, and language use. Most of the literature on culture change is oriented toward the North American experience.

CULTURE CHANGE AND QUALITY OF CARE

There is no doubt that the revolutionary medicalization of nursing homes in the United States, as discussed in Chapter 2, yielded benefits that raised standards and clinical outcomes. The imposition of an exclusively medical model, however, brought with it a hospital-based culture across all of its activities, including approaches to nursing. Treatment took primacy over care, and stories abound of heroic efforts to keep people alive rather than commence palliative and end-of-life care. Interestingly, a recent study of newly introduced Tyrollean nursing homes describes the challenges for nurses who have been prepared for hospital roles to adjust to a nurse-led nonmedicalized approach. There is much to learn from the experiences within the United States of the pitfalls of medicalization at the expense of other aspects of care. Also, there are lessons to be learned from the rejection of the medical model from

Table 4–2.   CHALLENGES TO PROVIDING QUALITY NURSING HOME CARE
Funding and Admissions
• The health and social care needs of older people admitted to nursing homes is becoming increasingly complex, and funding does not reflect the complexity of needs.
• Admission of people with the means to self-fund and pay higher fees creates inequality of access.
• The business need to fill beds can prompt inappropriate admissions.
Staffing Levels
• Shortage of registered nurses with appropriate expertise
• Shortage of care assistants
• Access barriers to expert physician input
Appropriate Skill Mix
• Lack of evidence-based guidance around skill mix given the changing needs of the care home population
Recruitment and Retention
• Transient management and leadership
• New starters often have to learn on the job
• Errors or poor approaches being overlooked in attempt to retain staff
• Reliance on agency staff
Low Levels of Morale
• Poor working conditions
• Disillusioned staff with the intention to leave
• Negative media
Lack of Training
• Statutory training being prioritized in the absence of funding for training essential to advance professional practice and practice improvement
• Lack of affordable or appropriate courses to skill up care assistants
• Difficulties with back fill when staff attends training courses
• Training is first thing to go when budgets are cut
Lack of Equipment
• Particularly medical equipment and medical supplies
Bureaucracy and Inspections
• Management driven by compliance agenda to satisfy minimum standard requirements for facility registration
• Administrative burden of inspections disproportionately high
Ethic of the Organization
• Business ethic and quest for profit undermining delivery of high-quality care
Working with Other Sectors
• Incompatible systems and poor communication between sectors (e.g., when residents are admitted to and from hospitals)
• Lack of respect for nursing home sector staff

countries such as the United Kingdom, where a social-nursing model of care predominates. Indeed, a recent review in the United Kingdom concluded that although the social model is central to life in nursing homes, it is insufficient, and expert healthcare administered by geriatricians, old age psychiatrists, and nurse experts in the care of older people is essential. Throughout the United States and United Kingdom, there are examples of failing nursing homes with poor standards that fail to consistently provide safe and dignified care. In contrast, there are also examples of centers of excellence where nursing home practice flourishes and care is personalized and aligned with the best available evidence.

A survey of nursing homes in the United States in 2001 suggested that nearly half of nursing homes had inadequate staff, that a quarter of staff were uninterested and nonresponsive to family concerns, and a quarter of residents had been treated badly or abused by staff. This led to an examination of the medical model of nursing home care and a broader definition of quality (Table 4–3), giving rise to new multidimensional approach to quality (Table 4–3).

Although adequate care for health conditions remained a component, more emphasis was placed on maximizing functional independence in a safe and clean environment. This should be done in a home-like environment that maintains residents' dignity and promotes positive feelings among residents, family, and caregivers. Above all, this approach to quality emphasizes the need of the resident to maintain as much control of their life needs and life spaces as possible.

Numerous barriers to improving nursing home care were identified. These include a top-down management organization; poor pay in a difficult environment, leading to high staff turnover and workforce shortages; a poor physical environment for family, caregivers, and residents to interact in; and a focus on the need for healthcare rather than focusing on creating a home-like environment and in the United States, an adversarial regulatory and legal system that inhibited movement away from a medical model.

The crucial central role of elderhood in long-term care communities was recognized in the 1970s by the Live Oak Regenerative Community. In 1994, Wellspring Innovative Solutions pioneered the concepts of collaboration among caregivers, family, and residents and staff empowerment. They also pointed out the value of consistent staff assignment to a resident. The Holistic Approach to Transformational Change (HATCH) created an approach in which the resident was placed in the center of a series of circles of staff with an emphasis on creating a place of home for the resident. More information regarding the

Table 4–3.   THE BASIC ELEMENTS OF QUALITY
• Care
• Staff attitude
• Environment
• Communication
• Family involvement

Table 4–4.   PIONEER NETWORK PRINCIPLES
• Every person makes a difference.
• Feelings of the person supersede the task.
• Spiritual feelings are equally important to the needs of the mind and body.
• Older persons have the right to self-determination.
• Living entitles persons to take risks.
• The environment needs to be shaped to its full potential to the benefit of the community.
• Involving persons is a key to happiness.
"Culture change and transformation are not destinations but a journey—always work on progress"

Adapted from Pioneer Network.

HATCH model can be obtained at http://www.health centricadvisors.org/hatch.html.

In 1997, the Pioneer Network (http://www.pioneer network.net) was founded to advocate for person-centered or person-directed care in nursing homes. This network includes a wide variety of partners, including policy makers, consumers, academia, and provider stakeholders. The Pioneer Network defines "culture change" as a transformation of nursing homes in which person-directed care hears and respects the voices of older persons and their direct caregivers. The core values are choice, respect, dignity, self-determination, and purposeful living. The Pioneer Network principles are outlined in Table 4–4.

It is well established that the way people talk to one another and the discourses among staff members reflect workplace culture. Furthermore, choice of language is mediated by powerful influences that reflect often taken for granted aspects of our practice and our value base. Part of transforming a culture starts with terminology, and it is important that nursing home staff think carefully about how they talk about residents and converse with them. It is generally acknowledged that residents should be addressed respectfully and called by appropriate titles and surnames (e.g., Mrs. or Mrs. Reed) unless they specifically request otherwise. Interestingly, in the American culture movement, euphemistic terminology is considered progressive. For example, a resident needing feeding should be termed one who enjoys company with meals, an agitated residents is an "active" person, and a resident with dementia is forgetful and "likes to walk" if he or she is at risk for elopement. Manipulative residents are clearly "resourceful." The acceptability of such practices might seem questionable in other cultures (e.g., Northern Europe), where this would not be appropriate and might be construed as disrespectful.

For culture change to work, it is necessary to recognize the paramount importance of the resident and the central role of the certified nurses' aides with the support of recreation therapists. All others, including the administrator, nurses, and physicians, need to provide support to this essential triad (Figure 4–1).

Culture change begins with the administrator recognizing the need to build a community of caregivers,

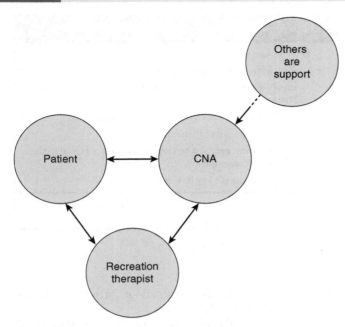

Figure 4–1. Keys to culture change.

residents, and family members. This requires empowerment of staff to make decisions and break rules when they will benefit the community. The environment needs to be deinstitutionalized (made more home-like). Staff are cross-trained to do multiple tasks. Residents choose their own schedules and are encouraged to be a part of the team. Family involvement is considered key, and family are expected to help with care. Finally, a diverse active recreation program is central to care.

The concept of culture change has become an important component in making nursing homes more "home-like." At present, there are limited data that culture change improves medical outcomes, but evidence indicates that it enhances residents' experience of care and satisfaction with care and promotes a sense of well-being.

KEY POINTS

1. Organizational cultures determine how things are done and reflect deeply felt values that shape the behaviors of staff and experiences of residents.
2. A negative culture is one is which different staff groups hold different understandings of each other and are unaware of these felt differences.
3. Improvement efforts will only succeed in a positive organizational culture that demonstrates valuing of staff and genuine concern for nursing home residents as individuals.
4. Improving standards requires culture change, and culture change requires insight into the prevailing culture and negotiation of persistent challenges to quality improvement.

5. Improving quality is most likely to succeed when service users (nursing home residents) and family caregivers are involved in the improvement process.
6. The key to culture change is to place the resident and primary caregiver (usually a nurse's aide) at the center of the process.

SUGGESTED READINGS

British Geriatric Society. *Quest for Quality. An Inquiry into the Quality of Healthcare Support for Older People in Care Homes: A Call for Leadership, Partnership and Improvement.* London: British Geriatric Society; 2011. http://www.bgs.org.uk. Accessed March 24, 2013.

Grol R, Grimshaw J. Evidence-based implementation of evidence-based medicine. *Jt Comm J Qual Improv.* 1999;25(10):503-513.

Hill NL, Kolanowski AM, Milone-Nuzzo P, Yevchak A. Culture change models and resident health outcomes in long-term care. *J Nurs Scholarsh.* 2011;43:30-40.

Jones CS. Person-centered care. The heart of culture change. *J Gerontol Nurs.* 2011;37:18-23.

Manley K, McCormack B, Wilson V (eds). *International Development in Nursing and Healthcare.* Oxford, UK: Blackwell Publishing; 2008.

Morley JE. Clinical practice in nursing homes as a key for progress. *J Nutr Health Aging.* 2010;14:586-593.

Rahman AN, Schnelle JF. The nursing home culture-change movement: recent past, present, and future. *Gerontologist.* 2008;48:142-148.

Royal College of Nursing. *Persistent Challenges to Providing Quality Care. An RCN Report on the Views and Experiences of Frontline Nursing Staff in Care Homes in England.* London: Royal College of Nursing London; 2012. http://www.rcn.org.uk. Accessed March 24, 2013.

Scott-Cawiezell J, Jone K, Moore L, Vojir C. Nursing home culture. *J Nurs Care Quality.* 2005;20(4):341-348.

Sterns S, Miller SC, Allen S. The complexity of implementing culture change practices in nursing homes. *J Am Med Dir Assoc.* 2010;11:511-518.

Tappeiner W. *Disclosing Nursing Worlds Within Nursing Homes: A Later Heideggerian Exploration.* Unpublished doctoral thesis, Glasgow Caledonian University; 2009.

Volicer L. Culture change for residents with dementia. *J Am Med Dir Assoc.* 2008;9:459.

White-Chu E, Graves W, Godfrey S, et al. Beyond the medical model: the culture change revolution in long-term care. *J Am Med Dir Assoc.* 2009;10:370-378.

MULTIPLE CHOICE QUESTIONS

4.1 Which of the following is *not* a principle of the Pioneer Network?

a. Involvement is a key to happiness.
b. Persons are entitled to take risks.
c. Feelings of the person supersede the task.
d. The voices of caregivers are less important than the voices of the residents.
e. Spiritual feelings are not to be ignored.

4.2 Which of the following is *not* a barrier to producing culture change in nursing homes?

a. Top-down management
b. High staff turnover
c. Poor physical environment
d. Focus on the medical model
e. Empowerment of staff to produce change on their own initiative

4.3 Which of the following is a universal truth regarding appropriate use of terminology in nursing homes?

    a. No resident should be addressed by his or her first name.

    b. Terminology depends on the cultural beliefs of a particular area.

    c. Use of euphemistic terms such as "likes to walk" for a resident who wanders is progressive.

    d. Residents should not be asked how they wish to be addressed.

4.4 Which of the following is *not* a component of the culture change movement in nursing homes?

    a. Ability of staff to break rules to the benefit of the resident

    b. Deinstitutionalization of the environment

    c. Staff are cross-trained to do multiple tasks

    d. All persons (staff and residents) in the nursing home are a centered focus of care

    e. Family involvement is an important component

4.5 Which of the following statements is true?

    a. Values are not determined by organizational cultures.

    b. In a negative culture, staff hold different understandings of each other and are aware of these differences.

    c. Culture change requires insight into the prevailing culture.

    d. A positive organizational culture requires valuing of staff.

    e. Family members are not a part of culture change.

Part 2
FUNDAMENTALS OF NURSING HOME PRACTICE

Chapter 5

PRINCIPLES OF NURSING HOME PRACTICE

The International Association of Gerontology and Geriatrics (IAGG) recommends nursing home practice that is evidence informed, safe, and delivered with respect and dignity by staff equipped with the necessary knowledge and competencies. This chapter introduces ethical dimensions of practice and issues related to protecting vulnerable individuals, including medication risks, elder abuse, falls prevention and restraints, accident prevention, fire risk management, and disaster preparedness. Some of the topics are further elaborated in subsequent chapters, and the principle of person-centred practice is a central tenant of this book.

VALUES-BASED CARE

The human rights movement, as embodied in 18 United Nations Principles for Older People (Table 5–1) promotes care that is dignified, personalized, and mindful of older people's entitlement (or right) to be free from constraints and from being restrained. So the moral imperative exits for nursing homes to be restraint-free environments; later in this chapter, we examine the evidence base to support this assertion in terms of physical and chemical restraints. Contemporary nursing home regulatory guidance in many countries reflects the fundamental right of older residents not to be harmed and their right to have their choices supported.

A tension, however, can develop when the rights of one person undermine the rights of another or a group of residents. Although considerations of individual rights is essential, rights-based decision making in isolation from other guiding frameworks is an insufficient moral compass for practice. It is recommended that setting out broader principles of care or a set of commitments to older people, aligned with human rights, helps staff to understand in practical terms the implementation of values-based care. Table 5–2 lists examples of research-based practice commitments to older people.

Such applied ethics helps staff to make sense of the value base, which should guide their day-to-day practice and interactions with residents. A value base that is shared across the staff team assists in the achievement of care that is compassionate and in the promotion of the ethic of equity (fair and consistent approaches to all residents) and the ethic of autonomy (enabling the recipient of care involvement in decision making). Application of agreed practice commitments or a shared value base is the cornerstone of person-centered care and a prerequisite to creating a positive culture and improving experiences of care.

International rights movements have highlighted the principles of fairness, respect, equality, dignity, and autonomy. Negotiated autonomy is the basis of person-centered care that is set within a caring dynamic between the practitioner and the person. Furthermore, it is a way as to preserve personhood in a process of shared decision making. When a person does not have capacity to make his or her views known, the practitioner is not the final arbiter of caring decisions but will engage family, friends, advocacy partners, and creative approaches in the pursuit of person centered caring. Hence, although we think about person-centered approaches as focused on the individual, they are contextualized within a web of relationships and interconnections among the person, his or her family and close community, and the nursing home staff.

It is important for nursing home managers to consider how the implementation of agreed practice values is demonstrated in practice in the ways that staff work with residents, speak to residents, and document their care. For example, if you claim commitment to person-centered care but residents have no choice about the food they consume, it is inconsistent, and ways to respond to satisfy food preferences need to be established.

PERSON-CENTERED CARE

There are four core concepts within person-centered care that are critical to good nursing home practice, which are founded on the development of reciprocity and trust between staff and the older person:

- Being in relation as concerned with relationships with people
- Being in a social world as highlighting the essential sociability of a person
- Being in place as the context in which personhood is articulated
- Being with self is about being recognized, respected, and trusted and its impact on our sense of whom we are (McCormack, 2003).

Table 5–1.   UNITED NATIONS PRINCIPLES FOR OLDER PEOPLE

Independence

1. Older persons should have access to adequate food, water, shelter, clothing, and healthcare through the provision of income, family and community support, and self-help.
2. Older persons should have the opportunity to work or to have access to other income-generating opportunities.
3. Older persons should be able to participate in determining when and at what pace withdrawal from the labor force takes place.
4. Older persons should have access to appropriate educational and training programs.
5. Older persons should be able to live in environments that are safe and adaptable to personal preferences and changing capacities.
6. Older persons should be able to reside at home for as long as possible.

Participation

7. Older persons should remain integrated in society, participate actively in the formulation and implementation of policies that directly affect their well-being, and share their knowledge and skills with younger generations.
8. Older persons should be able to seek and develop opportunities for service to the community and to serve as volunteers in positions appropriate to their interests and capabilities.
9. Older persons should be able to form movements or associations of older persons.

Care

10. Older persons should benefit from family and community care and protection in accordance with each society's system of cultural values.
11. Older persons should have access to healthcare to help them to maintain or regain the optimum level of physical, mental, and emotional well-being and to prevent or delay the onset of illness.
12. Older persons should have access to social and legal services to enhance their autonomy, protection, and care.
13. Older persons should be able to use appropriate levels of institutional care providing protection, rehabilitation, and social and mental stimulation in a humane and secure environment.
14. Older persons should be able to enjoy human rights and fundamental freedoms when residing in any shelter, care, or treatment facility, including full respect for their dignity, beliefs, needs, and privacy and for the right to make decisions about their care and the quality of their lives.

Self-Fulfillment

15. Older persons should be able to pursue opportunities for the full development of their potential.
16. Older persons should have access to the educational, cultural, spiritual, and recreational resources of society.

Dignity

17. Older persons should be able to live in dignity and security and be free of exploitation and physical and mental abuse.
18. Older persons should be treated fairly regardless of age, gender, racial or ethnic background, disability, or other status and be valued independently of their economic contribution.

Further information on United Nations Principles on Older Persons can be found at http://www.un.org/ageing/un_principles.html.

These dimensions highlight the centrality of staff behaviors and communication in promoting good experiences of care. Achieving resident-centered care is essential to the advancement of nursing home practice. Provision of resident-centered care does not require expensive equipment, but it does require organizational commitment to deliver. The rewards are high, and the reciprocity that is nurtured between residents and staff has been shown to improve residents' quality of life and to increase staff job satisfaction and team morale.

Table 5–2.   EXAMPLES OF PRACTICE COMMITMENTS TO OLDER PEOPLE
Commitment to person-centered care or relationship centered care
Commitment to negotiating care decisions in an atmosphere of trust
Commitment to provide care that is safe, dignified, and respectful
Commitment to evidence informed practice
Commitment to maximizing functional potential
Commitment to an enabling environment
Commitment to consistency of practice values by the multiprofessional team

TRUTH TELLING

Recognition of the ethical dimensions of conversations between practitioners and older people is pivotal to the relationships that can be formed with nursing home residents and their family caregivers. In general, we make judgments about the people who we can trust and those we cannot on the basis of whether we can trust what they say and their subsequent actions. In encounters with health professionals, truth telling is an important aspect of professional behavior and trust development.

Truth telling is related to information sharing and our decision to share or withhold information from a nursing home resident. This is often based on our notion of what the person can cope with or would want to know. Very often family members have strong views as to what an older person would want to know, whether or not they have discussed this with their relative. Truth-telling behaviors are a matter of conscience, and in general, people agree that it is appropriate to tell the truth. For some situations and cultures, telling a lie or withholding truth is seen as an expression of power. This denies people who do not know the truth the choices they would make had they been informed. It follows that in nursing homes, if a resident is not told the truth, this undermines his or her opportunity for self-realization and for autonomy. On the other hand, there are occasions when health professionals and family members genuinely believe that information disclosure will be harmful, although the basis of this subjective judgment might reasonably be challenged. Interestingly, if we turn to codes of professional conduct for health professionals for guidance, it is clear that the principles of truthfulness in care encounters are an expected professional standard.

The research basis to truth-telling practice in nursing homes is emergent and relies heavily on work from Australian and Dutch nursing home studies. An important finding from these studies is the recognition that nursing homes are places endowed with suspicious awareness and mutual pretence. What this means is that what older people know or think they know is thought to be different from what their relatives know and are willing to share with them. When information is rationed by well-meaning relatives or staff, it can have unintentional and negative consequences on the resident's well-being and sense of safety. Whether or not information nondisclosure constitutes a lie is debatable, and interpretations of the rights and wrongs of truth telling is an emotive subject that is culturally bound.

Studies of the cultural influences on the attitudes of healthcare professionals working with cancer patients and families toward truth-telling practices revealed that doctors in the United States, Northern Europe, and Anglo-Saxon countries tell the truth to both patients and their spouses. In contrast, doctors from Southern and Eastern Europe, Africa, France, Iran, Panama, Japan, Singapore, and Saudi Arabia have traditionally concealed the truth, although attitudes in these nations toward disclosure are changing. The familial influence in countries such as Spain, Italy, Greece, Saudi Arabia, Egypt, Singapore, China, and Japan means the family often sanctions truth telling by health professionals.

From our review of the research literature, we believe that it is important for practitioners not to assume:

1. What older people want to know
2. What is important for them; ask them
3. A resident's preferences for truth telling can be decided based on his or her cultural background race; ask the person how informed he or she wishes to be

PROTECTING THE VULNERABLE

As shown in Table 5–2, it is desirable that the value base for nursing home practice includes an atmosphere of trust in which older people can expect to receive care that is safe. The drive for evidence-based healthcare assists in the delineation of practices and treatments that are safe and effective. Such effective practices become recommended and perpetuated through quality-assured clinical and care guidance and governance strategies. However, there are many challenges to delivering evidence-based care within nursing homes. Older people who are dependent, frail, cognitively impaired, and without family support are particularly vulnerable to poor practices. Vulnerability arises for many reasons related to a range of organizational, system, and people factors. There are numerous examples around the world of media exposure of poor nursing home practices, and it is essential that all practitioners understand the boundaries of acceptable and unacceptable practice and acts that might be perceived of as abusive. Vulnerability within nursing homes is heightened because many residents are unable to report abuse or neglect, or they or their family are fearful that reporting will lead to greater problems.

An astute manager will be alert to indicators of possible abuse. Clear policies need to be in place to address all forms of abuse that might arise within staff-to-resident, family-to-resident, or resident-to-resident situations.

The World Health Organization (WHO) defines elder abuse as "a single or repeated act or lack of appropriate action, occurring within any relationship where there is an expectation of trust, which causes harm or distress to an older person."

A recent large-scale survey of more than 15,000 nursing homes in the United States suggests that 45% of facilities fail to provide safe environments for their residents. Another study of 32 nursing homes found that 70% of nursing aides had witnessed a colleague yelling at an older resident, and 33% of staff admitted having done this themselves. In a nursing home resident survey, 48% of the 80 respondents reported having been roughly handled by staff.

Several types of abuse might arise within nursing homes, including acts of neglect, physical abuse, emotional abuse, financial abuse, and sexual abuse. When any form of abuse is suspected, evidence should be collected and strategies put in place to protect vulnerable individuals. For example, when staff members are concerned about visitor behavior, a simple remedy might be to seat to residents in a public area for visits, which can be more easily observed than private visits undertaken behind closed doors.

ACTS OF NEGLECT

Two forms of neglect that might occur within nursing homes: passive neglect and intentional neglect. Passive neglect may arise when staff members do not have the capacity or competence to provide appropriate evidence-informed care. In this sense, the organization is responsible for providing staffing levels that are appropriate to the needs of the residents and for ensuring that all staff members have access to the training they need to keep pace with best practice. Examples of intentional neglect include deliberately leaving a resident in soiled bedding, failure to assist a dependent person to drink or eat sufficient fluids and food to maintain health, and failure to take actions to avert the development of preventable pressure and moisture lesions. Reviews shows that acts of neglect are more likely to occur when there is inadequate staffing and there is low supervision of staff.

SIGNS OF PHYSICAL ABUSE

Sometimes it can be difficult to determine whether or not abuse has taken place, and accurate and detailed record keeping that will explain legitimate occurrences is important. The sequelae of physical abuse and common age-related changes may appear the same. However, it is essential that when a staff member suspects abuse or cannot explain a physical injury that the cause of the injury is fully investigated by senior staff and detailed written records are kept of the investigation. The signs of physical abuse include:

- An older person telling you he or she has been hit, slapped, kicked, or roughly handled
- Cuts, lacerations, puncture wounds, open wounds, bruises, welts, discoloration, black eyes, or fractures
- Poor skin condition or poor skin hygiene
- Dehydration or malnourished without an illness-related cause
- Unexplained loss of weight
- Broken eyeglasses or frames, physical signs of being subjected to punishment, or signs of being restrained
- Inappropriate use of medication; overdosing or underdosing

It is the physician's and nurse's duty to recognize the reasonable possibility that abuse may have occurred and to alert the appropriate authorities (e.g., ombudsman or police). When making a report to the ombudsman or Adult Protective Services, it is important to provide a clear description of the resident, care setting, injury or incident, timing, and any inconsistencies in the causal stories. The key responsibilities of the physician and senior nurse are:

1. Prevention
2. Detection
3. Reporting (to authorities, next of kin, or legal guardian)
4. Management of the situation, including care of the resident and a corrective action plan

SIGNS OF PSYCHOLOGICAL ABUSE

Psychological abuse can be difficult to distinguish from other causes of behavior change and emotional upset. Signs include:

- A resident reporting verbal or emotional abuse
- Confusion or disorientation
- Anger without apparent cause
- Sudden change in behavior

- Emotionally upset or agitated
- Unusual behavior (sucking, biting, or rocking)
- Unexplained fear
- Extremely withdrawn and noncommunicative or nonresponsive.

FINANCIAL ABUSE

This includes taking someone's money or property without his or her permission. In the nursing home environment, theft of residents' belongings by visitors or staff is a real possibility. However, when property or cash disappears, it is important to consider whether the item has been taken or misplaced by the person or another resident. To reduce the problems associated with loss of valuable goods, most nursing homes discourage residents from bringing in items of high value. Abuse of finances is more difficult to detect, particularly when others have legal powers, and when concerns are raised, social workers are best placed to investigate and take steps to protect the vulnerable person. Financial abuse of older people is a criminal act whether it is undertaken by a stranger or a trusted person with legal power of attorney.

SEXUAL ABUSE

Sexual abuse is a crime, and in a nursing home, it may be the result of an opportunistic act or the continuation of domestic violence into old age. Some of the physical signs to watch for are bruises around the breasts, genital area, or buttocks and unexplained vaginal or anal bleeding. If rape is suspected, then it is important not to lose forensic evidence and to act swiftly in alerting the police and other authorities and in communicating with the family. Unfortunately, rape by a young staff member on an older resident is not as rare as one would expect. This has to be balanced against false allegations made by persons with dementia. A recent review highlighted the importance of undertaking background checks on staff before hiring them because several case studies report unsuspecting nursing homes recruiting new staff with a prior criminal record of rape or sexual abuse of residents at other facilities. Persons with dementia in facilities occasionally attempt to have a pedophilic relationship or to inappropriately touch young children visiting the facility.

MEANINGFUL ACTIVITIES

The broad vision encapsulated within the culture change movement (see Chapter 4) seeks a nursing home culture that is life affirming, satisfying, humane, and meaningful. The goal of making nursing homes a place to thrive, not just survive, is central to the IAGG-WHO Nursing Home Agenda. From an emotional state perspective, thriving may be considered a state of satisfaction or psychological well-being emanating from a positive balance between the expectations of the individual and the environment's capacity to meet the expectations. For many people, being active is a driving force for life. Few studies have specifically explored which factors contribute to thriving among nursing home residents. An important contribution is made by a Norwegian Study, which explored thriving from the perspective of 26 mentally lucid nursing home residents who had been residents for over 2 months. Thriving was a function of a number of core elements of which the quality of care was central. Other key factors identified by the residents were positive relationships with other residents, participation in meaningful activities in the nursing home, opportunities to go outside the nursing home, relationships with family, and qualities in the physical environment. Certain activities were described as pleasant and meaningful (e.g., musical events, religious services physiotherapy); others (e.g., bingo) were valued as pastimes. Residents who organized their own daily activities usually did this by reading or watching television. The importance of providing opportunities for older nursing home residents to continue with familiar activities and interests was highlighted by an occupational therapy study completed within the Netherlands. Importantly, this Dutch study found that although some participants had given up some activities because of old age, moving to the nursing home did not change their interests in activities such as reading, watching television, needlework, writing, having a drink, doing household activities, or attending church services. Unfortunately, a common experience for the residents was that they often had long waits before anyone would help them to do something purposeful. The most important finding in the Dutch study was that two forms of occupational performance were experienced: "doing" and "being in the atmosphere of the doing." A distinction must be made between staff-imposed activities that are seen by residents as ways of passing time and the meaningful activities that are of real interest to people as they affirm a sense of personal identity and are both satisfying and enjoyable.

The key messages for practice is that it is important that residents can perform one or more activities that are experienced as a continuation of familiar activities and occupations. Approaches that enable residents to gain a sense of self-determination and control in the ways they spend their time are particularly welcomed by older people.

Provision of group and individual activity programs is an important aspect of quality in nursing home life. Activity coordinators need to work in partnership with residents, family, friends, and practitioners to plan activities that are both meaningful and appropriate. It is important that activities and entertainment reflect the preferences of residents; assumptions should not be made about what will be of interest or enjoyable. With a little creativity and the help of volunteers, family, and technology, engaging activities can be provided that promote well-being and purposeful activity. Examples of innovative activities are shown in Table 5–3.

A failure to provide meaningful activity and psychosocial stimulation fuels low mood, restlessness, and boredom. For people with dementia, a lack of cognitive stimulation is harmful and is associated with decline greater than expected by disease process alone (see Chapter 12). An interesting innovation in Dementia Care is the Enriched Opportunity Programme, which involves a senior member of staff acting as a "locksmith." The locksmith has responsibility of discovering and developing "keys" to unlock the potential for well-being in the person with dementia. In this way, a personal program of stimulation through meaningful activities

Table 5–3.	EXAMPLES OF POTENTIALLY MEANINGFUL ACTIVITIES

- Craft work (e.g., artwork, sewing, knitting)
- Reminiscence around an anchor topic such as baseball or football, or cultural history
- Reading (e.g., newspapers, magazines, books)
- Online activities, including social networking, gaming, online shopping, and eLearning
- Phone calls to friends and family
- Baking or other cooking activities
- Outings
- Pet therapy
- Individual and group based entertainment, including performing arts, music, and seminars
- Selective contributions to the decision making within the nursing home (e.g., through resident committees or through recipe selection with the chef)

is crafted that focuses on using remaining capacities and compensating for deficits.

MEDICATION AND POLYPHARMACY RISKS

Older frail persons in nursing homes have many diseases, all of which potentially could benefit from drugs. This has resulted in multiple drugs being given to residents. A study in Ontario, Canada, found that 15.5% of persons in long-term care homes received nine or more drugs. The variation of polypharmacy between homes ranged from 7.9% to 26.7%. Excessive polypharmacy (10 or more drugs) in Europe was present in 24.3% of residents, with 49.7% receiving five to nine drugs (Table 5–4). In addition to

Table 5–4.	POLYPHARMACY IN NURSING HOMES IN EUROPE AND NORTH AMERICA	

Country	Criteria	Residents (%)
United States	≥9 medications	68.8
Ontario, Canada	≥9 medications	15.5
Italy	>10 medications	8.8
Israel	>10 medications	12.9
Germany	>10 medications	15.7
England	>10 medications	22.7
Holland	>10 medications	24.4
Czech Republic	>10 medications	25.2
France	>10 medications	30.2
Finland	>10 medications	56.7

Table 5–5.   EXAMPLE OF A PROGRAM TO TRACK MEDICATION CHANGES IN A NURSING HOME

Medications	Jan	Feb	Mar	Apr	May	June	July	Aug	Sept	Oct	Nov	Dec
Routine (average per resident)	7.48	7.35	7.41	7.47	7.55	7.64	7.77	7.63	7.62	7.66	7.59	7.80
PRN (average per resident)	1.73	1.97	1.83	1.94	1.82	1.82	1.87	1.42	1.87	1.89	1.87	2.01
Antipsychotics[a]	37	40	40	34	40	41	39	39	43	33	37	38
Antidepressants[a]	99	102	105	107	110	109	109	114	110	106	106	103
Anxiolytics[a]	55	53	58	61	60	56	63	65	70	70	71	66
Hypnotics[a]	3	8	7	6	5	6	7	8	6	5	6	4
Census[a]	198	199	200	197	204	200	197	199	206	205	203	203

	Nursing Home A (%)	Missouri (%)	United States (%)
Antipsychotics	18.7	28.2	25.2
Antidepressants	50.7	54.3	48.3
Anxiolytics	32.5	24.9	20.8
Hypnotics	2.0	7.7	7.4

[a]Total numbers being used.

polypharmacy, many nursing home residents take potentially inappropriate medicine (e.g., drugs on the "Beers" list, a list developed of potentially inappropriate drugs in nursing home residents; see http://www.americangeriatrics.org/files/documents/beers/PrintableBeersPocketCard.pdf). For example, one study in the United States found 38% of nursing home residents receiving one or more potentially inappropriate medicines. An alternative to the Beers criteria is the European STOPP (Screening Tool of Older Person's Prescriptions) and START (Screening Tool to Alert doctors to Right Treatment). This consists of 65 criteria for potentially inappropriate prescribing in older persons and 22 evidence-based prescribing indicators for commonly encountered disease in older persons (http://www.nature.com/clpt/journal/v89/n6/extref/clpt201144x1.doc). It has been validated in Europe and in the Veterans Administration in the United States.

It has been shown mathematically that when an older person receives more than five medicines, every medicine beyond that he or she receives has an equal chance of causing benefit or harm. For this reason, it is essential to carefully review medicines received by older persons in nursing homes.

A number of controlled studies have attempted to examine methods to reduce polypharmacy in nursing homes. A systematic review found that pharmacist medication reviews had little effect, but multidisciplinary team meetings were effective. On the whole, computerized clinical decision support systems had a minimal effect. Academic "detailing" has been successful in reducing medication use.

The starting point of a polypharmacy continuous quality improvement program is to track monthly changes in medications and detect variations (Table 5–5). These tracking charts should also include use of antipsychotics, anxiolytics, and hypnotics. Comparisons with national averages are also provided.

One approach to reducing medications is for all physicians to receive a list of their prescribing practices compared with others. This has proven highly successful in reducing polypharmacy (Table 5–6). This approach in one of the National Health Care (NHC) nursing homes has led

Table 5–6.   COMPARISON OF DIFFERENT PHYSICIAN PRESCRIBING PRACTICES IN A NURSING HOMES

Physician	Routine Medications	PRN Medications
A	7.26	1.38
B	6.91	2.22
C	8.19	2.35
D	7.59	2.29
E	11.75	4.75
F	11.67	4.30
G	8.75	2.00

PRN = as needed.

to 47% of residents receiving nine or more medications compared with the national average of 68.8%. In multidisciplinary meetings (pharmacist, medical director, director of nursing, and administrator) to discuss patients with polypharmacy, a logical approach to reducing the number of medicines a resident is given can be developed and then provided to the primary care physician (Table 5–7). These reviews focus on the patients with the highest number of medicines in the facility. A set of rules to approach medications reduction is given in Table 5–8.

Table 5–7.   EXAMPLE OF A MULTIDISCIPLINARY REVIEW OF A PATIENT WITH INAPPROPRIATE MEDICATIONS

Case Study, May 2012

LH (6481) is an 88-year-old woman on wing 300 who was admitted to the facility in April. She is receiving 13 routine medications.

Code: II **Allergies:** Bactrim (sulfa)

Estimated creatinine clearance: 28 mL/min using actual body weight

Diagnosis and Problem List

Alzheimer's dementia, degenerative joint disease, osteoporosis, urinary incontinence, constipation, hypothyroidism, hypo vitamin D, borderline B_{12} deficiency, peripheral vascular disease, bilateral heel wounds, bilateral edema

	Blood Pressure (mm Hg)	Pulse (beats/min)
4/6	128/68	91
4/7	148/78	88
4/8	98/68	64
4/9	108/64	74

Diet: Mechanical soft; MPS 120 mL/day (4/13)

Weight: 99.9 lb on 4/12/12; 94.2 lb on 5/3/12 94.2

Protein supplement: 30 mL/day

Current Medications

Amlodipine 2.5 mg/day (now discontinued)	9 AM	4/7/12 discontinued 4/11/12
Furosemide 20 mg/day	9 AM	
Alendronate 70 mg weekly	6:30 AM	4/7/12
Calcium 600 mg/day	9 PM	4/7/12
Levothyroxine 150 mcg/day	7 AM	4/20/12 (increased twice on same lab); MD aware
Mirtazapine 7.5 mg at bedtime	9 PM	4/7/12
Exelon patch 9.5/24 hr	9 AM	5/6/12 (increased by psychiatrist)
Depakote 250 mg sprinkles every morning	9 AM	4/17/12 (added by psychiatrist)
Omeprazole 20 mg/day	6 AM	4/7/12
Oxybutynin ER 5 mg/day	8 AM	4/7/12
Vitamin D 1000 units/day	9 AM	4/11/12
Multivitamin daily	9 AM	4/7/12
Ferrous sulfate 325 mg twice a day with meals	9 AM; 5 PM	4/18/12
Sorbitol 30 cc at night (hold for diarrhea)	9 PM	4/11/12

(continued)

Table 5–7.   EXAMPLE OF A MULTIDISCIPLINARY REVIEW OF A PATIENT WITH INAPPROPRIATE MEDICATIONS (CONTINUED)

PRN medications: Tramadol 50 mg every 6 hours PRN pain

Laboratory test results: 4/23/12: moderate arteriosclerotic occlusive disease of both lower extremities

4/20/12 CMP Calcium 7.9↓; Protein 5.4↓; Albumin 2.4↓ B12 302 (MMA 169); T4 3.9↓; TSH 20.85↑

4/18/12 CBC RBC 3.02↓; Hgb 8.8↓; Hct 26.3↓; MCV 87 (wnl)

Discussion

1. Consider iron studies because of low hemoglobin and hematocrit.
2. Consider H_2 antagonist rather than a proton pump inhibitor because of OP history.
3. Reevaluate oxybutynin use with Exelon patch (opposing MOA).
4. Decrease ferrous sulfate to once daily. Do not give with other medications.
5. Consider discontinuing Exelon patch because it is expensive and has questionable efficacy.
6. The dose of L-thyroxine is high. Is it being given with iron, or is it not being taken by the resident?
7. Is furosemide being used for peripheral edema because of stasis? The patient does not have elevated jugular venous pressure, so trial without furosemide may be reasonable.
8. The resident is eating well and not losing weight, so discontinue the multivitamin.
9. The sorbitol dose is too low if the resident is constipated and so may not be needed.

PREVENTING AND MANAGING FALLS

Frail older people are at risk of slips, trips, and falls. Older people who live in nursing homes are three times more likely to fall than those who live at home, and the falls are often injurious. U.K. statistics show that there are 10 times more hip fractures in nursing homes than in other environments. Many factors increase the risk of falls, such as physical frailty, multiple long-term conditions, physical inactivity, taking multiple medications, and the unfamiliarity of new surroundings. For these reasons, nursing homes should prioritize falls prevention and develop person-centered processes to manage and reduce injurious falls. Fear of falling can be as limiting as an actual fall because it leads to avoidance of physical activity, a lack of confidence when mobilizing, and adoption of sedentary behaviors.

A fall is nearly always caused by the presence of one or more risk factors that relate to the person's condition or surroundings (Table 5–9). On admission to a nursing home, a multifactorial falls risk assessment should be completed, and the person should be orientated to the new environment. Ideally, the assessment should include review of the person's bone health, and those with osteoporosis should be seen as being at high risk of injurious falls and fractures.

The risk of a person falling out of bed or slipping from a chair is an important consideration when planning resident's care. It is essential for staff to understand that devices intended to stop someone from rolling out of bed do not prevent a person from climbing over the rail, and the fall

Table 5–8.   RULES FOR REVIEWING MEDICATIONS IN NURSING HOMES

- Is there an indication for the drug?
- Is the drug causing side effects?
- Is the dose appropriate for an older or malnourished person?
- Is the patient receiving two drugs that antagonize one another (e.g., cholinesterase inhibitor and an anticholinergic)?
- Are the drugs causing hypotension or orthostatic hypotension?
- If the person is falling, is he or she taking a statin or excess hypertensive agents?
- Is the person receiving drugs to prevent diseases in which the time to prevention is longer than the person's expected survival?
- Does the drug have a clinical, not statistical, benefit?
- Is the drug the cheapest, most cost-effective drug available?

Table 5–9. INTRINSIC AND EXTRINSIC FALLS RISK FACTORS	
Intrinsic Risks (Person)	**Extrinsic Factors (Environment)**
• Previous falls	• Poor lighting
• Fear of falling	• Wet, slippery, highly polished floor
• Changes in the body caused by the aging process	• Uneven floor surfaces
• Certain long term medical conditions present	• Clutter
	• Chairs or beds being too high or low
• Being less physically active	• Unsafe or absent handrails
• Side effects of some medications	• Inappropriate use of bed rails for an agile person unaware of risks of falling
• Poor vision	• Loose-fitting or inappropriate footwear and clothing
• Wearing multifocal glasses	• Inadequate staffing levels
	• Lack of falls prevention strategies

is likely to be more serious than if the person rolled from a low bed onto the floor or a floor mat. Decisions about bed rails are a balance between competing and complex risks. The current evidence suggests that for mobile people who are confused, bed rails are more hazardous than protective. In person-centered care, the decision to use or not use bed rails should be negotiated when the individual has the capacity to understand the benefits and risks and express preference. Best practice would thus include a risk assessment and discussion with the person and his or her family on the most appropriate care plan.

Decisions about suitable chairs should ideally be undertaken with the physiotherapist taking account of posture, body mass and height, limb length, the resident's ability to support his or her head and neck, and comfort. An occupation therapist will be able to advise on appropriate designs of pressure-relieving cushions that can be used safely. When special seating or pressure-relieving surfaces are required, it is essential that all members of the nursing team and visitors are informed so that the personalized seating is reserved for that resident.

RESTRAINTS

The definition of restraint is the intentional restriction of a person's voluntary movement or behavior using either a physical device or drug that induces a restraining effect (chemical restraint).

Drugs are considered inappropriate chemical restraints when they are:

- Given without specific indications
- Prescribed in excessive doses that affects the resident's ability to function
- Used as a sole treatment without investigating an alternative nonpharmacologic or behavioral intervention
- Administered for purposes of discipline or convenience to staff

Examples of physical restraint used in nursing homes include body belts, restraining vests, cuffs, and bilateral bed rails. Chemical restraints are any medication used to manage what are perceived to be challenging behaviors such as agitation, aggression, or verbal abuse. The prevalence of restraint use varies in different regions of the world, and internationally, calls to reduce the use of restraints in nursing homes has been heralded by the IAGG in concert with the WHO. Although the use of restraining devices is often justified in terms of harm prevention, accumulating evidence indicates that restraint-free environments are associated with a reduction in the incidence of injurious falls. In nursing homes in the United States, after the Omnibus Reconciliation Act (OBRA) of 1987, there was a reduction in restraints from more than 40% to less than 5% with no increase in injurious falls. Therefore, the use of physical restraints cannot be justified in terms of accident prevention, and it is considered in many cultures to be a violation of human rights. The use of physical restraints within a nursing home should be considered only when all other alternative interventions have been explored.

Table 5–10. A FRAMEWORK FOR NURSING HOME PHYSICAL RESTRAINT USE POLICY

The policy should address the following:
- An understanding that there are very few uses for physical restraints except when being used for positioning or enhancing mobility (e.g., merry walkers, a device to allow mobility)
- Definitions of restraining devices with clear guidance on how and when they might be lawfully used and the associated risks
- The type of situations when a restraint may be appropriate to be used and other alternative management strategies
- The assessment procedure for using or discontinuing use
- Involving of the older person or family in all decisions regarding restraint
- Staff education and training schedule in the use of and risks associated with restraint use in practice
- Governance processes and permissions to authorize the use of restraints, documentation, clinical supervision, and monitoring
- Procedure if the resident or relative refuses restraint

A restraint policy that addresses the imperative to create restraint-free nursing homes for older people should be in place to guide staff in restraint-related decisions; a suggested framework for such a physical restraint policy is shown in Table 5–10.

Alternatives to using restraint should be integral to the person-centered care plan and include daily physical exercise, meaningful activities that are both enjoyable and cognitively stimulating, and involvement of family and friends.

ACCIDENT PREVENTION

Accidents by their very nature will happen. The role of a nursing home's administration is to have systems in place to decrease the incidence of accidents, to educate staff in how to decrease the number of accidents, and to develop an appropriate response to accidents when they occur. These approaches need to be coupled with documentation of accidents, a review of potential preventable factors, and a continuous quality improvement program looking for patterns of accidents that can lead to a decrease in accident rate. Accident prevention strategies need to focus not only on residents but also on staff and visitors. The major factors that limit high-quality approaches to accident prevention are poor management, high rates of staff turnover, staff quality, and a punitive system that inhibits reporting of accidents.

An environment of safety awareness requires that accident hazards are minimal in nursing homes and that residents receive "adequate supervision." Nursing homes need to identify hazards, modify them when possible, and monitor the effectiveness of interventions. Overall, many nursing homes are behind other workplace environments in creating a culture of safety, but increased vigilance by regulatory bodies is rapidly changing this.

In the United States in 2010, nursing homes had a lost workday injury and illness rate of 7.3 compared with 1.8 for other private industries. Nurses aides have a work-related musculoskeletal disorders of 249 for every 10,000 workers compared with 34 for workers in other industries.

Table 5–11.	COMMON ACCIDENTS THAT OCCUR IN NURSING HOMES
Residents	**Staff**
Falls	Chemical hazards
Burns	Biological hazards (e.g., bloodborne or airborne infections)
Pressure ulcers	Workplace violence
Infections (e.g., catheter induced or caused by other residents)	Ergonomic hazards
	X-ray hazards
Escape from facility	Environmental hazards
Injuries induced by other residents or staff	Heat stress
	Slips and falls
Medication errors	Electric shock
	Burns

Table 5–11 lists the most common accident hazards in nursing homes. Accident prevention for residents is covered in future chapters. The rest of this section will focus on accident prevention for staff.

The major approaches to preventing ergonomic injuries include:

- Education on appropriate lifting techniques
- Using two persons to lift residents
- Gait belts (although the evidence for their efficacy is minimal)
- Mechanical lifting equipment (e.g., Hoyer lifts)
- Wheelchair scales
- Shower chairs
- Floors kept dry
- Nonslip mats
- Workplace analysis
- Regular review of workplace injuries
- Adjustable bed height
- Use of mechanical aids to lift heavy objects

To protect staff from bloodborne pathogens, all staff should use universal precautions (i.e., assume all human blood and other materials are assumed to be potentially infectious); personal protective equipment (gloves, gowns, and masks) should be worn under appropriate situations. All employees need to be trained in appropriate infection avoidance procedures. Sharps should be handled appropriately and be contained and disposed of appropriately. Use of needle systems or built-in safety control devices for needles should be used. All staff needs to be offered hepatitis B vaccination series. Appropriate postexposure testing and prophylaxis together with monitoring in a private environment needs to be available to all staff.

FIRE PREVENTION AND MANAGEMENT

Fire safety within nursing homes is a priority because residents who are immobile, confused or medicated, or sleeping are particularly vulnerable if a fire occurs. In the 2004 Rosepark Care Home Fire in Scotland, 14 older residents perished. The fatal accident inquiry concluded that this tragedy could have been avoided with appropriate fire risk assessment and a number of simple precautionary steps. Had the single occupancy bedroom doors been closed and the closed bedroom doors been fitted with smoke excluders or detectors, residents who died of smoke inhalation would have most likely survived. The careless storage of combustible materials in cupboards without fire retardant doors was also contributory. The fatal accident report is available at http://www.scotcourts.gov.uk/opinions/2011FAI18.pdf.

In most regions, there is a legal framework and range of regulations and requirement concerning building design and maintenance, policies, and procedures in relation to fire prevention and the achievement of safety in the event of fire.

Fire risk assessment in a nursing home should seek to identify hazards associated with fire risk. For example, when cigarette smoking is permitted on the premises, careless disposable of a lighted cigarette is a known hazard. Action plans are required to reduce the risk that the hazards will cause harm. Table 5–12 provides a five-step assessment of fire risk in nursing homes.

Table 5–12.	FIVE-STEP ASSESSMENT OF FIRE RISK IN NURSING HOMES
1. **Identify residents at risk.**	
2. **Identify fire hazards.** • **Sources of ignition** (e.g., lighters, matches, fires, faulty electrical equipment, toasters, hair dryers) • **Sources of fuel** (e.g., flammable soft furnishings, paper stores, garbage) • **Sources of oxygen** (e.g., piped oxygen outlets, stored cylinders, portable oxygen equipment)	
3. **Evaluate the risk and decide if existing fire safety measures are adequate.** • Remove of reduce known hazards (e.g., supervised smoking areas for residents) • Fire alarm (test regularly and ensure staff, residents and visitors are informed of testing schedule and recognize the alarm) • Fire-fighting equipment (staff skilled in use) • Accessible fire exits and lighting • Signage and notices (clear for staff, visitors, and residents, including people with cognitive impairment) • Maintenance • Staff training • Evacuation drills (including horizontal and vertical building evacuation of mobile and immobile residents)	
4. **Record findings and create action plan.**	
5. **Review and update.**	

Adapted from Scottish Government. *Practical Fire Safety Guidance for Care Homes.* http://www.firelawscotland.org/files/CHG-rev2.pdf. Published 2008. Accessed May 16, 2012.

All staff working in nursing homes should be knowledgeable in fire response procedures, evacuation plans, and procedures and should be able to use fire-fighting equipment.

DISASTER PREPAREDNESS

Disasters can strike nursing homes at any time as is shown in Figure 5–1 of the aftermath of a tornado that struck a nursing home in Joplin, Missouri. Besides the potential devastating effects of the disaster, the psychological and social effects have been shown to markedly increase death rates over the next 3 months to 1 year in nursing homes. Posttraumatic stress disorder is common after disasters. The most common disasters that need to be prepared for include heat waves, fire, earthquakes, tsunamis, floods, landslides, thunderstorms, tornadoes, volcanoes, wildland fires, winter storms, and extreme cold and human-made disasters (nuclear, radiologic, chemical, and biologic).

Heat waves, which are often accompanied by blackouts (power shortages), are some of the most common disasters affecting nursing homes. Frail residents are particularly at risk. Nursing homes need to have a plan to deal with heat emergencies (Table 5–13).

Table 5–13. EMERGENCY PLAN TO PREVENT HEAT-RELATED DEATHS
• Backup power source to maintain air conditioning units
• Availability of fans
• Availability of fluids
• Increase fluid intake of residents
• Reduce activities
• Use cool showers
• Identify areas of nursing home that are cooler
• Wear lightweight clothing
• Monitor residents for heat stroke
• Develop an evacuation plan to use when appropriate

Emergency evacuation plans and a plan to move residents to a safe area in the nursing home during a natural disaster (e.g., tornado or hurricane) need to be in place. A recent study has suggested that maintaining residents in the nursing home rather than evacuation leads to fewer hospitalizations and fewer excess deaths. This suggests that the policy of universal evacuation needs to be carefully reconsidered.

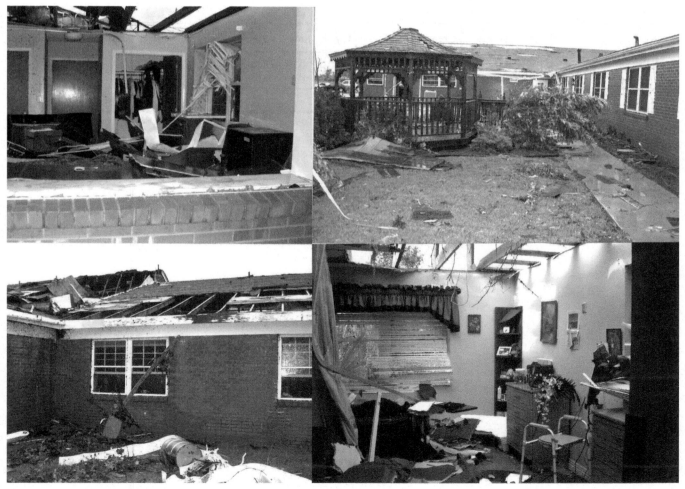

Figure 5–1. A weather ravaged nursing home and resident's room after the Joplin, Missouri, tornado of 2011. (Reprinted with permission from Mel Rector.)

KEY POINTS

1. Nursing home residents have a right to care that is dignified and personalized and mindful of their human entitlement (or right) to be free from constraints and from being restrained.
2. Person-centered care is critical to good nursing home practice and is founded on the development of reciprocity and trust between staff and the older person.
3. The vulnerability of older nursing home residents needs to be recognized, and staff needs to be alert to the signs of psychological, physical, financial, and sexual abuse.
4. Expression of sexuality is a fundamental aspect of personal identity. Safe and respectful opportunities for residents who wish to engage in intimate acts should be integral to personal care planning.
5. Taking more than five medications has a major chance of increasing side effects in residents.
6. Nursing homes should prioritize falls prevention and develop person-centered processes to manage and reduce injurious falls.
7. Both staff and residents are at risk of accidents in the nursing home, and all nursing homes need to develop an accident prevention program.
8. Older nursing home residents are particularly vulnerable during emergencies such as fire and natural disasters, and staff should be skilled in evacuation procedures and knowledgeable in the implementation of rehearsed action plans.

TOOLKIT

Medication Usage Review

Year_____

Month	Jan	Feb	Mar	Apr	May	June	July	Aug	Sept	Oct	Nov	Dec
Routine Meds (no. per resident)												
PRN (no. per resident)												

APPENDIX

Multifactorial falls risk assessment and management tool (includes an osteoporosis risk screen)

Name of resident: _____

DOB: _____   **Room no.:** _____

Name of assessor: _____

Date of assessment: _____

Record all risks and actions in the resident's care plan

Risk factor (Tick if applicable, then link with recommended actions)	Recommended actions (Select appropriate interventions and record in care plan)	Date and sign
1. History of failing: ☐ Has the resident had one or more falls in the past 12 months?	a. Obtain details about past falls, including how many, causes, activity at time of fall, injuries, symptoms such as dizziness, and previous treatment received. Determine any patterns and consider throughout assessment. Ask about/ observe for fear of falling. b. Discuss falls risk with family. c. Flag in care plan and at handover if resident is high falls risk. **Consider:** d. Contacting GP or falls prevention services to review resident's falls risks if at high risk **or** there have been unexplained falls **or** several falls in a short period of time. Give details of specific concerns. e. If recent falls, and the resident has a temperature (fever), consider checking for infection (with urine, sputum, and stool samples). f. Assess for postural or orthostatic hypotension (a drop in BP when standing up). Record in resident's progress notes and inform GP if hypotension found. g. Consider how the resident can be observed/supervised more easily.	
2. Balance and mobility: ☐ Is the resident unsteady/unsafe walking? ☐ Does the resident have – difficulty with transfers (getting on and off the toilet/bed/chair)?	a. Ensure mobility aid and rails are used correctly and consistently. Prompt, place within reach, and use visual cues if appropriate. (Seek advice if unsure of correct use of mobility aids). b. Provide supervision when walking or transferring if required. Record what assistance is required. c. Record and hand over recommendations from physiotherapist regarding mobility and transfer status (e.g., if supervision is needed). d. Review bathroom grab rails. Are they appropriate and in good condition? Refer to maintenance if necessary. e. Ensure brakes are on bed at all times. Ensure correct height of bed and chairs. f. Ensure that frequently used items are within easy reach i.e., glasses, drinks, walking aid. g. Ensure buzzer is within easy reach and the resident is able to use it. h. Ensure residents with poor mobility, who are known not to ask for assistance, are not left unattended on commodes, toilets, baths, and showers (consider/ discuss the balance between safety and dignity). i. Increase opportunity for appropriate exercise through Activities of Daily Living (ADL) and the activities program. **Consider:** j. If required, discuss concerns with the GP or physiotherapist to identify need for assessment of balance, walking and transfers, assessment for/ review of mobility aid. Record concerns in the resident's notes. k. Hip protectors – discuss suitability and funding with resident's care manager and family.	

(continued)

APPENDIX (CONTINUED)

Risk factor (Tick if applicable, then link with recommended actions)	Recommended actions (Select appropriate interventions and record in care plan)	Date and sign
3. Osteoporosis: ☐ Does the resident have osteoporosis (check transfer notes or ask GP) If not: ☐ Is the resident at risk of osteoporosis? • Ask the following: • Has he/she had fracture after a minor bump or fall, over the age of 50? • Is there a family history of osteoporosis or hip fracture? • Has he/she been on steroids for 3 months or more? • Is there loss of height and an outward curve of the spine?	a. If osteoporosis is diagnosed check the resident is taking medication for osteoporosis as prescribed. b. If at high risk speak to GP about osteoporosis risk and further investigation and/or treatment.	
4. Medication: ☐ Is the resident taking 4 or more medications? ☐ Is the resident taking any of the following? – Sedatives – Anti-depressants – Anti-Parkinson's – Diuretics (water tablets) – Anti-psychotics – Anti-coagulants – Anti-hypertensives ☐ Has there been a recent change in medication that may effect falls risk (e.g., changes involving any of the above?)	a. Check medications have been reviewed with respect to falls risk (within the last 12 months is good practice). b. Report side effects/symptoms of medication to GP. c. Read patient information leaflet that comes with the medication or speak to local pharmacist for information on medication side effects and interactions. d. Anticipate side effects and take appropriate measures: – Sedatives: toilet and prepare for bed before giving night sedation. Monitor at all times, but especially overnight, and supervise in the morning. – Anti-psychotics: can cause sedation, postural hypotension, and impaired balance. Anticipate and compensate and report to GP. – Inform GP if the resident is excessively drowsy or mobility has deteriorated. – Diuretics: anticipate immediate and subsequent toileting. Ensure easy access to toilet and assist if required. e. Write in progress notes and alert staff at handover. f. Report changes in alertness or mobility. g. Assess for postural hypotension before and one hour after morning medications, for 3 days. h. Anticipate side effects and take appropriate measures.	
5. Dizziness and fainting: ☐ Does the resident experience: • dizziness on standing • a sensation of the room spinning when moving their head or body • fainting attacks • palpitations?	a. Carry out a lying standing blood pressure reading to check for postural or orthostatic hypotension if staff trained to do so. b. Refer the resident to the GP for review of dizziness/fainting/blackouts/palpitations. c. If postural/orthostatic hypotension prompts resident to move ankles up and down before rising, then rise slowly and with care from lying to sitting, and sitting to standing.	
6. Nutrition: ☐ Has the resident lost weight unintentionally or do they have little appetite? ☐ Does the resident spend little time outside in daylight?	a. Refer to GP or dietician. b. In consultation with GP or dietician: – commence food record chart. – consider food supplements. Refer to GP for assessment of vitamin D levels.	

(continued)

APPENDIX (CONTINUED)

Risk factor (Tick if applicable, then link with recommended actions)	Recommended actions (Select appropriate interventions and record in care plan)	Date and sign
7. Cognitive impairment: ☐ Is the resident confused, disorientated, restless, or highly irritable or agitated? ☐ Does the resident have reduced insight and/or judgment and/or are they uncooperative with staff?	a. If there is a new change in cognitive status monitor for pain, signs of infection, or constipation. b. Monitor behavioral issues and discuss chart with GP. c. Include behavioral issues in care plan and follow with regard to falls prevention. d. Ensure the resident's GP has reviewed this condition. Report fluctuations and patterns to treating GP. e. Do not leave the resident unattended on commodes, in toilets, baths, or showers. f. Optimise environmental safety; remove clutter and hazards. g. Use visual cues (e.g., signs and symbols) as reminders or to aid orientation. h. Use routine practices when instructing/assisting the resident. i. Record useful practices in care plan. j. Investigate the resident's previous patterns and incorporate into care plan (e.g., usual time of showering or preferred side of bed). k. Ask family/relatives to visit at particular times of day to assist with management and care when able. l. Consider the need for falls prevention equipment in keeping with local policies and in discussion and agreement with family and principal carer.	
8. Continence: ☐ Do continence issues contribute to the resident's falls risk?	a. If no toileting routine is in place, carry out a continence assessment and/or review of continence chart. b. Agree on a toileting regime and use of continence products as appropriate. c. Optimize environment safety – remove clutter and hazards, consider night lighting, monitor floors for wet areas – clean or report as soon as possible. d. Ensure adequate hydration during the day, not excessive in late afternoon. e. Provide with commode chair or urinal as appropriate. **Consider:** f. If required, referral to district nurse or the continence service.	
9. Sensory impairment: ☐ Does the resident have poor vision? (Remember: following a stroke someone may have restricted vision on one side, some people with dementia experience visual problems?) ☐ Does the resident have poor hearing?	a. If vision has not been tested in last 12 months, refer to optometrist. b. Ensure room is free of clutter and obstacles. c. Ensure bedroom lighting is adequate; consider need for night lights. d. Ensure glasses are in good condition, clean (each morning), worn consistently (prompting, note in care plan), kept within reach when not worn, and appropriate (e.g., reading vs. distance) e. If hearing has not been assessed in last 12 months, discuss options, including referral to audiologist with GP. f. Ensure hearing aid is worn, clean, and batteries are working. g. Use common gestures/cues/instructions. h. Minimize excess noise.	

(continued)

APPENDIX (CONTINUED)

Risk factor (Tick if applicable, then link with recommended actions)	Recommended actions (Select appropriate interventions and record in care plan)	Date and sign

10. Night patterns:
To be completed by night staff
☐ Does the resident often get out of bed overnight?
   If yes:
☐ Is the resident able to get in and out of bed safely on their own?
	a. Provide night lighting appropriate to vision.
	b. Optimize environmental safety – remove clutter and hazards.
	c. Check bed height is suitable for the resident.
	d. Ensure spectacles and buzzer are within easy reach.
	e. Discuss with family if nightwear is not appropriate – consider especially slippers (should be good fit, with back and heel support) and length of nightgowns.
	Consider:
	f. Treaded bed socks.
	g. Alert pad if resident is likely to fall while moving around the room.
	h. Hi-low bed. Keep in a position to suit the resident's needs overnight.
	i. Provide with commode or urine bottle for night toileting.
	j. If agitated at night:
	   – Ensure calm environment and follow advice in the behavioral plan for settling the resident.
	   – Observe every 15 to 30 minutes overnight.
	   – Engage in regular activity during the day to aid sleep at night and/or reduce agitation during the day.
	k. Refer to GP for review of evening or night medication.	

11. Feet and footwear: ☐ Does the resident have corns, ingrown toe nails, bunions, fungal infections, pain or loss of the sensation in their feet? ☐ Does the resident wear ill-fitting shoes, high-heel shoes, or shoes without grip?	a. Refer to podiatrist (or GP if fungal infections). Start foot care regime. b. Liaise with family to provide shoes with thin hard sole, enclosed heel, fastening mechanism. c. Do not walk with socks only. If shoes are too tight or loose fitting, walk with bare feet. d. Consider rubber tread socks if shoes are often removed.	
12. New or respite resident: ☐ Is the resident oriented to their new environment? ☐ Does the resident have suitable clothing and footwear?	a. Orientation to facility/unit including their room, the bathroom, communal areas, and outdoor areas. b. Optimize environmental safety – remove clutter and hazards. c. Inform and discuss with family/visitors as appropriate. d. Refer to preadmission information to identify specific issues. e. Liaise with family and principal carer to provide suitable clothing and footwear. Refer to information sent in from carer with regard to safety and falls risks.	
Other: Are there other factors that you consider relevant in considering this resident's falls risk, e.g., alcohol intake, pain, low mood/depression?	• Identify suitable action/s.	

(*continued*)

APPENDIX (CONTINUED)

Consider the relevance of the following risk factors:

Perceptual/Cognitive	Physical	Environment	Activities
Insight/judgment	Balance	Footwear	Mobility
Cognitive status	Strength	Aids	Transfers
Memory	Vision	Equipment	ADL
Orientation	Hearing	Clothing	Opportunity for exercise
Psychiatric condition	Continence	Lighting	High-risk activity
Anxiety	Nutritional status	Floor surface	Inactivity
Depression	Time spent outside	Location of bedroom	Fitness
Motivation	Medical condition	Seating	
Medication effects	Medication effects	Bedroom furniture	
Communication	Sensation	Signage	
Nocturnal patterns	Range of movement	Contrasting colors	
	Foot health		
	Constipation		

Action plan:

Risk Factors Identified	Intervention Strategies and Referrals

Intervention listed in:

☐ Care plan   ☐ Hand-over sheet

Date: _____   **Signature:** _____

Review date: _____

Adapted from a tool developed by Westerlands Care Home, Stirling.

SUGGESTED READINGS

Akabayashi A, Taylor Slingsby B. Informed consent revisited: Japan and the US. *Am J Bioethics*. 2006;6:9-14.

Alexander GL, Rantz M, Skubic M, et al. Evolution of an early illness warning system to monitor frail elders in independent living. *J Healthc Eng*. 2011;2(2):259-286.

American Geriatric Society. 2012 Beers Criteria Update Expert Panel. American Geriatrics Society updated Beers criteria for potentially inappropriate medication use in older adults. *J Am Geriatr Soc*. 2012;60:616-631.

Australian Nursing and Midwifery Council. *Code of Ethics for Nurses in Australia*. Australia: Dickson: ANMC; 2008.

Bergland A, Kirkevol M. Thriving in nursing homes in Norway: contributing aspects described by residents *Int J Nurs Stud*. 2006;43:681-691.

Brooker D, Woolley R, Lee D. Enriching opportunities for people living with dementia in nursing homes: an evaluation of a multi-level activity based model of care. *Aging Mental Health*. 2007;11:361-370.

Dosa D, Hyer K, Thomas K, et al. To evacuate or shelter in place: implications of universal hurricane evacuation policies on nursing home residents. *J Am Med Dir Assoc*. 2012;13:190.e1-190.e7.

Fitzgerald SP, Bean NG. An analysis of the interactions between individual comorbidities and their treatments—implications for guidelines and polypharmacy. *J Am Med Dir Assoc*. 2010;11:475-484.

Gallagher P, Baeyens JP, Topinkova E, et al. Inter-rater reliability of STOPP (Screening Tool of Older Persons' Prescriptions) and START (Screening Tool to Alert doctors to Right Treatment) criteria amongst physicians in six European countries. *Age Ageing*. 2009;38:603-606.

Gallagher P, Lang PO, Cherubini A, et al. Prevalence of potentially inappropriate prescribing in an acutely ill population of older patients admitted to six European hospitals. *Eur J Clin Pharmacol*. 2011;67:1175-1188.

Gruneir A, Mor V. Nursing home safety: current issues and barriers to improvement. *Annu Rev Public Health*. 2008;29:369-382.

Hertogh CM, The BA, Miesen BM, Eefsting JA. Truth telling and truthfulness in the care for patients with advanced dementia: an ethnographic study in Dutch nursing homes. *Social Sci Med*. 2004;59:1685-1693.

Lindbloom EJ, Brandt J, Landon D, et al. Elder mistreatment in the nursing home: a systematic review. *J Am Med Dir Assoc*. 2007;8(9):610-616.

Loganathan M, Singh S, Franklin BD, et al. Interventions to optimise prescribing in care homes: systematic review. *Age Ageing*. 2011;40:150-162.

McCormack B. A conceptual framework for person-centred practice with older people. *Int J Nutr Pract*. 2003;9:202-209.

Monroe T, Carter M, Parish A. A case study using the beers list criteria to compare prescribing by family practitioners and geriatric specialists in a rural nursing home. *Geriatr Nurs*. 2011;32:350-356.

Morley JE. Polypharmacy in the nursing home. *J Am med Dir Assoc*. 2010;11:296-297.

Morley JE. Transitions. *J Am Med Dir Assoc*. 2010;11(9):607-611.

Mosqueda L, Heath J, Burnight K. Recognizing physical abuse and neglect in the skilled nursing facility: the physician's responsibilities. *J Am Med Dir Assoc*. 2001;2(4):183-186.

Mystakikdou K, Parpa E, Tsilika E, et al. Cancer information disclosure in different cultural contexts. *Support Care Cancer*. 2004;12:147-154.

Nursing and Midwifery Council. *The Code: Standards of Conduct, Performance and Ethics for Nurses and Midwives*. London: Author; 2008.

Onder G, Liperoti R, Fialova D, et al; for the SHELTER Project. Polypharmacy in nursing home in Europe: results from the SHELTER study. *J Gerontol A Biol Sci Med Sci*. 2012;67(6):698-704.

Ouslander JG, Berenson RA. Reducing unnecessary hospitalizations of nursing home residents. *N Engl J Med*. 2011;365(13):1165-1168.

Ouslander JF, Lamb G, Tappen R, et al. Interventions to reduce hospitalizations from nursing homes: evaluation of the INTERACT II collaborative quality Improvement project. *J Am Geriatr Soc*. 2011;59: 745-753.

Pyszka LL, Seys Ranola TM, Milhans SM. Identification of inappropriate prescribing in geriatrics at a Veterans Affairs hospital using STOP/ START screening tools. *Consult Pharm*. 2010;25:365-373.

Smith M, Kolanowski A, Buettner LL, Buckwalter KC. Beyond bingo: meaningful activities for persons with dementia in nursing homes. *Ann Long Term Care*. 2009;17.7:22-30.

Social Care and Social Work Improvement Scotland. *Managing Falls and Fractures in Care Homes for Older People. Good Practice Self Assessment Resource*. Scotland: Communications SCWIS. Available at http://www.scswis.com/index.php?option=com_content&task=view&id=7906&Itemid=725. Published 2011. Accessed March 24, 2013.

Stone RI, Reinhard SC. The place of assisted living in long-term care and related service systems. *Gerontologist*. 2007;47(special issue III):23-32.

Tak SH, Benefield LE, Mahoney DF. Technology for long-term care. *Res Gerontol Nurs*. 2010;3(1):61-72.

Tuckett A. Registered nurses' understanding of truth-telling as practiced in the nursing-home: an Australian perspective. *Health Sociol Rev*. 2006;15:179-191.

Van't Leven N, Jonsson H. Doing and being in the atmosphere of the doing: environmental influences on occupational performance in a nursing home. *Scand J Occup Ther*. 2002;9:148-155.

Vognar L, Buhr G. Elder abuse in long term care: a growing problem. *J Am Med Dir Assoc*. 2011;12:(3):B10-B11.

MULTIPLE CHOICE QUESTIONS

5.1 Which of the following is not one of the five major areas of the United Nations' Principles for Older People?

a. Independence
b. Care
c. Freedom from illness
d. Self-fulfillment
e. Dignity

5.2 Which of the following is true about "truth telling?"

a. Family members need to be allowed to decide if relatives should be told about a poor prognosis.
b. Truth telling undermines the opportunity for self-realization and for autonomy.
c. All cultures accept truth telling as being appropriate.
d. When a resident cannot expect to be told the truth, this creates a level of suspicious awareness, leading to unintentional negative consequences.

5.3 Which of the following is an example of intentional neglect?

a. A resident falls because the staff member has not been trained in appropriate transfer techniques.
b. A resident falls while the staff member is helping another resident.
c. A resident is not provided appropriate care because the staff member believes it will hurt the resident.
d. A resident is knowingly left lying in soiled bedding.
e. A resident is hit by a staff member.

5.4 The risk of side effects when a person taking five drugs receives another drug are

a. Equal chance of causing benefit or harm
b. Minimal chance of causing harm
c. Half chance of causing benefit or harm
d. Double chance of causing benefit or harm
e. Depends on the type of drug

5.5 Physical restraints lead to

a. A reduction in injurious harms
b. Less agitated behavior
c. No harm to the resident
d. On occasion, death of the resident
e. Abuse of the resident

Chapter 6

MODELS OF CARE DELIVERY

Older people are comparatively high users of health and social care, and as the demand for long-term care rises, it is important that models of care delivery are reviewed and refreshed. Challenges to the delivery of high-quality and effective nursing home care are numerous and involve workforce issues, professional role development, and expansion of practice in addition to the well-known challenge of funding and affordability. There is a global shortage of health professionals, and the historic low status afforded to those who choose a career in nursing homes compounds problems and gives rise to the need to develop new and advanced practice roles that can function effectively within a given model of care.

As outlined in Chapter 2, nursing home services vary by region, extending from hospital-styled facilities to those that operate toward the social care end of the spectrum. Care delivery models understandably reflect the specific contributions made by the nursing home sector within the regional wider health and social care system. The economic challenges of delivering nursing home and other long-term care solutions are a universal, and as we plan for the future, our consideration of models of care must embrace affordable innovative workforce, operational, and technological advances. As new models of care are embraced, it is imperative that they maintain or enhance the quality of the care experience and keep the person at the heart of our practice and operations. With this person-centered focus, staff must understand the interface between the person's care within the nursing home and other services such as hospital care to ensure optimal quality during transitions. Our consideration of models begins with a brief examination of the practical implications of person-centered approaches, issues involved in transitional, and a range of selected models extending from subacute through to end-of-life care.

MODELS OF CARE

The desire to provide practitioners with theoretical frameworks has yielded numerous nursing and to a lesser extent interdisciplinary models. We recognize that opinions are divided on the merits of what some describe as theoretical abstractions and their practical utility. However, if nursing home practice is to evolve, theoretical influences must be embraced, albeit with an understanding of what they offer practitioners and what they offer in terms of quality

enhancement and augmentation of the resident's experience. It is beyond the scope of this book to review models in depth, and we will confine our theoretical meanderings to a few salient observations before focusing on person-centered thinking. Over the years, theoretical challenges to the way we think about aging and the social constructions of old age have played pivotal roles in the advancement of geriatric medicine and gerontologic practices and attitudes toward the care of older people. For example, cognitive and psychological models opened the door to the development of cognitive and behavior adaptation therapies just as disease control models and biologic models have underpinned diagnostics and treatment development. If we follow this logic, then it is reasonable to suggest that embracing some of the thinking within models of care within our nursing home delivery models can assist us to bring about progress on culture change, practice development, and other quality improvements that require staff to change their practice along with the organizational mindset and systems.

PERSON-CENTERED CARE

In person-centered approaches to care, the relationship between staff members and the older person is the key to successful care outcomes. Being person-centered relies on staff knowing the older person as an individual and planning personalized approaches to care. To do this involves appreciating who the person is in the wider context of his or her former, current, and future lives. Four additional factors must also be addressed to achieve person-centered care within nursing homes:

1. The nursing home practitioner must believe in the value of person-centered practice and understand what this means in terms of day-to-day work with older residents and their family caregivers.
2. The environment of the nursing home must be receptive to person-centered approaches. There needs to be an appropriate skill mix and systems that align with the person-centered ethos (e.g., shared decision making, permissible risk taking, reciprocity between staff, reciprocity between the staff and residents).
3. Person-centered processes are required that allow a resident's preferences, values, and beliefs to shape care decisions; influence planning and approaches

to delivery; and, of course, be central to the evaluation of the care experience and outcomes.

4. Person-centered outcomes such as resident satisfaction, quality of life, and perceptions of well-being must be valued alongside more clinically focused outcomes.

Although person-centered care is the mantra of modernity, it is not simple to implement in practice, and conceptual frameworks can be off-putting. However, nursing home teams need to develop clarity as to what person-centered care or personalization of care means in terms of their day-to-day interactions and ways of working with older people.

Interest in life plans and life history as methods for staff to get to know the person and integrate this personal knowledge is most well advanced in the nursing and social care literature. The key ingredients of person-centered care include knowing the person, understanding the person's values and preferences, viewing the person in the context of his or her social history and future perspectives, and partnership working between the staff and the person throughout the journey of care. The interdependence of the myriad of relationships that are forged among older people, the staff, and the community must also be recognized and valued within person-centered thinking. Thus, reciprocity and relational aspects of care need to be nurtured as much as individual perspectives. These humanistic values should serve as a guide for practitioners intent on positioning the older person at the center of care and can be applied across the spectrum of delivery models that are found within the nursing home sector.

TRANSITIONAL CARE

Almost a quarter of persons admitted to a nursing home in the United States are readmitted to the hospital within 30 days. Nearly half of these hospitalizations are unavoidable or potentially unavoidable. In many situations, these persons could have been clinically cared for in the nursing home. Studies have suggested that three quarters of potentially avoidable hospitalizations involve five conditions. These are pneumonia, congestive heart failure, urinary tract infection, dehydration, and chronic obstructive pulmonary disease. A lack of a "do not hospitalize" order also played a role in increasing avoidable transfers. Feeding tube complications accounted for a major component of avoidable transfers to the emergency department. This is important because it is clear that numerous problems in delivery quality care occur during transitions with approximately one in five patients discharged from the hospital having an adverse event. At least 60% of these are caused by inappropriate drugs being taken after discharge. Transitions are extraordinarily complex and can occur during changes in physicians or specialists as well as movement between different domiciliary sites (Figure 6–1).

The key to decreasing the negative effects of transitions resides both in reducing transitions and enhancing communication between different sites. Medication reconciliation between sites represents a major step in decreasing transition problems. This requires both improved

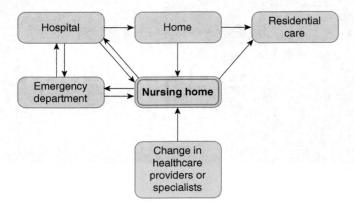

Figure 6–1. Complexity of transitions.

medication documentation in writing on discharge but also personal communication between providers at different sites explaining the rationale for the medications. A follow-up visit by a nurse from the hospital or nursing home within 24 hours of transfer allows identification of erroneous transfer of orders.

A major issue in transitions is the failure of advanced directives to transfer with the person. After a transfer, many abnormal laboratory results come back, but the results are not made available to the new facility. Transfers often fail to include patient preferences or triggers for agitated behavior.

All nursing homes should have rapid cycles in place to ensure that communication between the facilities with which they interact is complete. Methods for reducing inappropriate transfers have been explored by programs such as Interventions to Reduce Acute Care Transfers (INTERACT; http://www.interact2.net). This program emphasizes development of advanced directions and early recognition of new onset illness (Figure 6–2). Their change in condition information is supplied in the Toolkit. Figure 6–3 gives INTERACT's STOP AND WATCH tool for nurses' aides to recognize a change in condition. A preliminary study suggested that use of this tool reduced hospitalizations. A simple approach to improving the quality of transfers is given in Table 6–1.

Another intervention to reduce transitions is the Hebrew SeniorLife intervention. This relatively simple intervention has three components:

- A template to create a standard physician admission procedure
- A palliative care consult for all residents who have had three or more hospitalizations in the previous 6 months
- Bimonthly conferences to determine the reasons for problems with the transitions

This program resulted in approximately a 20% decline in rehospitalization and a 4.5% increase in discharges to home.

A number of transition programs that do not focus on nursing homes also have developed some potentially useful resources, such as the Coleman Care Transition Tools

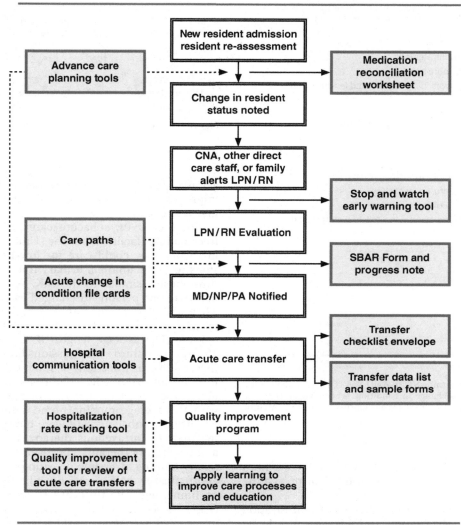

Figure 6–2. Overview of the Interact II program. SBAR, situation, background, assessment, recommendation. (Permission received to reprint Interact 3.0 materials from Joseph Ouslander, Florida Atlantic University.)

(http://www.caretransition.org) and Naylor Transitional Care Model (http://www.transitionalcare.info).

In the United States, Life Care Corporation is placing a full time physician in each facility to try to decrease transitions back to hospitals. The Centers for Medicare & Medicaid Services has funded a number of novel advanced practice nursing programs to reduce transitions.

INTERMEDIATE AND SUBACUTE CARE

In the United Kingdom, it was recognized that approximately 20% of hospitalized older persons do not need to be in the hospital. This led to the development of intermediate care, which can bridge care between the community and the hospital. It has three purposes:

1. Prevent unnecessary hospital admission
2. Facilitate earlier discharges from the hospital
3. Reduce unnecessary admissions to long-term care

Overall, it is expected to provide intermediate care for 2 to 6 weeks. Intermediate care can occur in the acute hospital, community hospital, dedicated facility, or day hospital. Approximately one third of intermediate care occurs as "the hospital in home." The concept was first developed in 1982 at the Lambeth Community Care Center. In 1992, a key version of the model was developed by Pearson and his

If you have identified a change while caring for or observing a resident, please **circle** the change and notify a nurse. Either give the nurse a copy of this tool or review it with her/him as soon as you can.

S	Seems different than usual
T	Talks or communicates less
O	Overall needs more help
P	Pain – new or worsening; Participated less in activities
a	Ate less
n	No bowel movement in 3 days; or diarrhea
d	Drank less
W	Weight change
A	Agitated or nervous more than usual
T	Tired, weak, confused, or drowsy
C	Change in skin color or condition
H	Help with walking, transferring, toileting more than usual

Name of Resident

Your Name

Reported to   Date and Time (am/pm)

Nurse Response   Date and Time (am/pm)

Nurse's Name

Figure 6–3. The early warning STOP AND WATCH tool to help nursing assistants recognize a change in condition. (Permission received to reprint Interact 3.0 materials from Joseph Ouslander, Florida Atlantic University.)

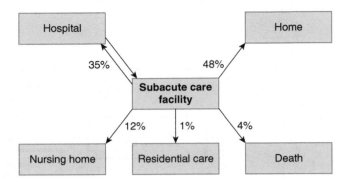

Figure 6–4. Outcomes for residents admitted to subacute care.

colleagues in Oxfordshire. Most intermediate care facilities provide care after hospitalization rather than preventing hospital admissions.

In the United States, the Veterans Administration developed Geriatric Evaluation and Management Units (GEMUs). These GEMUs in their optimum function took persons who were at high risk of nursing home admission because of complex medical disease and treated them with geriatric principles and intensive rehabilitation. This led to improved function, more days at home, and less cost in the first year of care.

In the 1990s, subacute care facilities flourished as freestanding facilities in the United States. Although in theory they could care for low-level hospital admissions (e.g., pneumonia, urinary tract infection, deep vein thrombosis), similar to the U.K. version, they predominantly served persons discharged early from the hospital. They accepted persons after 3 midnights in the hospital and provided medical and rehabilitation care 7 days a week. The average length of stay was approximately 20 days. Two thirds of admissions had medical conditions (heart, lung, or infection) or functional impairment. One in five had orthopedic conditions. Stroke and pressure ulcers accounted for the rest of admissions. Compared with the average nursing home admission, the patients admitted to subacute care were more likely to be receiving dialysis, intravenous therapy, injections, antibiotics, and respiratory therapy. They were less likely to have difficulty bathing, dressing, or eating. In the United States, approximately half of patients admitted to subacute care go home, and one third are readmitted to the hospital (Figure 6–4). In the twenty-first century, there has been a move to a lower acuity of subacute care because of alterations in federal reimbursement. This has led to a blending between subacute care and the skilled nursing facility. The potential advantages of intermediate and subacute care are summarized in Table 6–2.

Table 6–1.	EFFECTIVE APPROACHES TO ENHANCING TRANSITIONS

- A clear medication list
- Advanced directives
- Direct communication between health professionals at both sites
- Delineated lines of responsibility for transitions
- Clear knowledge of patient and family concerning the purpose of the transition
- A universal electronic record accessible by all sites
- Rapid cycles to regularly investigate successfulness of communication and outcomes

Table 6–2.	ADVANTAGES OF INTERMEDIATE OR SUBACUTE CARE OVER HOSPITALIZATION

- Less costly
- Focus on functional status and rehabilitation
- Residents involved in recreation activities
- Focus on pressure ulcer prevention
- Comprehensive geriatric assessment
- Residents eat in dining room, not bed
- Prevention of weight loss a priority

IMPROVING FUNCTION

All nursing homes need to focus on improving or at least maintaining function. This requires an active rehabilitation program with recognition that resistance exercise as well as walking programs can produce major improvements. All nursing homes need to offer regular exercise programs focusing on resistance exercise, aerobic exercise, and balance exercise. Restorative aides need to be available to help residents maintain function that they have gained from rehabilitation programs.

END-OF-LIFE AND HOSPICE CARE

Approximately one in five persons in the United States die in nursing homes. Hospice care has existed since ancient times. Its modern formulation was created by Madame Garnier, who, in the 1800s, established a Calvaire in Lyon, France, to care for dying people. Cicely Saunders, as a nurse in England, thought physicians failed to show adequate compassion for dying patients. She became a physician and at St. Christopher's Hospice in London (Figure 6–5) developed the hospice movement in England and then, working with nurses at Yale University, the American hospice movement. The other major change in approach to dying was Elizabeth Kübler-Ross' book *On Death and Dying*, which was published in 1969. This book enhanced the importance of "the good death" and established the psychological stages of dying (Table 6–3).

The major change in the hospice movement has been to move from the medical model to an end-of-life model of

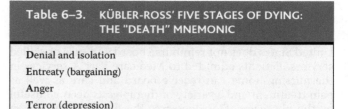

Table 6–3. KÜBLER-ROSS' FIVE STAGES OF DYING: THE "DEATH" MNEMONIC
Denial and isolation
Entreaty (bargaining)
Anger
Terror (depression)
Hopeful for the "afterlife" (acceptance)

care (Figure 6–6). This requires a shift from cure-focused care to one of a focus both on disease and symptoms. Early in the process, both spiritual and psychological supports are introduced. After death, bereavement care is provided for the family.

Five components of end-of-life care that are important to dying persons have been identified:

- Control of symptoms, especially pain
- Maintenance of locus of control for the person
- Decreasing the burden associated with dying
- Strengthening relationships with family
- Avoiding inappropriate extension of the dying process

Originally, most hospice deaths in the United States were caused by cancer. Now, although cancer is still the most common diagnosis, accounting for 40.1% of hospice deaths, other diagnoses are also commonly seen, including unspecified disability (13.1%), heart disease (11.5%), dementia (11.2%), and lung disease (8.2%). Two recent studies have clearly shown that appropriate end-of-life hospice care actually extends life compared with regular care. In one of these studies, survival was extended by 29 days and in another by 2.7 months.

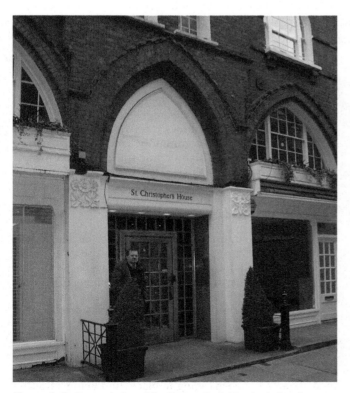

Figure 6–5. External view of St. Christopher's Hospice in London.

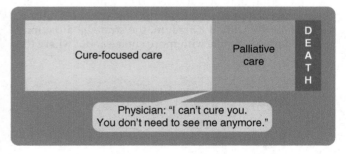

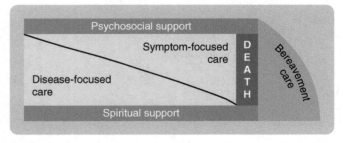

Figure 6–6. Comparison between the medical model and the end-of-life model.

In the United States, hospice care is paid for by the government for persons who are certified by a physician as having less than 6 months to live. Hospice care in the United States does not reimburse board and care or skilled services. Patients admitted to Medicare Part A services in the nursing home can receive board and care as well as pain treatment and a variety of therapies as deemed useful by the physician. This decreases the financial burden on the family.

Services provided by hospice in the nursing home in the United States include consultation by a hospice-trained nurse and the hospice medical director as well as variety of comfort services such as aromatherapy, massage therapy, volunteer visits, and physical and occupational therapy. Spiritual and psychological support are provided for both the patient and family. After death, the hospice provides follow-up bereavement care. Hospice staff also provides education regarding care of the dying for the long-term care staff. In Europe, a number of hospice houses have opened to provide end-of-life care (Figure 6–7).

Hospice care in the United Kingdom is dominated by independent sector provision and partnership models with the National Health Service. As in the United States, the movement began in response to the needs of people dying with cancer. Today many people are still admitted for hospice care with cancer, but people are also admitted with other life-limiting diseases although rarely for age-related conditions that lead to physical frailty and dementia. In people age 75 years and older, in 2006 to 2008, 58.4% of deaths were in hospitals, 12.1% were in nursing homes, 10.0% were in old people's homes, 15.5% were in the person's own residence, 0.9% were elsewhere, and 3.1% were in hospices. The trend is that an increasing number of older people are dying within nursing homes compared with the fairly constant number who die within a hospice.

Persons admitted to hospices are normally expected to die within 3 months or less; those who require longer term palliation may be admitted to care homes or receive community support supplemented by specialist nursing services. In the United Kingdom, the strategic direction is to provide older people with more choice about where they

Table 6–4.	STAGE 7C OF THE FUNCTIONAL ASSESSMENT STAGING SCALE

- No more than five words in vocabulary
- Cannot walk
- Fecal incontinence
- Cannot dress or bathe without assistance

live in their final years and where they would like to die. An important innovation improving the standards of end-life-care is the introduction of the Liverpool Care Pathway. The Pathway is for people with a known diagnosis when death appears inevitable. Symptoms are monitored and treated expectantly with an emphasis on comfort, preparation for death, and spiritual support.

The Department of Health in the United Kingdom has also developed a useful toolkit the Gold Standards for Care Homes to enhance end-life-care care provided within care homes. Such approaches have had a demonstrable impact on end-life-care care of residents in specialist dementia units within care homes.

In some countries, there is an increasing desire to include patients with dementia in hospice care. For entry to hospice, the Functional Assessment Staging Scale has been used. Level 7C correctly identifies 55% of persons who will die in the next 6 month (Table 6–4).

A recent study found that the Advanced Dementia Prognostic Tool was more successful in identifying persons liable to die within 6 months. Good care for persons with dementia at the end of life demands attention to the ABCDs of end-of-life dementia care:

- **A**cknowledgement of the authenticity of the person's life experience and maintaining awareness of his or her life history
- **B**lessings are counted for both the resident and the persons taking care of the resident. In particular, this requires limiting depression in the resident, family members, and caregivers.
- **C**onnectedness allows the resident to remain involved in the community and with his or her family as well as maintaining spiritual relationships. This means that the resident is not isolated.
- **D**ignity maintains the self-respect of the person. Respect for the individual is maintained by caregivers and family members.

Table 6–5 summarizes the principles of end-of-life care. Healthcare providers need to be aware of distressing symptoms and their management (Table 6–6). The St. Louis University approach to management of end-of-life symptoms is included in the Toolkit. The toolkit also provides charts for monitoring care of the resident.

ASSISTED LIVING

In the United States, assisted living has emerged as an intermediate area between "aging in place" and being admitted to a nursing home. In general, assisted living represents

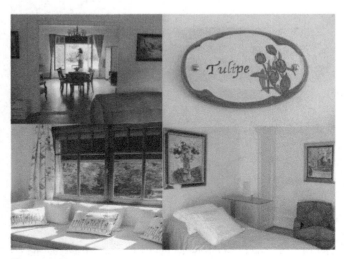

Figure 6–7. A hospice house in Geneva, Switzerland.

Table 6–5.	PRINCIPLES OF END-OF-LIFE CARE

- Enhance the quality of life of the person.
- Reduce the burden of the dying process.
- Do not inappropriately prolong the dying process.
- Treat distressing symptoms.
- Allow the dying person to keep their locus of control.
- Do not forget to provide comfort for existential ("psychic") distress.
- Enhance communication for all involved.
- Attend to spiritual needs for dying person and family.
- Coordinate the healthcare team to focus on the needs of the dying person.
- Provide bereavement care for the family.

individual rooms clustered in a senior housing apartment complex. It serves predominantly people independent on activities of daily living (ADL) or minimally ADL impaired. The level of disability and general health of persons in assisted living is much higher than that of persons living in nursing homes. Although cognitive impairment is common in assisted living, residents need to be able to find their own pathway to safety during emergencies.

A total of 92% of facilities provide medications, 79% provide medical care, and 40% have a full-time registered nurse. More than 60% of residents of assisted living are eventually discharged to nursing homes. Within some buildings funded by the U.S. Department of House and Urban Development, residents are provided with housekeeping, personal care, medication management, and an ability to provide emergency response systems. Most of these systems are publically funded. Adult day care is often co-located, and a house calls program using predominantly nurse practitioners with physician supervision may also exist.

The majority of assisted living facilities are privately funded. The major perceived advantage of assisted living is maintenance of independence compared with institutionalization in a nursing home. The tradeoff is often inadequate

levels of care. Cognitive impairment, incontinence, and increased level of care often lead to discharge of residents who are suitable for care in assisted living. Privately funded residential care facilities are often relatively expensive and because of minimal regulation offer inferior services compared with nursing homes.

EDEN ALTERNATIVE

William Thomas, MD, A Harvard graduate, suggested that cultural change in nursing homes would improve the outcomes of residents. He believed that deinstitutionalizing the culture and environment of nursing homes was a key to this improvement. He advocated an enlivened environment of pets and gardens (Figure 6–8). He also wanted residents and staff to have ownership of nursing home function, thus enhancing their locus of control. In addition, children were introduced into nursing homes (e.g., using after-school care and summer camps). In 1991, he called this the Eden alternative. Although he and others have attributed multiple improved resident outcomes, these were uncontrolled studies. The outcomes of controlled studies have been disappointing. This does not negate the effect of this approach for many, but not all, residents and family members. In our experience, parakeets (relatively large birds) have become particularly good companions for nursing home residents. More information about the Eden alternative can be found at http://www.edenalt.org.

MULTISENSORY ENVIRONMENT (SNOEZELEN ROOM)

The use of a multisensory environment was based on psychological studies showing that healthy young people in a sensory-deprived environment became anxious, but in a sensory stimulating environment, they had enhanced mental performance. Subsequently, the multisensory environment has been used for persons with autism, developmental disability, pain, and dementia. Dutch workers at the Haarendael Institute coined the term "Snoezelen," meaning sniffing and dozing.

Table 6–6.	END-OF-LIFE SYMPTOMS THAT SHOULD BE MANAGED

- Fatigue
- Depression
- Anorexia and cachexia
- Nausea and vomiting
- Insomnia
- Anxiety
- Delirium
- Pain
- Diarrhea and constipation
- Dyspnea
- Loneliness

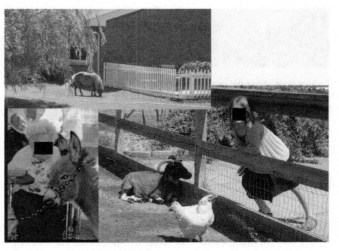

Figure 6–8. Eden alternative examples with children and animals.

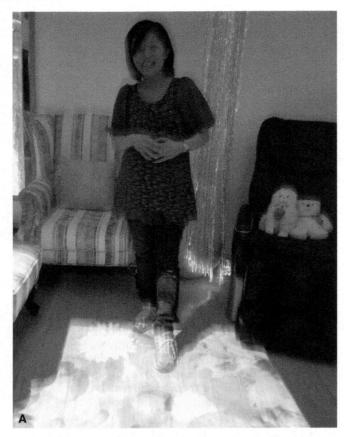

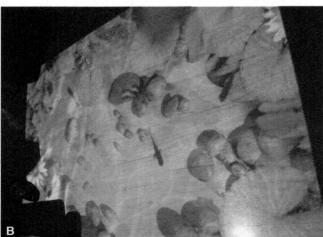

Figure 6–9. Example of a Snoezelen room. (Permission by Dr. Jenny Lee.)

Table 6–7.	DIFFERENT TYPES OF SENSATIONS USED FOR MULTISENSORY STIMULATION	
Visual	Room dimly lit	
	Rotating colored lights	
	Mirrors	
	Changing scenes on ceiling, wall or floor	
	Bubble tube	
	Lava Lamps	
Tactile	Vibrating or rocking chair	
	Soft seating	
	Boards with different textures	
	Sand box	
	Soft balls	
	Hanging material to walk through	
	Bead necklaces	
OLFACTORY	Oils with different smells, e.g., lavender oil from a burning candle, or hand oils for massage with different smells	
	Aromatherapy	
AUDITORY	Ocean sounds	
	Sounds of children playing	
	Nature sounds	
	Unusual music (new age or classical)	

The "Snoezelen" room should be the size of an average resident's room (Figure 6–9). It is a "failure-free" environment in which residents have the opportunity to explore and be exposed to multiple sensations. Residents with dementia share the experience with a caregiver (facilitator), usually a trained CNA or volunteer. The goal of the room is to produce enjoyment by the participants leading to relaxation. Examples of different kinds of stimuli are given in Table 6–7. A number of small mainly anecdotal studies support the use of a multisensory environment for the management of persons with agitation or apathy in nursing homes.

TECHNOLOGY AND CARE

Although high technology has become a norm in hospitals, its adoption by long-term care facilities has been slow. Nursing homes at present are bastions of low technology. Only in the past 5 years have computers begun to infiltrate nursing homes, being predominately used for financial reasons and the recording of the minimum data set. Charts in most nursing homes are paper. Given the large amount of data collected on residents by certified nursing assistants and the oversight required, a computerized medical record using an iPad would appear to be a logical early uptake of technology. Similarly, nursing, therapy, and physician notes would be much more accessible. Clearly, the computerized medical record in nursing homes will become a fact of life within the next few years.

Many nursing homes have introduced computers for residents to email their relatives or to talk to them on Skype. Thus, the personal computer represents the beginning of high-technology encroachment into nursing homes.

Technologies are being developed that will allow older persons to be able to perform basic and instrumental activities at higher levels. These technologies will also improve safety and allow less invasive monitoring of health problems. Technology should enhance the sense of control of seniors in long-term care and enhance their quality of life. Technology should be unobtrusive and can be in the environment as part of clothing or embedded in the resident. Examples of future nursing home technology are given in Table 6–8.

Table 6–8.	EXAMPLES OF FUTURE NURSING HOME TECHNOLOGY

Area	Technology
Health	Telemedicine
	Monitoring toilet activities
	Monitoring vital signs
	Sleep monitors including for apnea episodes
	Continuous glucose monitoring
	Dehydration monitoring
	Monitoring urine ketones
	Biosensors to monitor pressure areas
	Medication dispensers
Safety	Gait and motion monitors
	Fall sensors
	GPS location tracking for wanderers
	Motion sensors to detect resident getting out of bed
	Personal wireless help button
Recreational	Robotic companions
	Virtual reality scenes
	Communication with family and friends
	Clergy visits and virtual church attendance
	Allowing family to "look in" and "check up" on residents
	Automated email to family concerning health and happiness of residents
Mobility	Ceiling mounted lifts which can be easily controlled
	Exoskeletons to allow walking
	Intelligent walkers
	Computer operated wheelchairs to reduce accidents
	Treadmills that allow stroke patients to use without assistance
	Vibrating platforms designed to be safe for persons with balance problems
Communication	Computers for aphasic and deaf to communicate
	Computers to allow blind to have descriptions of their environment
	Use of brain waves to provide communication
Medical Devices	Computerized retinal implants
	Computer assisted upper and lower limb prostheses.

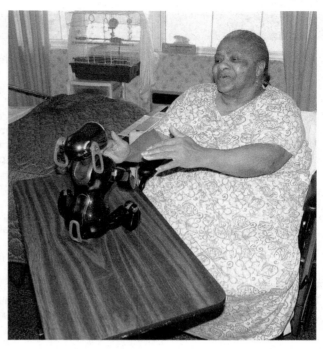

Figure 6–10. Robodog makes a nice companion for a long-term care resident. (Photos are provided by RIKEN-TRI Collaboration Center for Human-Interactive Robot Research.)

for soldiers are now well on the way to being available for individuals with paraplegia. Robotic arms for feeding persons are in existence. Telemedicine has been used in both the home and nursing homes. In nursing homes, it has been especially useful for obtaining consultations when a view of a skin lesion is necessary. Robotic nurses to help with lifting residents from bed and assisting with transfers to the toilet exist (Figure 6–11). Sensors to act as early illness warning systems have been developed at the University of Missouri and already tested at Tiger Place. Thus, as baby boomers enter nursing homes, we can expect to see a technological transformation of the nursing home.

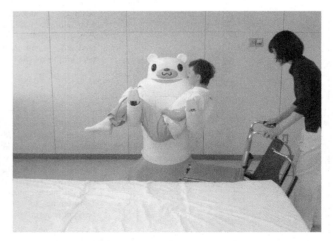

Figure 6–11. Example of a robotic nurse (RIBA) assisting with a transfer. These robots are safer for the resident and avoid back injuries among staff. (Photos are provided by RIKEN-TRI Collaboration Center for Human-Interactive Robot Research.)

Although much of the long-term technology has a "science fiction" feel to it, some is already infiltrating the long-term care arena. Computerized animals are being used for entertainment and as companions (Figure 6–10). Robotic companions such as "Kompai" have been developed by a French company. Exoskeletons developed originally

KEY POINTS

1. Approaches to care that are person centered and delivered with dignity and compassion are central components of best nursing home practice.
2. Relationships among older people, family members, staff, and the community must also be recognized and valued within person-centered thinking.
3. Transitions in care to and from the nursing home are complex, and effective communication strategies and rapid transfer systems to and from acute care should be place to optimize outcomes.
4. Avoidance of unnecessary hospitalization should be prioritized including for end-of-life care.
5. INTERACT II is a program that is readily available and proven to reduce transfers back to the hospital when it is properly implemented.
6. Intermediate or subacute care allows persons to be discharged from a hospital to a facility with a focus on rehabilitation. This is a cost-effective approach.
7. Hospice care can improve the quality of end-of-life for residents and their families.
8. Implementation of end-of-life care pathways can enhance the quality of care for nursing home residents who are dying.
9. The Functional Assessment Staging Scale can identify more than half of persons with dementia who will die in the next 6 months.
10. Person-centered approaches and deinstitutionalization of nursing homes are desirable.
11. Technological advances need to be embraced within nursing home practice, and the contribution of new technologies to person-centered nursing home care, experiences of care, safety, and impact on staff and workload should be evaluated.

TOOLKIT

St. Louis University Approach to Management of End-of-Life Symptoms (Modified from *Aging Successfully*)

	NONPHARMACOLOGICAL	PHARMACOLOGICAL		NONPHARMACOLOGICAL	PHARMACOLOGICAL
FATIGUE	Consider medication effect. Provide help at home. Provide emotional support. Utilize energy conservation strategies. Check sleeping patterns. Physical/Occupational therapy. Exercise.	Treat depression/If anemic, use Erythropoietin or Darbopoietin alpha. Testosterone. Dexamethosone (4-6 week benefit)/Methylphenidate.	**DYSPNEA**	Sit upright (may need armchair). Reduce room temperature. Maintain humidity. Avoid activities that increase dyspnea. Avoid irritants, *e.g.*, smoke. Elevate head of bed. Utilize oxygen when wanted. (Remember, cannula/mask can be irritating.) Use a fan.	Treat anxiety with benzodiazepines (Lorazepam). Dronabinol for CO_2 retainers. Opiates. Low-dose nebulized morphine. Steroids. Scopolomine/atropine/glycopyrollate (dries secretions, prevents death rattle).
DEPRESSION	Provide psychological support and regular visitors/outings.	Trazodone if associated with poor sleep. Mirtazapine if associated with anorexia. Desipramine/Nortriptyline. Selective serotonin reuptake inhibitors (SSRIs).	**CONSTIPATION**	Consider drugs as cause. **Increase fluid intake.** Exclude fecal impaction. Toilet after meals with **gastro-colic reflex.**	Use mainly osmotic laxatives: sorbitol, lactulose, polyethylene glycol. Methylnatrexone for opiate-induced impaction. Lubiprostone.
ANOREXIA/ CACHEXIA	Provide emotional support. Encourage small, frequent meals with calorie supplements between meals. Consider multivitamin. Consider glass of wine/beer.	Megestrol acetate (if anorexic, use nano formulation to enhance absorption). Dronabinol (causes munches, use only when weight gain is not a major concern). Testosterone (effectiveness uncertain).	**DIARRHEA**	Check to make sure it is not due to osmotic laxative. Rehydrate.	Use Kaopectate, Loperamide, prostaglandin inhibitors, or Octreotide (somatostatin analog).

(continued)

TOOLKIT (CONTINUED)

St. Louis University Approach to Management of End-of-Life Symptoms (Modified from *Aging Successfully*)

NAUSEA/ VOMITING	Check to make sure it is not due to drugs.	Dopamine antagonist. H₂ blockers. Serotonin antagonists. Prokinetic agents. Low-dose dronabinol.	**DELIRIUM**	Supportive nursing. Consider drugs as possible cause. Ensure adequately lighted room. Avoid illusional objects. Have someone in room (*e.g.,* use delirium ICU).	Avoid drugs. If essential: Trazodone (25-50 mg, 2-4 times/day), for agitation. Haloperidol (0.5-1 mg daily). Respiridol (1-2 mg daily) for paranoia, hallucinations, and rarely for agitation. IV Lorazepam (0.25-1 mg) for sedation to allow for medical procedures.
INSOMNIA	Avoid sleeping all day. Increase daytime activity. Control pain. Indulge in warm milk before sleeping. Get out of bed during the daytime. No reading or television in bed.	Treat depression. Treat anxiety. Treat pain. Trazodone. Melatonin (ramelteon). Zaleplon. Zolpidem. Eszopiclone.	**PAIN**	Make use of massage therapy. Try heat/cold, transcutaneous electrical nerve stimulation (TENS), lidocaine patch, and activity/distraction therapy.	Use WHO Analgesic Ladder. Try acetominophen, NSAIDs, weak opioids, strong opioids, adjuvant drugs, *e.g.,* Neurontin® (Gabapentin). All drugs scheduled by the clock and use PRNs for breakthrough pain. DO NOT USE MEPERIDINE due to seizure potential.
ANXIETY	Try supportive therapy and/or relaxation therapy. Consider various causes such as pulmonary embolus or myocardial infarction.	Lorazepam. Buspirone. Trazodone.	**GENERAL END-OF-LIFE ISSUES**	Provide psychological support, help with social issues, and spiritual support. Limit loneliness. Increase activities within patient's limitations. Keep out of bed.	Treat depression and anxiety. Consider dronabinol for general end-of-life care (enhances food intake and sleep, decreases nausea and pain, improves general well-being). Use low doses and introduce first dose at bedtime to limit delirium.

INTERACT
Version 3.0 Tool

Change in Condition: *When to report to the MD/NP/PA*

Immediate Notification

Any symptom, sign, or apparent discomfort that is:
- **Acute** or **Sudden** in onset, <u>and</u>:
  - **A Marked change** *(i.e., more severe)* in relation to usual symptons and signs, <u>or</u>
  - **Unrelieved** by measures already prescribed

Nonimmediate Notification

- **New or worsening symptoms that do not meet above criteria**

Nursing Home to Hospital Transfer Form

INTERACT®

Version 3.0 Tool

Resident Name *(last, first, middle initial)* _____

Language: ☐ English ☐ Other _____   Resident is: ☐ SNF/rehab ☐ Long-term

Date Admitted *(most recent)* ____/____/____   DOB ____/____/____

Primary diagnosis(es) for admission _____

Sent To *(name of hospital)* _____

Date of transfer _____/_____/_____

Sent From *(name of nursing home)* _____ Unit _____

Who to Call at the Nursing Home to Get Questions Answered

Name/Title _____

Tel (_____) _____

Contact Person _____

Relationship *(check all that apply)*

☐ Relative   ☐ Health care proxy   ☐ Guardian   ☐ Other

Tel (_____)

Notified of transfer?   ☐ Yes   ☐ No

Aware of clinical situation?   ☐ Yes   ☐ No

Primary Care Clinician in Nursing Home   ☐ MD   ☐ NP   ☐ PA

Name _____

Tel (_____) _____

Code Status   ☐ Full Code   ☐ DNR   ☐ DNI   ☐ DNH   ☐ Comfort Care Only   ☐ Uncertain

---

Key Clinical Information

Reason(s) for transfer _____

Is the primary reason for transfer for diagnostic testing, not admission?   ☐ No   ☐ Yes   Tests: _____

Relevant diagnoses   ☐ CHF   ☐ COPD   ☐ CRF   ☐ DM   ☐ Ca *(active treatment)* ☐ Dementia   ☐ Other _____

Vital signs   BP _____   HR _____   RR _____   Temp _____   O2 Sat _____ Time taken *(am/pm)* _____

Most recent pain level   _____ (☐ N/A)   Pain location: _____

Most recent pain med   _____ Date given ____/____/____   Time *(am/pm)* _____

Usual Mental Status:

☐ Alert, oriented, follows instructions

☐ Alert, disoriented, but can follow simple instructions

☐ Alert, disoriented, but cannot follow simple instructions

☐ Not alert

Usual Functional Status:

☐ Ambulates independently

☐ Ambulates with assistive device

☐ Ambulates only with human assistance

☐ Not ambulatory

Additional Clinical Information:

☐ SBAR Acute Change in Condition Note included

☐ Other clinical notes included

For residents with lacerations or wounds:

Date of last tetanus vaccination *(if known)* ____/____/____

Devices and Treatments

☐ O₂ at _____ L/min   by ☐ Nasal canula ☐ Mask (☐ Chronic ☐ New)

☐ Nebulizer therapy   (☐ Chronic   ☐ New)

☐ CPAP   ☐ BiPAP   ☐ Pacemaker   ☐ IV   ☐ PICC line

☐ Bladder (Foley) catheter (☐ Chronic   ☐ New) ☐ Internal defibrillator

☐ Enteral feeding   ☐ TPN   ☐ Other _____

Isolation Precautions

☐ MRSA   ☐ VRE

Site _____

☐ C. difficile   ☐ Norovirus

☐ Respiratory virus or flu

☐ Other _____

Allergies

_____

_____

_____

_____

_____

Risk Alerts

☐ Anticoagulation   ☐ Falls   ☐ Pressure ulcer(s)   ☐ Aspiration   ☐ Seizures

☐ Harm to self or others   ☐ Restraints   ☐ Limited/non-weight bearing: (☐ Left ☐ Right)

☐ May attempt to exit   ☐ Swallowing precautions   ☐ Needs meds crushed

☐ Other _____

Personal Belongings Sent with Resident

☐ Eyeglasses   ☐ Hearing Aid

☐ Dental Appliance   ☐ Jewelry

☐ Other _____

Nursing Home Would be Able to Accept Resident Back Under the Following Conditions

☐ ER determines diagnoses, and treatment can be done in NH   ☐ VS stabilized and follow-up plan can be done in NH

☐ Other _____

Additional Transfer Information on a Second Page:

☐ Included   ☐ Will be sent later

Form Completed By *(name/title)* _____ Signature _____

Report Called in By *(name/title)* _____

Report Called in To *(name/title)* _____ Date ____/____/____ Time *(am/pm)* _____

Nursing Home to Hospital
Transfer Form *(additional information)*

INTERACT
Version 3.0 Tool

Not critical for emergency room evaluation; may be forwarded later if unable to complete at time of transfer.
RECEIVER: PLEASE ENSURE THIS INFORMATION IS DELIVERED TO THE NURSE RESPONSIBLE FOR THIS PATIENT

Resident Name *(last, first, middle initial)* _____
DOB _____ / _____ / _____   Date transferred to hospital _____ / _____ / _____

Contact at Nursing Home for Further Information
Name / Title _____
Tel (_____) _____

Social Worker
Name _____
Tel (_____) _____

Family and Other Social Issues *(include what hospital staff needs to know*
about family concerns) _____
_____
_____

Behavioral Issues and Interventions
_____
_____
_____

Primary Goals of Care at Time of Transfer
☐ Rehabilitation and/or medical therapy with intent of returning home
☐ Chronic long-term care
☐ Palliative or end-of-life care
☐ Receiving hospice care   ☐ Other _____

Treatments and Frequency *(include special treatments such as dialysis,*
chemotherapy, transfusions, radiation, TPN)
_____
_____
_____

Diet
Needs assistance with feeding?   ☐ No ☐ Yes
Trouble swallowing?   ☐ No ☐ Yes
Special consistency *(thickened liquids, crush meds, etc...)*? ☐ No ☐ Yes

Enteral tube feeding? ☐ No ☐ Yes *(formula/rate)* _____

Skin/Wound Care
Pressure ulcers *(stage, location,*
appearance, treatments)
_____
_____
_____

Immunizations
Influenza:
Date _____ / _____ / _____
Pneumococcal:
Date _____ / _____ / _____

Physical Rehabilitation Therapy
Resident is receiving therapy with goal of returning home?   ☐ No ☐ Yes
Physical therapy: ☐ No ☐ Yes
interventions _____
Occupational therapy: ☐ No ☐ Yes
interventions _____
Speech therapy: ☐ No ☐ Yes
interventions _____

ADLs Mark I = Independent D = Dependent A = Needs Assistance

Bathing _____   Dressing _____   Transfers _____

Toileting _____   Eating _____

☐ Can ambulate independently _____
☐ Assistive device *(if applicable)* _____
☐ Needs human assistance to ambulate _____

Impairments – General
☐ Cognitive   ☐ Speech   ☐ Hearing
☐ Vision   ☐ Sensation
☐ Other _____

Impairments – Musculoskeletal
☐ Amputation   ☐ Paralysis   ☐ Contractures
☐ Other _____
_____

Continence
☐ Bowel   ☐ Bladder
Date of last BM _____ / _____ / _____

Additional Relevant Information _____
_____
_____
_____

Form Completed By *(name/title)* _____
If this page sent after initial transfer: Date sent _____ / _____ / _____   Time *(am/pm)* _____

Signature _____

SUGGESTED READINGS

Alexander Gl, Rantz M, Skubic M, et al. Evolution of an early illness warning system to monitor frail elders in independent living. *J Healthc Eng.* 2011;2(2):259-286.

Ball J, Haight BK. Creating a multisensory environment for dementia: the goals of a Snoezelen room. *J Gerontol Nurs.* 2005;31:4-10.

Brownie S, Horstmanshof L. Creating the conditions for self-fulfilment for aged care residents. *Nurs Ethics.* 2012;19(6):777-786.

Givens JL, Selby K, Goldfeld KS, Mitchell SL. Hospital transfers of nursing home residents with advanced dementia. *J Am Geriatr Soc.* 2012;60:905-909.

Gruneir A, Mor V. Nursing home safety: current issues and barriers to improvement. *Annu Rev Public Health.* 2008;29:369-382.

Hamilton N, Tesh AS. The North Carolina Eden Coalition: facilitating environmental transformation. *J Gerontol Nurs.* 2002;28:35-40.

Hockley J, Dewar B, Watson J. Promoting end of life care in nursing homes using an integrated care pathway for the last days of life. *J Res Nurs.* 2005;10:132-152.

Kidd L, Cayless S, Johnston B, Wengstrom Y. Telehealth in palliative care in the UK: a review of the evidence. *J Telemed Telecare.* 2010;16:394-402.

Loganathan M, Singh S, Franklin BD, et al. Interventions to optimise prescribing in care homes: systematic review. *Age Ageing.* 2011;40:150-162.

Makowski TR, Maggard W, Morley JE. The Life Care Center of St. Louis experience with subacute care. *Clin Geriatr Med.* 2000;16:701-724.

McCormack B, McCance T, Slater P, et al. Person-centred outcomes and cultural change. In Manley K, McCormack B, Wilson V (eds). *International Practice Development in Nursing and Healthcare.* Oxford, UK: Blackwell Publishing; 2008.

Monroe T, Carter M, Parish A. A case study using the beers list criteria to compare prescribing by family practitioners and geriatric specialists in a rural nursing home. *Geriatr Nurs.* 2011;32:350-356.

Morley JE. Transitions. *J Am Med Dir Assoc.* 2010;11(9):607-611.

Morley JE. End-of-life care in the nursing home. *J Am Med Dir Assoc.* 2011;12:77-83.

Morley JE. High technology coming to a nursing home near you. *J Am Med Dir Assoc.* 2012;13:409-412.

National End of Life Care Intelligence Network. *Deaths in Older Adults in England.* http://www.endoflifecare-intelligence.org.uk. Published 2010. Accessed March 24, 2013.

Onder G, Liperoti R, Fialova D, et al; for the SHELTER Project. Polypharmacy in nursing home in Europe: results from the SHELTER study. *J Gerontol A Biol Sci Med Sci.* 2012;67(6):698-704.

Ouslander JG, Berenson RA. Reducing unnecessary hospitalizations of nursing home residents. *N Engl J Med.* 2011;365(13):1165-1168.

Ouslander JF, Lamb G, Tappen R, et al. Interventions to reduce hospitalizations from nursing homes: evaluation of the INTERACT II collaborative quality improvement project. *J Am Geriatr Soc.* 2011;59:745-753.

Rantz MJ, Skubic M, Koopman RJ, et al. Automated technology to speed recognition of signs of illness in older adults. *J Gerontol Nurs.* 2012;38:18-23.

Rubenstein LZ, Joseph T. Freeman award lecture: comprehensive geriatric assessment: from miracle to reality. *J Gerontol A Biol Sci Med Sci.* 2004;59:473-477.

Stone RI, Reinhard SC. The place of assisted living in long-term care and related service systems. *Gerontologist.* 2007;47(special issue III):23-32.

Tak SH, Benefield LE, Mahoney DF. Technology for long-term care. *Res Gerontol Nurs.* 2010;3(1):61-72.

Walsh EG, Wiener JM, Haber S, et al. Potentially avoidable hospitalizations of dually eligible Medicare and Medicaid beneficiaries from nursing facilities and home- and community-based services waiver programs. *J Am Geriatr Soc.* 2012;60:821-829.

Weiner M, Callahan CM, Tierney WM, et al. Using information technology to improve the health care of older adults. *Ann Intern Med.* 2003;139(5 Pt 2):430-436.

MULTIPLE CHOICE QUESTIONS

6.1 Which of the following is *not* a component of person-centered care?

a. Knowing the person's values
b. Understanding the resident's preferences
c. A partnership between staff and resident
d. Focusing on the medical needs of the individual
e. Understanding the person's social history

6.2 Which of the following is a component of the INTERACT II program?

a. STOP AND WATCH tool
b. Direct physician training
c. Having an advanced practice nursing in the nursing home
d. Reducing polypharmacy

6.3 Which of the following is *not* one of the five conditions that account for three quarters of potentially avoidable hospitalizations?

a. Acute renal failure
b. Pneumonia
c. Dehydration
d. Urinary tract infection
e. Congestive heart failure

6.4 Which of the following is *not* a component of the Stage 7c Functional Assessment Staging Scale that identifies 55% of demented persons who will be dead within 6 months?

a. Cannot walk
b. Cannot dress or bathe without assistance
c. Fecal incontinence
d. Urinary incontinence

6.5 Which of the following is *not* one of Kübler-Ross' five stages of dying?

a. Denial
b. Depression
c. Happiness
d. Anger
e. Acceptance

Chapter 7

MULTI-PROFESSIONAL TEAMS: WORKING TOGETHER

You can do what I cannot do.
I can do what you cannot do.
Together we can do great things.

—Mother Teresa

The benefits of effective teamwork are well established and are central to culture change. It is particularly important to understand individual contributions and the influence of nursing home teams on experiences of care, quality, and resident-centred outcomes. Knowing who does what, defining and understanding roles, effective communication, and shared decision making that reflects agreed values are prerequisites to quality resident centred experience and an enriched environment of care.

Geriatric team models combine expertise from several disciplines that strive to work collaboratively with older persons and their family caregivers. The key disciplines contributing to nursing home practice include generalist and specialist physicians, nurses, social care professionals, and physical therapists. Interestingly, certified nursing aides and unregulated care assistants make up the largest staff group in most nursing homes around the world. This chapter focuses mainly on optimizing the collaborative working of the "on-staff team" employed by the nursing home providers. This discussion is mindful of the essential contributions of in-reach specialist services and practitioners from a range of allied health and social care disciplines who will periodically be involved and may be considered a part of the wider care team. Although we touch on elements of team leadership, leadership per se is more fully examined in Chapter 8.

COLLABORATIVE CARE

The success of geriatric team models is testimony to the benefits of collaborative interprofessional practice that in combination works to improve health and social care outcomes for older people and their families. In nursing home practice, such collaborative approaches must be inclusive of managers and administrators. Regulators and inspectors might also consider that they are also part of the team, but not all practitioners would agree with this view! The complexity of older nursing home residents needs require periodic expert inputs from a range of external specialist doctors, nurses, physiotherapists, occupational therapists,

psychiatrists, psychologists, pharmacists, dieticians, speech and language therapists, dentists, audiologists, and podiatrists to name but a few of the disciplines who act on a consultancy basis. Nursing home care is thus complex and interfaces with other agencies and across sectors. The vulnerability and high dependency of many older nursing home residents means that it is imperative that within the nursing home team that there is clarity as to who is responsible for:

- Promoting resident-centered approaches, including shared decision making
- Collaboratively determining what care and treatment is provided
- Overseeing the process of specialist consultations
- Ensuring that capacity to consent and standard consent processes are lawfully and sensitively implemented
- Providing advocacy when required.

To coordinate the care of individual residents, a senior nursing home practitioner often assumes the role of case manager or key worker. For families, it is helpful to know who is in charge of the nursing home and the name and contact details of the case manager coordinating the care of their relative. The key practitioner should adopt proactive communication strategies with the resident, and with the resident's approval, the communication strategy to be used with the family. It is helpful if one family member can be identified to act as the key point of contact for staff who will know who to call to share progress news and if appropriate to act as the family spokesperson.

Collaborative working patterns vary according to the type of facility, skill mix, and the duty schedule on the shift. It is important that staff who are familiar with the older person keep the resident informed of who is involved in their day-to-day care and to explain changes and why they have arisen. Residents can understandably become resentful or anxious if they are not informed of staff changes that directly affect them and their sense of continuity and security. Ideally, the case manager will explain treatment plans, the reasons for specialist referrals, and follow-up details and when appropriate will advocate for the resident. It is preferable that someone who knows the resident should escort him or her to outpatient appointments and be on hand to assist, support, and if necessary interpret meaning.

Because it may not always be possible for a staff member to escort an individual, it may be helpful to alert family and friends to appointment times and encourage them to go with the resident. Always remember to include the accompanying person when making transport arrangements and to provide them with a contact number in case of problems.

THE CONTRIBUTIONS OF PHYSICIANS AND NURSES

Physicians and nurses in many countries make a major contribution to the healthcare of older people. In the nursing home sector, medical and nursing roles vary in accord with the different services provided by facilities, which is to a large extent regionally determined. Internationally, most medical care within nursing homes is provided through generalist primary care physicians with consultations from geriatricians and other specialists. The Netherlands is the only country in the world with a 3-year specialist training program that leads to a certification as an elderly care physician with a focus on nursing home medicine.

As Table 7–1 suggests, physicians contribute clinical leadership in a variety of ways, as medical directors, medical coordinators, attending physicians, and others on a consultancy basis. In facilities that are structured around a social model of care, the primary care physician or family doctor attends residents, when requested to do so, much as he or she would any member of the community. The influence and leadership of the physician appears to be most established within the Netherlands and within medicalized nursing homes such as in the United States. In France, to keep primary care physicians (PCPs) involved with their own patients, nursing homes have physician coordinators. These physicians must have specific training in geriatrics and are responsible for the "gerontologic politics" of the nursing homes, including geriatric assessment, prevention practices, and prevention of infections. They do not have to prescribe any medications if the resident has his or her own PCP. The interest of the physician coordinator is for the care coordination. Their major limitation is the ability to develop a respect of the PCP and a good working relationship.

As discussed in Chapter 4, evidence suggests that the presence of physicians in a nursing home raises standards. In terms of nursing, there are a range of roles extending from advanced nurse practitioners (North America) who work collaboratively with physicians, nurse directors, and registered nurses who administer direct care and oversee the wider nursing team of certified nursing aides (United States) and unregulated healthcare assistants. Chapter 10 takes a close and critical look at the educational preparation of practitioners within the nursing home team.

THE NURSING CONTRIBUTION

Chapter 3 describes professional nursing as an activity encompassing curative and rehabilitative dimensions and long-term condition management through to palliative and end-of-life care. Nurses who become expert in working with older people draw on knowledge derived from medical and nursing sciences in addition to their knowledge of the older person and his or her family and life circumstances. The exact contribution that nurses make to residents' care will depend on a number of factors, not least the scope of practice set out by their registering authority and on the acquisition of postqualifying gerontologic knowledge and practice know-how. The legitimacy of nursing older people as a specialist area of nursing practice has long been debated, and nursing home careers have historically been afforded low status. The Nursing and Midwifery Council of the United Kingdom now recognizes that nursing older people is a specialty that requires highly skilled nurses who can respond to the complexity of health and social care needs of older people (Nursing and Midwifery Council, 2009, p. 6). Few countries mandate postregistration qualifications for nurses who work with older people. In Ireland, for example, where gerontologic nurses are required to complete a postregistration qualification in gerontologic nursing, this has been difficult to implement. Descriptions of the gerontologic nursing role from American and European discipline alliances highlight that it is essential that nursing home nurses can differentiate normal ageing from illness and disease processes and assess for syndromes and constellations of symptoms that may be manifestations of other underlying health problems in addition to administering technically competent care with dignity and compassion. Specific nursing interventions are explored in Parts 3 and 4, where we describe multi-professional management of age-related conditions and syndromes and diseases.

Many countries report nursing workforce shortages, including poor recruitment and retention within nursing homes. The ratio of registered professional nurses to nursing assistants is often low, and in these situations, the functional role of registered nurses is to assess nursing need, plan care, and supervise the wider nursing team.

Nurses who practice within nursing homes need knowledge derived from clinical subjects and social sciences, including the arts and humanities, so they can understand both what to do in a technical clinical sense and to convey their caring in ways that are safe and compassionate.

With the rapid development of nursing homes throughout the developing world and a shortage of physicians trained in nursing home care, there is clearly an increasing role for nurses working at an advanced level of practice. Although the role of advanced nurse practitioners is a relatively new and emerging role, accounts of their contributions to improving the quality of care within North American nursing homes is overwhelmingly positive.

WORKING IN PARTNERSHIP WITH OLDER PEOPLE

The spirit of resident- (person-) centered care should pervade all team practices within nursing homes. In such approaches, relational aspects of care and reciprocity within caring relationships need to be recognized. Working in partnership is about working with the recipient of care

Table 7–1.   KEY CONTRIBUTIONS AND ROLE FUNCTIONS MADE BY PHYSICIANS AND NURSES WORKING WITH NURSING HOME RESIDENTS

Discipline	Role within Medical Model Nursing Homes	Role within Nursing Model Nursing Homes	Role within Social Model Nursing Homes
Physician			
Geriatrician[a] / Internist[a] / Family practitioner[a] (general practitioner) / Other specialists	Medical director or physician coordinator (France) (administration) / Attending physician or consultant can be full-time attending skilled nursing facility-ist (SNF-ist) or as in Holland where family practitioners work fulltime in NH or part time	Consulting	No formal role
Geriatric (old age) psychiatry	Consulting	Consulting	No formal role
Nurse			
Advanced practice nurse (or nurse practitioner) or physician assistant	Collaborative practice with physician	Can have a primary care role if legislation permits	No formal role
Nurse consultant	Specialist in education or specific areas (e.g., incontinence, wound care, infection control, research leader)	Strategic / Leadership / Advanced practice / Practice development / Research and education	Strategic / Leadership / Advanced practice / Practice development / Research and education
Registered nurse (RN)	Nursing assessments, care planning and interventions within an agreed scope of practice, and supervision of nursing aides. May include aspects of case management	Nursing assessments, care planning and interventions within an agreed scope of practice, and supervision of nursing aides. Referrals to primary care team including physician when appropriate	There is usually no formal nursing, but in some homes, the manager may have a nursing qualification
Community nurse			Nursing assessments and interventions within an agreed scope of practice, including nurse prescribing
Licensed practical nurse (LPN)	Does many roles of RN under RN supervision		
Certified nurse's aide (CNA)	Provides day-to-day care for ADLs	Provides ADL care	Provides ADL care
Certified medical technician	Can dispense medicines		

ADL, activity of daily living.

[a]Can be AMDA certified as a medical director in the United States.

and working with his or her family and the wider health and social care teams. Nursing home staff frequently deal with complex situations in which they must negotiate and integrate clinical and social aspects of care while being mindful of individual residents' preferences and choices. All aspects of staff behavior, including teamwork, contributes to the environment of care that in turn influences the experience of care. Research from the United Kingdom has identified that an enriched environment of care contributes to staff well-being; job satisfaction; improved teamwork; and, most importantly, enhanced resident quality of life. An enriched care environment requires six senses to be experienced by residents, family, staff, and students: a sense of security, belonging, continuity, purpose, achievement, and significance.

For staff to work effectively, individuals and teams need to feel confident that they can make decisions and, if necessary, complain without fear of reprisal (sense of security). They need to experience a sense of belonging and being a valued team member. Continuity is important but difficult to achieve when facilities rely on agency staff or experience high staff turnover. To experience a sense of purpose, staff need to set appropriate goals, and a sense of achievement requires feedback from residents or colleagues about a job well done and signals that their efforts are valued and recognized. Significance is experienced through being valued within the nursing home itself but it is also about being valued by society and their own professional communities.

Becoming more resident focused is central to the culture change movement; it involves becoming more responsive to individual preferences and less preoccupied with routines. To do this requires strong relationships between staff and residents and new ways of team working. Creating effective teams is an imprecise science that requires buy-in from all of those involved. Good teamwork nurtures positive attitudes among staff and positivity reinforces the team spirit. For culture change to succeed, strategies are required to build and sustain teamwork.

SELF-MANAGED TEAMS

Interest in participatory management approaches has created opportunities for the emergence of self-managed staff teams within nursing homes rather than reliance on top-down, more directive management. The arguments for such an approach are compelling; self-managed teams have been shown to encourage self-expression, respect, and independence, which in turn lead to increased morale, satisfaction, and commitment and reduced staff turnover and absenteeism. The enhanced flow and use of information that is a feature of self-managed team approaches allows staff to fully participate in decision making, which is known to improve performance. Thus, it makes sense to nurture teamwork within nursing homes, particularly when it empowers staff groups such as nursing aides, who have a wealth of practice experience to share. Teamwork is not as intuitive or simple as it might appear, and the nursing home management team needs to be proactive in supporting team formation, provide timely feedback on progress, and demonstrate a commitment to teams as they evolve and develop their skills and contributions. Teams can grow

substantially by being allowed to make mistakes, recognize them, and build on this through problem solving.

UNDERSTANDING TEAMS

The hub of a successfully functioning nursing home is high-function interprofessional teams. Teams are not committees but rather small (2 to 5) or medium (6 to 12) groups that focus on solving a particular problem or set of problems. Larger teams can be successful when they are informational or educational, such as communities of practice (see Chapter 10). Multiple teams form the basis for making the nursing home function. Examples of teams in nursing homes could be a falls team, a pressure ulcer group, an incontinence team, or a rapid cycle team put together to solve a single problem. Within the nursing home, the customers (residents and family members) should be included as part of the team. Well-constituted teams include members from all levels of nursing home staff and need to include certified nurse aides and housekeepers if they are going to see the complete picture.

Teams should develop a mission statement to more clearly define their task; however, mission statements do not define a team. Team behavior is defined by the behavior of all the members all the time. Functional teams require integrity and, to perform at the highest level, "a soul." Examples of team roles can either be hard end products (e.g., decrease hospitalizations) or soft products (e.g., resident or family happiness, which are subjective). Tasks can be simple such as monitoring pain scores or improving medication to deliver to complex such as reducing polypharmacy or identifying and correcting the causes of falls. Within a nursing home, a set of overarching team goals can be defined (Table 7–2). In the modern era, "virtual teams" that do not meet in person but use computer or smartphone communication are becoming very successful and are particularly useful when the team needs input from staff working different shifts or if the teams are working in different institutions and working to standardize outcomes.

Teamwork is about *us* instead of *me*. As the American College basketball coach Bud Wilkinson said, "If a team is to reach its potential, each player must be willing to subordinate his goals to the good of the team."

Within a team, one member needs to be a leader to keep the team on task while a facilitator sees that all members of the team are heard and work as a team. One member needs

Table 7–2. TEAM GOALS IN A NURSING HOME
• Improve resident function.
• Maintain maximum resident independence.
• Enhance resident well-being.
• Increase resident and family satisfaction.
• Reduce unnecessary transitions to hospitals.
• Reduce healthcare costs.
• Increase satisfaction of employees.
• Reduce turnover of nursing staff at all levels.

Table 7–3.   PROBLEMATIC TEAM MEMBERS
• Talk consistently without listening
• Always annoyed or negative
• Want to take credit but not do their share
• Loners
• Excessively slow
• The skunk: smells like a problem, but the reason is not readily apparent.

Table 7–5.   ROLES OF A GOOD TEAM MEMBER
• Have a set of skills that is useful to the team.
• Believe that you can make a difference.
• Recognize your role in helping the team reach its goals.
• Trust the person leading the team.
• Be motivated to help the team.
• Be friendly with other team members; avoid making enemies.
• Listen to feedback from other team members and give feedback in a nonjudgmental way.

to be tasked with recording the team's decisions. Content experts can come from different disciplines, and the team then melds their content into a cohesive whole. Team members can and should be encouraged to play different roles such as exploring possibilities, providing innovating concepts, sculpting ideas into a plan, looking after the team's mission (a curator), and coaching and conducting the team's efforts. There are a number of potentially problematic team members who need coaching to retreat from their positions to allow a team to function (Table 7–3). It should be remembered that good teams are as good as their weakest member. Bad attitudes are the result of selfishness and guarantee a team's failure.

In teams, team members need to recognize the skills of each team member. Each team member may make a list of his or her skills, and they can be shared publically with the team. Teams should do some cross-training so there is a backup for each task. Highly functional teams are better than the sum of the whole. Functional teams share success and blame, laugh together, and play together.

Communication is the key to a team being successful. Listening is the golden rule of communication. Teams need to acknowledge and explain their perceptions. Differences and similarities in the team's viewpoints need to be clearly expressed. Finally, agreement needs to be negotiated to allow the team to find the appropriate solutions to problems. Successful teams are very rewarding to work in, but it is important that team members complement one another and that administrators complement the team and its members regularly. As Mark Twain said, "I can live for two months on one good complement."

There are four stages to the birth of a team (Table 7–4). The behaviors of a successful team member are outlined in Table 7–5. For teams to succeed and survive, change is mandatory. There is magic in a successful team, and there is no blueprint that says any one team should look like another. The leader of the team needs to watch for the five basic elements of a team's becoming dysfunctional. These are the failure of the team to trust one another, failing for members to engage in friendly conflict, team members lacking commitment to the mission of the team, failing to be results oriented, and not taking chances and recognizing that the team is accountable for its successes or failures. In the end, successful teams look to the future, do not get upset by short-term failures, and use not only all their own brains but also any brains they can borrow.

SKILL MIX

Another important dimension of multi-professional teamwork is skill mix, which perhaps might be more accurately described as "grade mix." In the earlier discussion of the different role functions, we highlighted the overlap between the work of some physicians and expert nurses within nursing homes. In regions that operate medicalized nursing homes, for example, role substitution (nurses with advanced practice skills selectively substituting for physicians) is an important consideration with an unrealized scope for development. There is still much to learn about the impact of skill mix within the nursing team and the nurse–doctor balance, registered practitioner, and less qualified staff balance and the opportunity cost of this within the different service delivery models. Skill mix formula and staffing needs differ between day and night shifts, and this has important quality, safety, and cost implications. The evidence base informing minimum staffing requirements is, to say the least, unclear. Research on nursing home skill mix is difficult to interpret because studies tend to be small scale and do not fully map the issues and relationships among care quality, teamwork, and skill mix. What we can say with confidence is that most studies conflate practice competence and skill with grade, and assumptions are made that grade is indicative of a practitioner who is an effective team worker. Most published projects that have evaluated skill mix in nursing homes focus on cost and quality implications of initiatives that are often organizational responses to staffing shortages and retention challenges. These studies make an interesting read but should be interpreted with caution because of methodologic and

Table 7–4.   CHARACTERISTIC STAGES OF THE FORMATION OF A TEAM
Forming: Getting to know one another
Storming: Discussing and agreeing on the mission and the roles of the team members
Norming: Defining the expectations of the team's outcomes and of the individual members
Performing: Working together to enhance the quality of life of the residents in the nursing home

conceptual limitations, noting that findings may be organizationally specific and may not be transferable to different contexts. Determining appropriate skill mix, defining and advancing roles within the nursing home workforce presents a major challenge and is part of the International Association of Gerontology and Geriatrics improvement imperative.

KEY POINTS

1. Effective teamwork is key to a positive care environment and enriched culture of care.
2. Geriatric team models are testimony to the benefits of collaborative interprofessional practice, and in a nursing home, the team should include administrators and managers.
3. Physicians and nurses with expertise in the care of older adults make a major contribution to nursing home teams and nursing home leadership.
4. Collaborative multiprofessional teams are essential to the provision of high-quality nursing home care.
5. Partnership working means that staff has to work collaboratively with internal and external colleagues from a range of disciplines and most importantly in partnership with residents and their family caregivers.
6. Teamwork is about *us* instead of *me*.
7. Teamwork is best when there are explicit goals to be met through collaborative actions and learning between colleagues who trust each other and respect each other's contributions.
8. There is a lack of strong evidence to inform skill mix decisions within nursing homes.

SUGGESTED READINGS

American Association of Colleges of Nursing. *Nurse Practitioner and Clinical Nurse Specialist Competencies for Older Adult Care.* Hartford Geriatric Nursing Initiative. http://www.aacn.nche.edu/Education/dpf/APNCompetenceis.pdf. Published 2004. Accessed May 23, 2012.

Buchan J, Dal Poz MR. Skill mix in the health care workforce: reviewing the evidence. *Bull World Health Organ.* 2002;80(7):575-580.

Koopmans RT, Lavrijsen JC, Hoek JF, et al. Dutch elderly care physician: a new generation of nursing home physician specialists. *J Am Geriatr Soc.* 2010;58(9):1807-1809.

Kratz P. An international perspective on long term care: focus on nursing homes. *J Am Med Dir Assoc.* 2011;12:487-492.

Milisen K, De Geest DE, Schuurmans M, et al. Meeting the challenges for gerontological nursing in Europe: the European Nursing Academy for Care of Older Persons (ENACO). *J Nutr Health Aging.* 2004;8:197-199.

Nolan M, Allan S, McGeever P, et al. The aims and goals of care: a framework promoting partnerships between older people, family carers and nurses. In Reed J, Clarke C, MacFarlane A (eds). *Nursing Older Adults.* UK: Open University Press; 2011.

Philpot C, Tolson D, Morley JE. Advanced practice nurses and attending physicians: a collaboration to improve quality of care in the nursing home. *J Am Med Dir Assoc.* 2011;12(3):161-165.

Tolson D, Booth J, Schofield I. Principles of gerontological nursing. In Tolson D, Booth J, Schofield I (eds). *Evidence Informed Nursing with Older People.* Oxford, UK: Wiley Blackwell; 2011.

Tyler DA, Parker VA. Nursing home culture, teamwork and culture change. *J Res Nurs.* 2011;16(1):37-49.

Yeatts DE, Cready C, Ray B, et al. Self-managed work teams in nursing homes: implementing and empowering nurse aide teams. *Gerontologist.* 2004;44(2):256-261.

MULTIPLE CHOICE QUESTIONS

7.1 Which of the following determinants underpins effective teamwork?

   a. A dedicated development budget
   b. Clarity about staff roles within the team
   c. An authoritarian leader
   d. An explicit and shared value base

7.2 The largest staff group within nursing homes are registered nurses; is this true or false?

   a. True
   b. False

7.3 Which of the following is the role of the medical director in the United States?

   a. Meets regularly with director of nursing and administrator
   b. Attends quality improvement meeting
   c. Monitors the performance of other physicians in the facility
   d. All of the above

7.4 Which of the following defines a rapid cycle?

   a. A regular quarterly meeting
   b. Data collection
   c. A very large team
   d. Teams without physicians
   e. A team that comes together to solve a specific problem over a short period of time

7.5 Which of the problems is a problematic team member?

   a. Content experts
   b. Loner
   c. Recorder
   d. Facilitator
   e. Leader

Chapter 8

NURSING HOME LEADERSHIP

There are three key dimensions to an exploration of nursing home leadership. To begin, it is important to consider the basic elements of leadership and followership. Leaders and followers come in many shapes and sizes; all disciplines involved in nursing home care are potential leaders and also followers; and all need to understand the practicalities of leading teams, leading staff through change, and driving quality improvement. Equally, as followers, all staff need to be aware how their behavior either facilitates or undermines what the project lead or overall nursing home leader is trying to achieve. At times it will be appropriate for the senior administrator or senior practitioner to lead; other times it will be more helpful if a leader is identified from a particular staff group or specific discipline. Sometimes a distributed leadership model with shared responsibilities across a group may be more appropriate. What will work in one nursing home may not work in another, and a skillful leader will select from a repertoire of approaches depending on the culture and leadership capacities and capabilities of the team mindful of the task in hand. Just as there is diversity in nursing home delivery models (see Chapter 6), there is diversity in the leadership roles and models found within nursing homes, each creating its own leadership dynamic and influences.

The terms *management* and *leadership* are often used interchangeably, and both words evoke multiple meanings. Many staff members are critical of their bosses and complain about the absence of good leadership in practice. A simple explanation for this is that some managers do not demonstrate great leadership because they do not think enough about the situation that they and their people are in; instead they rush in and get things wrong or fail to act when people are looking for leadership because they fear the consequences of failing to respond quickly enough. In defense of nursing home leaders and managers, leading people is not easy; people are complex and have different needs, motives, abilities, and expectations. Human flexibility and adaptability are great strengths, but staff members can also be unpredictable and changeable; their moods may alter, reflecting whether they are happy, sad, enthusiastic, angry, or depressed. People's emotional states affect their approach to work and their performance at work and at work emotional influences arising from their interactions with colleagues, residents, and visitors to the nursing home have a cumulative impact on behaviors. In other words, positive and negative experiences both in the workplace and beyond work influence individuals, and in turn individuals

influence the team. A major determinant of successful leadership is followership, and people follow leaders who they respect and who display emotional intelligence and value them as individuals and important contributors to the nursing home team and collective practice know-how.

Good nursing home leaders are often good managers, and many managers exhibit leadership qualities. In the highly regulated environment of the nursing home sector, where compliance agendas are mandated, it is understandable that sometimes management approaches overshadow leadership. There are, however, important differences and outcomes between the leaders and managers who master the context and those who surrender to the system and get by. Of course, there is a need for some bureaucracy and governance processes, but to thrive and excel in their work, nursing home practitioners also need to feel inspired and have permission to innovate.

At the risk of oversimplification, we suggest that nursing home leaders create and drive change, leading to reform, and managers manage the present, creating stability through rationality and control. Nursing homes require both management and leadership to deliver safe care and to respond to new evidence and embrace the demands of culture change.

> *Management without leadership is sterile; leadership without management is disconnected and unsustainable.*

The conscious task of the nursing home manager is to manage the environment of care; the unconscious task is to manage the emotions and expectations of the staff group. Theorists argue that unless the unconscious tasks are managed, conflict and destructive behaviors will result.

A recent review of the literature identified five leadership impacts demonstrated within long-term care facilities (Table 8–1).

Nursing home leadership is a contentious topic rich with stories of failures in care quality, insolvent businesses, and major struggles to retain and grow high-caliber personnel. As acknowledged by International Association of Gerontology and Geriatrics (IAGG), some of the difficulties arise because of poorly developed leadership career pathways and low reward compared with other sectors. This is compounded by the challenge of the required fusion between clinical and practice leadership skills with business acumen and administrative leadership requirements.

Table 8–1.   LEADERSHIP IMPACTS

1. Staff job satisfaction and retention
2. Successful change and positive workplace culture
3. Staff productivity and unit performance
4. Care quality and resident outcomes
5. Associated costs

LEADERSHIP APPROACHES

There are several recognized leadership styles, which include the controlling figure of authority, the therapist leader with high emotional awareness, and the visionary messiah. Each of these leadership discourses has strengths and weaknesses, and in their own ways, the different leadership personalities exert power and influence over subordinates. Different situations within nursing home practice require different leadership responses. For example, emancipatory approaches can be helpful in working through value reconciliation phases of culture change but would be completely inappropriate in a medical emergency in which decisive clinical action is required.

Nursing home leaders traditionally fit within the paradigm of transactional leadership, where following rules and maintaining the status quo are motivating factors. This problem is compounded by a highly regulatory environment coupled with multiple changes resulting from government regulations year after year. Many NH leaders focus on regulatory compliance and command and control approaches to management, which are counter to the desired culture change approach fostering communication, relationships, and teamwork, as explained in preceding chapters. Staff members want to be led by a leader who inspires them to do the best they can. Inappropriate leadership can reduce staff motivation and organizational loyalty, leading to poor standards of care.

A major part of a leader's role is to get the best from the nursing home staff, and this involves deciding how best to lead individuals and teams today, tomorrow, and in the longer term.

Leadership has been traditionally defined in terms of actions intended to influence the behaviors of staff toward effective ways of working. Contemporary views on leadership approaches emphasize the benefits of relationship-oriented approaches with approachable leaders who have the skills and aptitude to foster self-managing staff teams (see Chapter 7). Interestingly, several studies have demonstrated better resident outcomes from transformational leadership approaches than from top-down leadership approaches with their emphasis on traditional clinical process and hierarchical command structures. Such studies suggest that nursing management practices characterized by communication openness, participation in decision making, relational leadership, and formalization are associated with a range of improved resident outcomes, including reduction in restraint use, promotion of physical activity, and falls prevention.

There is widespread acceptance that effective leadership includes:

- Looking to the future, planning ahead, and anticipating future demands
- Communicating a powerful vision, which provides a sense of direction, inspiring and uniting people with a shared sense of commitment
- Adapting leadership styles to suit particular circumstances, and developing a high performing senior management team
- Driving change and managing communication effectively during periods of change.

Figure 8–1 shows the key leadership domains involved in improving practice within nursing homes.

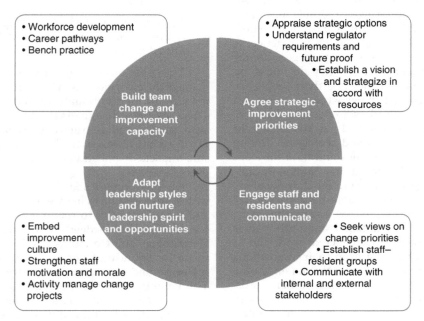

- Workforce development
- Career pathways
- Bench practice

Build team change and improvement capacity

- Appraise strategic options
- Understand regulator requirements and future proof
- Establish a vision and strategize in accord with resources

Agree strategic improvement priorities

Adapt leadership styles and nurture leadership spirit and opportunities

- Embed improvement culture
- Strengthen staff motivation and morale
- Activity manage change projects

Engage staff and residents and communicate

- Seek views on change priorities
- Establish staff–resident groups
- Communicate with internal and external stakeholders

Figure 8–1. Key leadership domains involved in improving practice within nursing homes.

DEMOCRATIC LEADERSHIP AND PARTICIPATIVE STYLES

The human relations movement advocates the merits of democratic and participative leadership styles. In this approach, democratic leadership involves shared decision making, giving employees responsibility and a degree of autonomy in the workplace. Much is written about transformational leadership in healthcare in relation to culture change and practice development approaches. Leaders and democracy are always in tension in clinical and quasi clinical environments, and some would argue that behavior, not position, matters. Others favor clear hierarchy control and order. There are also discipline-specific views of leadership, and tensions can arise between transformational aspirations within nursing home leadership and traditional views as to medical superiority over nursing and social care. Group dynamics can be complex, and sometimes in nursing homes, an informal leader unconsciously elected by staff groups may become a powerful opinion leader with greater influence on colleagues than the official leader. Follower resistance can take many forms from the subtle ways staff can undermine change to groups taking a stance to object to a change in the nursing home. In short, the power of the nursing home leader is a consequence of the actions of the followers rather than the cause of it. All members of the nursing home team have the potential to influence leadership. Those tasked with formal leadership responsibilities face many challenges, and their effectiveness can be enhanced through participation in leadership networks.

Mindful that all staff members have leadership contributions to make within nursing homes, there are four key questions that should be asked when decisions about working practices and change need making (Table 8–2).

Much can be learned about leadership and power influences in nursing homes by observing formal staff meetings. Voices that are easy to overlook are those of the resident and family, yet in discussions about care standards, for example, these are voices that need to be heard. Strategies that are helping in promoting user involvement include resident-led committees. For example, in France, many nursing homes have a "social life committee" in which a representative from a resident's family is elected to represent them and is in charge of bringing their point of view to managers and the leader. In the United Kingdom, most care homes have similar groups and encourage all stakeholders to contribute their views through written postings and participation in consultation events.

Table 8–2. IMPORTANT LEADERSHIP QUESTIONS
1. Who is sitting at the leadership table?
2. Whose voices are being heard, and whose voices are not being heard? Why?
3. Whose values are being represented and on whose behalf?
4. Who is absent from the decision-making process, and what would be gained from their involvement?

Table 8–3. ATTRIBUTES OF POOR MEETING LEADERSHIP
• The meeting started late because of people waiting for someone to arrive.
• There were too many or few people around the table.
• Key stakeholders such as residents or key staff groups were excluded.
• Attendees were not briefed in advance.
• The conversation drifted off the subject.
• Subjects or issues were discussed, but no decisions were made.
• Decisions were made, but it was not clear who would take action.
• Deadlines were not set for actions to be taken.
• People were unsure of the finish time and began to leave before meeting closure.
• There was no written record of what was discussed or agreed or the actions to be taken.
• Some attendees did not think they had an opportunity to contribute.

CHAIRING MEETINGS

Staff meetings take many forms and address a variety of topics. The person who instigates the meeting is responsible for planning, setting the agenda, inviting attendees, and briefing attendees as to what to expect. Meeting leadership may seem commonsense, but it is not always easy to hold a productive meeting in a nursing home. The lack of formal education on leading meetings is an important deficit in this regard. Table 8–3 summarizes features of a poorly led meeting at which participants may consider to have wasted their time.

INSPIRING COLLEAGUES

An important leadership charge is to inspire staff and encourage them to deliver the best care to residents. The leadership style needed within different situations in a nursing home requires a balance between doing the right thing for the resident, resolving tensions among different views as to what the right thing is, and developing the skills of the staff team without demotivating individual members. It is widely accepted now that the most successful leaders are those that inspire their followers to perform well rather than terrify or coerce them into doing something they do not understand.

Hence, the nursing home leader, irrespective of his or her discipline, has a responsibility for promoting mutual respect among staff groups and ensuring that all understand the importance of their own specific contributions to the experience of nursing home life. Leaders inspire others using a variety of strategies, including role modeling. Leaders should be positive and enthusiastic about new ideas and talk in ways that demonstrate respect and valuing of staff and their many contributions. Whereas a leader's enthusiasm rubs off on the team, a leader's disregard or disapproval undermines individual confidence and commitment and dispirits the team. The interpersonal skills of the leader are a major determinant of the staff response to that leader, more so than the leader's clinical knowledge and status. If a nursing home leader wishes to improve the staff's behavior or performance and sustain that improvement, the leader needs to be skilled in engaging the staff and opinion leaders within the staff group to gain their commitment to the workplace or practice change; when staff reluctantly comply, performance eventually deteriorates. Both staff and leaders need to be confident in each other's knowledge and behavior. Without this mutual respect, improvement will not be sustained, and staff turnover is likely to be high.

PREPARING FOR CHANGE

To achieve high standards within nursing homes and to keep pace with developments in evidence-based practice, nursing home leaders need to be skillful at change management. Perhaps the most important questions that any leader can ask are how to engage the staff and empower them to rise to the challenge of delivering better care. There are a number of well-established change theories to draw upon in planning change. For our purposes, let it suffice to say that there are some simple principles of change to consider no matter how small or large the project in terms of planning and empowering nursing home practitioners.

First, a safe space needs to be created for staff to voice concerns about "change pain" and to prepare to let go of entrenched ways of working or old practice ideals. Many change projects fail because this simple step is overlooked. Yesterday's practice has to be set aside for newer ways. Empowering staff means involving them in all stages of the change journey and giving them voice, listening to their ideas and concerns and acting on them, or at least providing feedback and information to explain why suggestions cannot be implemented. Honest communication is essential.

Staff members have to recognize the benefits for residents of the new approach and believe it is achievable where they work and not simply aspirational. This may require some educational support and opportunities to see for themselves how best practice can be delivered. There are a range of innovative ways to help nursing home practitioners prepare for change, including real-time or virtual visits to demonstrate "best practice" nursing homes, adopting bespoke learning materials, inviting speakers to talk to staff, and so on. A range of multimedia resources, online approaches, and group-based methods are also available. For example, Chapter 10 explores a learning framework to augment change leadership through communities of practice.

Regardless of the approach, it is important that staff members have opportunities to rehearse their own solutions to change programs rather than imposed top-down approaches. By developing their own understandings and problem solving, staff will feel a sense of ownership of the change. Arguably, one of the keys to embedding culture change is that nursing home practitioners believe they are asked what they think and not simply told what they should do. Table 8–4 presents 10 activities and key challenges to leading collaborative change within nursing homes.

A central feature of nursing home leadership and management is the pursuit of excellence in the standards

Table 8–4.	COLLABORATIVE APPROACH TO CHANGE PROJECTS	
	Activity	**Key Challenge**
1	Create an environment that facilitates staff buy-in.	Achieving buy-in of staff opinion leaders
2	Share the change vision.	Creating a sense of vision ownership across all staff groups and disciplines
3	Provide opportunities for staff to voice their concerns and prepare to let go of current ways of working.	Influencing the opinion leaders and moving forward
4	Create shared understanding of the rationale for the change in terms of resident benefits or other relevant outcomes	Reaching consensus on the benefits of change
5	Identify barriers to reaching the desired goal.	Finding ways to overcome the barriers
6	Nurture the belief that the desired change is achievable in the current workplace.	Staff lack confidence or are resistant to change
7	Develop the capacity and capabilities of the staff to deliver the change project; this may require technical skills and competency development.	Resourcing staff development
8	Create a sense of urgency to achieve the change within a realistic time plan.	Perceived change capacity and work load implications
9	Involve teams in the development, implementation, and evaluation of action plans.	Sustaining effort and providing feeding in a way that encourages perseverance
10	Review and reward success.	Involving residents and other stakeholders in progress reviews and responding to criticism

of care provision and user experiences of care. The quest for continual betterment of nursing home practice is at the heart of the IAGG's improvement agenda. To achieve this, leaders and operational managers need to understand and be skilled in driving quality improvement.

QUALITY IMPROVEMENT

Continuous Quality Improvement

The concept of collecting outcome data to establish the effectiveness of a healthcare intervention began with

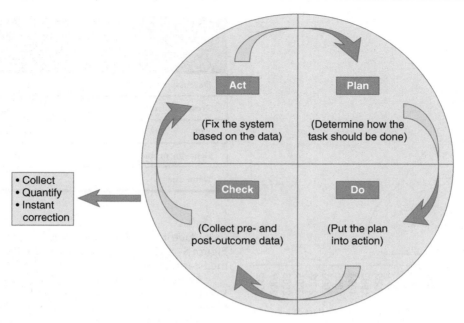

Figure 8–2. The Deming cycle.

Florence Nightingale during the Crimean War. She collected data on her outcomes in the barracks hospital, which she presented to the generals as Nightingrams. This was the beginning of the concept that data should drive recommendations.

In Japan in the 1950s, Dr. W. Edwards Deming introduced his approach to improving quality, which he believed would lower the costs of work. He pointed out that quality depended on the individual, and thus through transformation and empowerment of the individual with knowledge and the ability to fix the system, the quality of the system will improve. Pride in workmanship at the individual level is a key to success. Although Deming recognized that the most important things are not measurable and that "you can expect what you check," he also believed that workers should measure their quality output and be able to react to produce improvement. This resulted in what has become known as the Deming cycle. The components of the cycle are plan, do, check, and act (PDCA) (Figure 8–2). In essence, one plans how to do the work (e.g., decrease agitation in residents with dementia or decrease falls); then the plan is carried out by the individuals who helped plan, thus establishing their pride in ownership; then the change in behavior or in falls is measured, and problems are identified; finally, the revision of the plan is acted on. Deming recognized that most simple tasks such as those carried out by nursing aides are at continuous risk to deteriorate, so the cycle must be continuous. Deming believed we lived in a world of mistakes, so to improve outcomes, we need to adopt a new philosophy in which management cedes a substantial proportion of their control to workers and created true team work. In France, workers are usually asked to come to different workshops related to quality to get them involved in the process. Moreover, they decide whether or not an indicator is relevant. Then they are more receptive during the resulting presentation even

if the result is bad or negative. However, the whole process is as new in nursing homes as the obligation regarding quality (external certification) is for 2015 in France. It is also crucial to create a bridge between the medical sector and the nursing sector to bring the expertise of the medical sector to the nursing home. Many groups use this way to achieve not only a resident flow but also to ensure quality improvement and prepare the nursing home sector for the big challenge to come.

The Deming approach revolutionized the old-fashioned quality assurance approach to one of total quality management (Table 8–5).

Table 8–5.	COMPARISON BETWEEN TOTAL QUALITY MANAGEMENT AND QUALITY ASSURANCE	
	Total Quality Management	**Quality Assurance**
Data collection	Workers	Specialized staff
Data reviewed	Real time	Retrospective
Statistical methods	Sophisticated	Minimal
Graphics	High level	None
Feedback	Rapid to all staff	Irregular, limited
Employee training	At work	Classroom
Employee involvement	High with ability to make changes	Minimal
Employee motivation	Have control over system	"Carrot and stick"

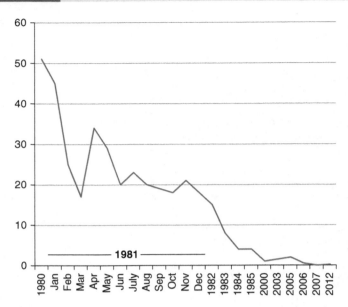

Figure 8–3. Quality control chart demonstrating the effect of a quality improvement program on reducing physical restraints in a U.S. nursing home. By comparison, in 2012, the U.S. national average was 2.3%, and in 2003, it was 8.5%.

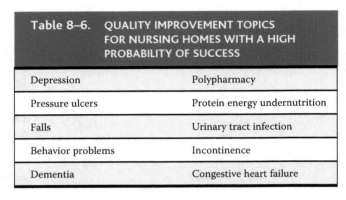

Table 8–6.	QUALITY IMPROVEMENT TOPICS FOR NURSING HOMES WITH A HIGH PROBABILITY OF SUCCESS
Depression	Polypharmacy
Pressure ulcers	Protein energy undernutrition
Falls	Urinary tract infection
Behavior problems	Incontinence
Dementia	Congestive heart failure

To allow visualization of the outcomes of a process, Juran developed quality control charts (Figure 8–3). These allow workers to easily visualize improvement while at the same time providing statistically accepted upper and lower limits of acceptable care levels.

Pareto points out that although there are often many reasons why something goes wrong, usually two or three of these factors will be responsible for the majority of cases. Figure 8–4 gives examples of Pareto diagrams for falls and medication errors.

An expert panel at St. Louis University and the Veterans Administration developed a list of the 10 areas in the nursing home most likely to be responsive to continuous quality improvement techniques (Table 8–6).

THE ROLE OF THE ADMINISTRATOR (CARE MANAGER)

The nursing home administrator is the key person in the nursing home. She or he has to balance the needs of multiple different groups while ensuring that the facility provides the best quality care for residents and maintains profitability for the company (Table 8–7). A nursing home administrator is a licensed health professional who acts as

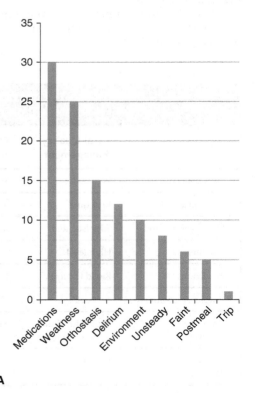

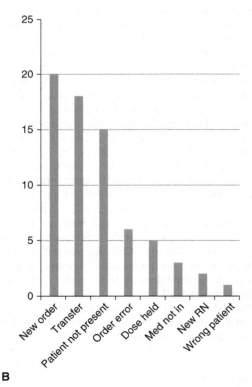

A   B

Figure 8–4. Examples of Pareto diagrams for falls (**A**) and medication errors (**B**).

Table 8–7.	FORCES TO WHICH THE ADMINISTRATOR NEEDS TO BE RESPONSIVE

- Residents
- Families
- Staff
- Company
- Regulators and surveyors

Table 8–8.	DUTIES OF A NURSING HOME ADMINISTRATOR

- Maintain fiscal responsibility for their employers and employees.
- Supervise hiring, training, and firing of staff and contractors.
- Develop policies and operating procedures in accordance with government regulations.
- Direct quality assurance programs.
- Supervise the development of new programs to enhance quality of life of residents.
- Compile, analyze, and prepare reports.
- Interact with residents and families.
- Attend staff and corporate meetings.
- Interact with third-party payers and regulators.
- Provide advertising and public relations for the facility.
- Ascertain that the facility provides high-quality healthcare while maintaining a home-like environment.
- Handle legal suits brought against the facility.
- Provide resident care or services dependent on his or her background training.

the chief executive officer of a nursing home. He or she plans, organizes, directs, and controls the nursing home functions. In the United States, most administrators have a bachelor's degree and have passed state and federal board examinations. Many have undergone an administrator-in-training internship as well.

Administrators require high leadership skills. They are responsible for managing the managers of the different departments (nursing, social services, food service, medical services, recreational activity programs, medical records program, pharmaceutical program, rehabilitation program, housekeeping, and building maintenance) as well as maintaining the fiscal integrity of the facility and managing residents' funds. The administrator leads the monthly quality assurance meeting. The administrator is responsible for all policies within the facility and appoints the managers of the different departments, including the medical director. Within contractual obligations, the administrator decides whether or not the managers are performing adequately and whether to retain their services.

The nursing home administrator plays a major role in setting the tone of the nursing home both by communicating expectations and acting as a role model for the staff. The administrator is responsible for maintaining satisfaction of the residents and families, which includes meeting with them to solve disputes. Staff satisfaction is another role for which the administrator plays a primary role. In many nursing homes, more than 100% of the nursing staff turn over every year. Low nursing home turnover is an index of the quality of the administrator. The administrator also is the first point of contact for surveyors and is responsible to respond to survey findings and make sure that appropriate corrections and improvements are made to the care process. Administrators also interact with lawyers when a lawsuit is filed against the facility. The administrator needs to see that adequate staffing to provide quality care is in place at all times (Table 8–8). A forceful administrator who is visible throughout the facility greatly improves the quality of care.

INTERNATIONAL EXAMPLES OF NURSING HOME LEADERSHIP ROLES

International diversity in nursing home models has led to the emergence of a number of leadership models and roles. In most countries, nursing homes are regulated and must adhere to national health or social care policies and national standards. National regulatory systems and processes exert a major force across the sector through monitoring quality and the power they have to mandate provider responses.

All nursing home leaders have to address the requirements of the legislative, policy, and regulatory systems. In the United States with the medicalization of nursing homes, a tripartite model of leadership has emerged, which includes medical, nursing, and administrative directors. In U.K. care homes, which are predicated on a social model, the medical director is absent from the leadership team. In other parts of Europe such as France, the organization is similar to that of the United States since the well-established medicalization of the nursing home in early 2002. The director is in charge of the administrative task but is still responsible for everything (vision, technical part of the building, investment, accounting, human resources, relation to national regulatory system, and so on). She or he usually works with a small team of administrators. In the administrative staff, the director has a nursing director in charge of care and a medical coordinator in charge of admission. A physician medical director works with the nursing director to assure quality care. As challenges for improvement among nursing homes rise, more and more nursing homes join financial groups because expertise is very expensive. Financial groups may provide a kind of added value. Nursing homes will experience big upheaval in the years to come with the economic environment emphasizing this change.

Although in many parts of the world, where the social model of nursing homes predominates, physicians are minimally involved in nursing home leadership, we strongly believe that involvement of physicians in the leadership structure can greatly improve the quality of nursing homes. This has been demonstrated both in Holland and the United States.

DIRECTOR OF NURSING

The director of nursing (DON) is a key player in the leadership structure of nursing homes. The DON reports directly to the administrator, although in some leadership

Table 8–9.	AREAS OF RESPONSIBILITY OF THE DIRECTOR OF NURSING

- Organize nursing coverage 24 hours a day
- Development of care plans
- Quality of nursing care
- "Medical" continuous quality improvement
- Developing and updating nursing standard operating procedures
- Maintaining the knowledge of nursing staff
- Training certified nursing aides (assistants)
- Feedback to nursing staff and maintaining appropriate care for residents
- Maintenance rehabilitation
- Interacts with medical staff and other health professionals
- Safe dispensing of medications

structures, the DON may also be the administrator. The major role of the DON is to oversee the nursing staff and to be responsible for having appropriate nursing coverage for all shifts. The areas for which the DON has direct responsibility are outline in Table 8–9.

In nursing home chains, the DON may also have to report to a regional nursing supervisor. In many ways, the DON is the lynchpin of quality care provided in the nursing home. The DON sets the tone of care in the nursing home. The DON intercedes with physicians, other health professionals, and nursing home staff (e.g., kitchen, cleaning, laundry) and the nursing staff while acting in a primary role as the advocate for the residents. The DON has responsibility for ensuring that the records of care are meticulously maintained and investigating all injuries and complaints concerning nursing care. As the nursing leader, the DON ensures that nursing staff are cheerful and happy in their jobs. A number of nursing homes have staff turnover in excess of 100% per year. The DON has a major responsibility for reducing staff turnover. Low staff turnover is directly related to quality of care.

THE ROLE OF THE MEDICAL DIRECTOR

In the United States, the physician as the medical director, working closely with the DON and administrator, brings a different perspective to care issues. Because most of nursing home residents have multiple comorbidities necessitating regular, and often urgent, interaction with the medical system, this perspective is key. It is particularly important that the physician who is the medical director has had special training in either geriatrics or by a course such as the Certified Medical Director's (CMD) Course offered by the American Medical Directors Association (AMDA). Nursing homes using such a trained physician have significantly improved outcomes. In the United States all nursing homes are required to have a medical director.

There are multiple roles for the medical director, and they vary depending on the sophistication of the nursing

home and the medical needs of the residents. The medical director's role is primarily an administrative one, and whether or not she sees residents as patients is a secondary role. Some believe that the medical director should organize the medical staff but should not serve as the primary care physician for residents except in emergencies. In small facilities (fewer than 100 beds), the medical director should be present for a monthly quality assurance meeting and spend between 2 and 4 hours on at least 1 other day a month in the facility to observe and discuss problems. In larger facilities (>200 beds), the medical director should be employed to work at least 15 hours a week in the facility.

The roles and responsibilities of the medical director have been outlined by the AMDA and the U.S. Centers for Medicare and Medicaid Services (CMS).

- Coordination of physician and licensed practitioner services
- Clinical leadership
- Quality of care
- Education
- Employee health
- Community relations
- Interact with surveyors

The CMS has outlined the responsibilities for coordination of physician and licensed practitioner services (Table 8–10). The medical director needs to guide physician and healthcare practitioner services to help residents attain and maintain their highest practicable level of functioning consistent with regulatory requirements. A process needs to be in place on to review basic credentials on a regular basis. A minimum is that the physician or healthcare practitioner is on staff at a local hospital or the nursing

Table 8–10.	ROLE OF MEDICAL DIRECTOR IN PROVISION OF PHYSICIAN AND LICENSED PRACTITIONER SERVICES

- Availability of physician services 24 hours a day
- Practitioner reviews and documents resident's condition, program of care, medications, and treatments
- Frequency of visits as required (in the United States, monthly for the first 3 months and then every second month; patients are also seen when an urgent condition arises)
- Signing and dating all progress notes, medications, and admission and re-admission orders
- Appropriate responses to consultant recommendations are carried out
- Licensed practitioners (e.g., advance practice nurses, physician assistants, podiatrists, optometrists) perform delegated tasks within regulatory requirements
- Ensure that practitioners (including specialists who visit the facility) are appropriately credentialed to carry out their medical tasks
- Ensure that all residents have a primary attending physician and backup coverage
- Be available to make medical decisions if the primary attending cannot be contacted in a reasonable time period

home needs to maintain its own credentialing including peer review of the practitioners. The medical director addresses and resolves concerns among physicians, healthcare practitioners, and facility staff members. The medical director also reviews a selected number of charts of physicians in the facility to ensure quality care. Issues related to continuity of care and transfer of medical information among facilities and other care settings need to be resolved by the medical director. A system should be in place to provide feedback on performance to physicians working in the facility. This includes intervening when the care does not meet current standards of care.

Clinical leadership includes participating in administrative decision making and policies and procedures for admission and care processes. The medical director must be prepared to discuss with the leadership when a resident's care needs cannot be met by the facility and work with the facility to find alternative placement. Specific attention should be paid to ascertaining that residents are aware of and have the opportunity to have appropriate advanced directives and end-of-life care and that these are appropriately carried out. The medical director needs to review the radiologic, laboratory, and pharmacy services. She or he should also make sure that physical, occupational, and speech therapy are providing appropriate services. The medical director needs to ascertain that the residents are involved in decision making when possible. The medical director has to evolve a system to be aware of and resolve issues related to medical care. If research is being conducted in the facility, the medical director is responsible to see that it was approved by the appropriate institutional review board or ethics committee and is carried out as approved.

The medical director should work with the administration to develop systems for quality and appropriateness of care within the facility. She or he should participate in the continuous quality improvement meetings on a monthly basis. The medical director should advise on infection control issues and specifically monitor need for isolation, special care, and appropriate hand washing. This involvement of the medical director should lead to a safe and caring environment.

The medical director should remain up to date on evolving approaches in the care of persons in nursing homes. There should be a learning culture in the facility that is promoted by the medical director. The medical director should provide updated resources for the facility from recognized medical care societies (e.g., AMDA guidelines) and ensure that updated education is provided to all staff members in the nursing home.

Employee health programs should be in place. The medical director needs to help organize "health fairs" or other mechanisms by which employee physicians can be done.

The medical director is a part of the external face of the facility. She or he needs to champion the facility in the community and with referral sources. The medical director should be available to provide lectures to the public and family members on nursing home care.

The medical director needs to be available to meet with inspectors during the survey process and communicate with them afterward to clarify clinical questions or information concerning the care of the residents. The medical director should, when possible, attend the exit conference and ask inspectors to clarify citations on clinical care. The medical director works with the facility to draft corrective actions in response to the inspectors.

In the United States, the nursing home inspectors can site either the nursing home (for not having a designated physician medical director) or the nursing home or medical director for failure to involve the medical director or for the medical director not having performed his or her roles and function related to coordination of medical care or implementation of resident care policies. This citation is known as F-tag 501. When directed at the medical director, this citation requires the establishment of another citation for deficiency of medical care. Approximately 1.7% of nursing facilities have received a citation for problems with medical directorship. The CMS guidelines and its investigative protocol are included in the Toolkit.

NURSING HOME LEADERSHIP IN THE UNITED KINGDOM

Care homes in the United Kingdom operate within a social model of care, and the leadership model rarely involves a medical director. A recent survey of members of the British Geriatric Society found that 56% of consultant geriatricians thought care home medical work was important but more than 90% spent less than 10% of their time seeing care home residents. A full discussion of the state of medical care in English nursing homes is available within the 2011 British Geriatrics Society's report "Quest for Quality," which can be accessed at http://www.bgs.org.uk.

Care homes operate as part of a large corporate organization, a small company, individually owned facility, local council, or voluntary sector-owned care home. The exact leadership configuration within each facility varies; nursing homes that provide 24-hour nursing care often have a Manager (akin to the administrator in the United States) or a matron or senior nurse (equivalent to the United States' DON). In care homes providing residential style care, the senior practitioner may be a nurse or social worker. Staffing levels must comply with those set out by statutory regulators across the four U.K. nations, which vary with the category of the care home (e.g., old age or specialist dementia care).

Based on the Care Standards Act 2000, the respective National Minimum Standards set out regulations for record keeping, planning, and health monitoring in all four U.K. countries, and it is a requirement that care home residents are enabled to register with a general practitioner of their choice. At the time of writing, the Care Quality Commission for England was conducting a special review into meeting the medical and healthcare needs of older care home residents. The manager is responsible for staff appointments and for ensuring that all staff members complete mandatory training in topics such as lifting and handling and fire evacuation. There is no obligation to provide continuing professional development for registered nurses or social workers; the onus is on the individual (see Chapter 10). However, the manager is responsible for ensuring that all staff members have the minimum level of required skills, training, and supervision to provide care to the residents.

Table 8–11.   SCOTTISH CARE HOME CONSULTANT PRACTITIONERS

Nurse Consultant for Older People in Care Homes	Rehabilitation Consultant Post	Nurse Consultant Infection Control
This strategic nursing leadership post works in partnership with services and other national organizations and supports care homes to improve the quality of care and standards of nursing care.	This improvement post works in partnership with services and other national organizations and supports care homes and day services to improve the quality of care in relation to aspects of rehabilitation.	This improvement post works in partnership with services and other national organizations and supports care homes and day services to reduce the risk of transmission of avoidable infections, therefore improving overall quality of care and safety for older people in care.
Role functions include practice development and workforce development and learning for nursing teams across the care home sector. Examples of national leadership include nutritional care and end-of-life care projects.	Includes falls prevention and management, promoting day-to-day activity, encouraging a culture of enablement, and improving aspects of care for residents with dementia.	

Staffing levels and skill mix are a major leadership challenge, and necessity dictates that there is a high proportion of care assistants to registered nurses, although there is no evidenced-based formula to guide staffing decision, and the regulators minimum requirements must be satisfied. Recruitment and retention challenges are well known, and a recent survey by the Royal College of Nursing highlighted the transient nature of managers, particularly nurse managers.

The care home manager plays a central role in financial considerations in respect of new admissions because funding comes from a mix of set local authority fees, which tend to be lower than those that can be secured from self-funding clients. The senior nurse will assess the appropriateness of the admission based on nursing needs and the capacity of the home to meet the needs of the individual. Often the senior nurse will undertake an initial assessment visit with the older person and family caregivers to determine the appropriateness of the potential admission from the care home's perspective but also to answer questions from the person and his or her family to help them with placement decisions.

An additional and possibly unique national leadership resource has been introduced in Scotland in the form of Consultant Practitioners, who are employed by the Scottish Care Home Regulators and are centrally funded. To date, three consultant posts have been established with national responsibilities to support strategic developments across the sector. These national appointments provide leadership across the 900 registered care homes throughout Scotland. Funding for these new leadership roles is providing by the Scottish Government Health Department, and lead consultant practitioners (nurse and Allied Health Professionals [AHP]) work collaboratively with care home providers, national agencies, and education providers to deliver and embed improvements. Examples of national projects include improving nutritional care and reducing healthcare-associated infections within care homes. The Care Home Nurse Consultant for Infection Control plays a key leadership role working with care home providers to address common healthcare-associated infections such as *Clostridium difficile*, *Staphylococcus aureus*, and methicillin-resistant *S. aureus*. The role involves working in partnership with national organizations such as Health Protection Scotland to coordinate surveillance, identify and support outbreak management, and implement evidence-based guidance and National Education Scotland to develop educational initiatives aimed at driving improvement in practice and reducing healthcare-associated infections.

Table 8–11 provides an overview of the three consultant practitioner roles. Only one formal evaluation has been completed of the inaugural Nurse Consultant Post, which indicated a range of positive strategic and operational impacts.

KEY POINTS

1. A central feature of nursing home leadership and management is the pursuit of excellence in the standards of care provision and resident experiences.
2. An important question for leaders to ask is how to engage the nursing home staff and empower them to rise to the challenge of delivering better care.
3. All staff members are potential leaders and followers, and their individual and group behavior serve to either facilitate or impede change.
4. An essential initial step in any change project is to create space for staff to voice their views, concerns, and regrets about perceived losses and threats of the change project.
5. An effective leader recognizes change pain and takes actions to empower staff and to equip them with the belief that the change is achievable and the confidence that they have necessary knowledge, skills, and resources to deliver.
6. Quality improvement is an important leadership tool; it is a complex and continual process that involves a cycle of planning, action, and responsive evaluation.
7. Involvement of physicians in nursing home leadership has demonstrably improved the healthcare of older residents in United States and Netherlands.
8. Nursing makes an important contribution to nursing home leadership as registered nurses leading teams, as nurse directors, through advanced practice roles, and through the recently introduced national strategic leadership of the Scottish Nursing Home Nurse/AHP Consultant.

TOOLKIT

Medication Usage Review												
Year_____												
Month	Jan	Feb	Mar	Apr	May	June	July	Aug	Sept	Oct	Nov	Dec
Routine meds (no. per resident)												
PRN (no. per resident)												
Antipsychotics (%)												
Antidepressants (%)												
Anxiolytics (%)												
Hypnotics (%)												
Census for nursing home (number)												

Adapted from http://www.cms.gov/transmittals/downloads/R386CP.pdf.

SUGGESTED READINGS

American Medical Directors Association. Roles and responsibilities of the medical director in the nursing home: Position statement A03. *J Am Med Dir Assoc.* 2005;6:411-412.

Anderson RA, Issel LM, McDaniel RR. Nursing homes as complex adaptive systems: relationship between management practice and resident outcome. *Nurs Res.* 2003;52(1):12-21.

British Geriatric Society. Quest for Quality. An Inquiry Into the Quality of Healthcare Support for Older People in Care Homes: A Call for Leadership, Partnership and Improvement. http://www.bgs.org.uk. 2011 by British Geriatric Society, London. Accessed March 24, 2013.

Crecelius C. F-tag 501 medical director: where are we now? *J Am Med Dir Assoc.* 2009;10:221-222.

Jones D, Orsolini-Hain L. *Collaboration and Developing Partnerships in "101" Global Leadership Lessons for Nurses: Shared Legacies from Leaders and Their Mentees.* Rollins Gantz N (ed). Sigma Theta Tau Indianapolis, USA: International Nursing Society; 2010.

Rice A. *Learning for Leadership.* London: Tavistock; 1965.

Royal College of Nursing. *Persistent Challenges to Providing Quality Care. An RCN Report on the Views and Experiences of Frontline Nursing Staff in Care Homes in England.* London: RCN Publishing; 2012.

Tolson D, Rolland Y, Andrieu S, et al. The IAGG WHO/SGFF (World Health Organization/Society Français de Gérontologie et de Gériatrie). International Association of Gerontology and Geriatrics: A global agenda for clinical research and quality of care in nursing homes. *J Am Med Dir Assoc.* 2011;12(3):185-189.

Tolson D, Schofield I, Brown J. *Evaluation of Nurse Consultant for Older People. Care Commission Scotland* [unpublished report]. Glasgow: Glasgow Caledonian University; 2009.

Western S. Leadership power and authority. In *Leadership: A Critical Text.* Los Angeles: Sage Publications; 2008:41-56.

MULTIPLE CHOICE QUESTIONS

8.1 Leadership and management are the same.

   a. True
   b. False

8.2 Which of the following leadership approaches should be adopted within nursing homes?

   a. Transformational leadership
   b. Authoritarian leadership
   c. Distributed leadership

8.3 Which of the following is *not* essential when leading change projects?

   a. Clarity of project goals
   b. Medical leadership
   c. An action plan
   d. Feedback
   e. Staff empowerment

8.4 Which of the following is *not* a component of the Deming action cycle?

   a. Plan
   b. Check
   c. Do
   d. Control
   e. Act

8.5 Which of the following is *not* the responsibility of the director of nursing?

   a. Organizing 24-hour-a-day nursing coverage
   b. Medical continuous quality improvement
   c. Providing oversight of physician prescribing practices
   d. Training certified nursing assistant
   e. Responsible for safe medication dispensation

Chapter 9

ADMISSION TO A NURSING HOME

Many studies have explored the views and concerns of older people about moving into long-term care. Findings consistently highlight the negative impacts and fears associated with myths, realities, and the legacy of institutional suspicion. A relatively small number of studies present admission as a welcome relief and sanctuary from recent struggles. Nonetheless, the introduction of evidence-based practice and culture change movement means that the modern nursing home is capable of providing an affirming life experience whether it is for a short rehabilitative stay, long-term care, or end-of-life care. Whatever the reason for the admission, strategies to make the admission experience as positive and reassuring as possible should be prioritized. The more positive the early experiences of the nursing home, the greater the sense of worth experienced by the individual and the family caregiver. The best relationships among a resident, staff, and family feature open and respectful communication; this should begin on admission or during the preadmission phase. It has been shown that personal relationships influence perceptions of the quality of care. Family members who recognize that staff members are doing their best for their relative and care about them as individuals tend to trust staff and be more understanding of the constraints and challenges faced by staff within the nursing home.

PREPARING FOR ADMISSION: OLDER PERSON AND FAMILY PERSPECTIVES

Admission to a nursing home, particularly when it is for long-term care or an extended stay, is a major and stressful life event, and reassurance is an essential ingredient of the admission process. Although "routinized care" has frequently prompted pejorative reactions from onlookers who argue that it is impersonal, a recent U.K. study has suggested that some level of routine and familiarization with daily routines assists new residents in their adjustments to life in a nursing home. Anticipation of the daily routine and some structure to the day may alleviate anxieties and certainly enable staff to plan without compromising the goal of resident-centered approaches. Indeed, some residents and family positively welcome the markers of routine, which provide a sense of coherence to what is happening. The ability to anticipate and sense familiarity with the structure of the day can help to preserve a sense of being in control of oneself. For visitors, it also creates opportunity to plan visits and activities to punctuate the day and allow for quality time.

Preadmission screening and admission assessment procedures are critical to the determination of healthcare needs, diagnosis, and the formalization of treatment and care plans. In addition to the formal assessments of health and social needs, new residents, just like new staff members, need to be orientated to how things are done in the nursing home and supported through their probationary period as they adjust to nursing home life. Residents and their visiting family members need to be guided in relation to local policies and practices that will influence their day and be made aware of emergency procedures (see Chapter 5).

Admission decisions should be taken carefully; they should be based on a comprehensive assessment of the individual's health and social care need, care preferences, self-care capacity, and family capacity to care and weighed against the suitability of community care packages and aging in place alternatives (for a fuller discussion, see Chapter 1). In the ideal situation, nursing home admission for long-term care should be a positive choice and a shared decision that is carefully planned. An interesting observation recently made by a U.K. relative of a newly admitted resident was that in all other aspects of healthcare, much is made about informed consent and consent procedures, yet the decision about where to end your days can feel disempowering and at best a forced choice of the worst alternatives when you are most vulnerable and ill informed.

In the rush to complete admission procedures and paperwork, the emotional impact and symbolism of admission for long-term care on the individual can easily be overlooked. Equally, for an exhausted family caregiver, admission involves relinquishing caring responsibilities and reframing relationship with a partner, parent, or other loved one. Learning to become a visitor of the person you have spent your life with, as discussed in Chapter 3, can and often is a stressful and emotional time requiring major adjustments. There are many considerations involved in choosing a nursing home, and often the individual and family require assistance. A social worker or nurse with case management responsibilities should provide information and advice on the type of care home best suited for the person's needs, local availability, waiting lists, and contact information. Sometimes involving an independent advocate who will represent the wishes of the person with dementia without being emotionally involved can be helpful. For non-urgent admissions and in the spirit of person-centered care, the older person should feel central to decisions and believe that he or she has choices. Table 9–1 sets out a checklist of considerations for individuals and families to use when selecting a nursing home.

When possible, it is useful for the individual and family to visit several nursing homes so they can compare the facilities and care being offered. There may be a waiting list, and it is important that individuals understand this and have a list of preferred facilities that includes first and second choices and absolute rejections. In this way, if admission becomes necessary and a place is unavailable at the first choice of facility, then the reserve list can be used. It is preferable not to transfer people between homes because this can be unsettling, but sometimes there may be justifications for doing so.

Nursing home brochures are helpful but may give a slightly misleading impression, and it is important that a member of the nursing team welcomes and dedicates time to spend with prospective residents, showing them around and giving them time to ask questions. It is helpful to provide printed information concerning frequently asked questions. Sometimes a trial stay is useful, or an opportunity to eat a meal or take refreshment with the accompanying person can be reassuring and allow time for reflection. Introducing people to other residents may or may not be helpful, although it is important for individuals to meet their potential neighbors.

In addition to the many considerations set out in Table 9–1, it is important that the fees and methods of payment are made clear. Different administrations have a range of direct payment, copayment methods, and insurance systems to fund long-term care placements. Where state funding is available, often it supports the minimum acceptable standard of care, but when people have personal resources, a superior quality of "hotel" and other services can be secured. For brevity, we will not attempt to debate the rights and wrongs of different systems, but it is important to recognize that funding for nursing home care is limited and that this inevitability reduces the choices and options available. Across the world, the funding of nursing home places and the sustainability of funding is a contentious and emotive issue, and the International Association of Gerontology and Geriatrics recognizes the inherent inequalities in the resourcing and variability of the quality of nursing home care around the world. Nursing home staff members have a responsibility to explain the options that are available to individuals and families and to do their best to deliver the best possible care with dignity and compassion within given resources. Good housekeeping is an essential part of nursing home management, and residents need to know how and in what ways they might supplement and enhance standard care provision.

Each nursing home has its own admission procedures, which include policies for the residents' personal belongings, including money. When possible, family members should be asked to label belongings, including all items of clothing, with a permanent marker or embroidered name tag. In some nursing homes, a preadmission list of what is recommended in terms of the numbers and types of garments may be useful, particularly if there is limited storage space. On admission, it is relatively easy to make a list of personal belongings and ask the family member or resident to sign a disclaimer form; however, it can sometimes be difficult to keep track of new items brought into the home, and losses and breakages do occur. For residents wishing to bring in valuable items, the family would be well advised to take out insurance.

As part of the preadmission processes, it may be helpful to alert individuals and family members to the sorts of questions they will be asked on admission or during the first few days of admission. The list shown in Table 9–2 should be adapted depending on local cultures and customs.

ADJUSTMENT TO A NURSING HOME

Entry into a nursing home is stressful both for the resident and his or her family members. On the whole, persons do not choose to live in a nursing home but are forced to enter the home either because of a catastrophic illness requiring entry to the nursing home for rehabilitation or because they or their relative(s) can no longer manage the burden of care at home. In the latter case, incontinence (urinary, fecal, or both) or dementia with behavioral abnormalities or requiring a large amount of help with activities of daily living (ADL) precipitates the need for nursing home admission. Admission and adjustment to nursing homes is stressful for both the new resident and the family caregivers.

New residents in nursing homes display a number of behaviors in response to admission to the nursing home (Table 9–3). Studies in the Netherlands have suggested that adjustment to the nursing home depends on four privacy issues:

- Building design to allow privacy
- Attitude of staff and other residents to allowing privacy
- Ability to have choice and control one's environment
- Lack of disturbance by other residents.

The last two items are the most important in allowing a smooth adjustment to a nursing home.

Although nursing homes have been accused of promoting conformity, apathy, and submissiveness ("social breakdown behavior"), the development of a patient-centered care approach has gone a long way toward changing this situation. Studies from countries as diverse as Korea and the United States have found that effecting adaptation to the nursing home is based on similar factors (Table 9–4). In many developed countries, the inability to deal with rules and schedules is a major difficulty during the adjustment period. However, in Hong Kong, this was found to be a minor inconvenience. In Asian nursing homes, making new friends in the nursing home has been considered to be

Table 9–1.   CONSIDERATIONS FOR THE OLDER PERSON AND FAMILY IN CHOOSING A NURSING HOME

Reputation for Quality

- How do the quality ratings (inspection reports) for the local nursing homes compare?
- Does the description in the brochure reflect the quality reports?
- What is the on-the-street reputation of the nursing home? It may be helpful to speak to local caregivers, support groups, or families of current residents.

Location and Setting

- Is this locality appropriate for the person, and is the home convenient for relatives and friends to visit?
- If the person is religious, is there a suitable place of worship nearby?
- What are the views like from the bedrooms, the lounge, or dining room when residents are sitting?

Outdoor Space

- Is there a safe, attractive outdoor area, and is it well maintained and accessible to residents?
- Is there outdoor furniture such as tables, chairs, and benches for residents to use?

First Impressions

- Is the atmosphere friendly, welcoming, and homely?
- Is the home clean without being too tidy, and is it pleasantly furnished and decorated?
- Do you notice any unpleasant smells?
- How do the staff talk with residents? Are they respectful and attentive?

Visitors

- Are visitors welcome at any time?
- Can they join the resident for a meal or make snacks?
- Are children welcome in the home?
- Are visitors able to take the resident out if they want to?
- Can animals or pets come to visit residents? Does the home or unit allow residents to keep pets, or are there any resident pets owned by the home?

Bedrooms and Personal Possessions

- Can the person have a single room? This is important in retaining dignity and privacy.
- Can residents bring some of their own furniture and possessions? This can be very important in helping the person to settle in and feel at home.
- Can residents go to their rooms when they want to be alone, and do staff respect the need for privacy and always knock on bedroom doors?
- Does the laundry system make sure that clothes do not get lost or returned to the wrong person?
- Are there en suite facilities?
- Are pets allowed to visit?
- Does staff try to ensure residents use their spectacles and hearing aids?

Living Areas

- Is there more than one room where residents can sit?
- Is there a designated smoking room for residents?

Meals

- Does the home cater for special diets, and do they take into account residents' likes and dislikes?
- Is there any choice at meal times?
- Can residents choose to eat at different times or in their rooms?

Activities

- What opportunities are there for meaningful activities, including hobbies?
- Are birthdays and special events celebrated?
- Do people come in from the community to visit, to help with activities, or to entertain?
- Does the level and variety of activity appear to be too stimulating or too boring for your family member?

Cultural

- If the person you care for comes from a different background or culture than most of the other residents, will his or her particular needs be catered for in an understanding and sensitive manner?
- Does staff seem interested in and respectful of differences such as diet, religious observances, hygiene practices, clothing, and ways of relating to other people?

Staff

- How many staff members are on duty at night and day, and for how many residents?
- How many registered nurses are on duty during the day and overnight?
- Is there a medical director or medical coordinator in the home, and if not, how are the medical needs of the residents addressed?
- How often does the home use agency staff? A lot of new faces can be difficult for residents, and agency staff will not get to know them.
- Is there much staff turnover? Ask a few individuals how long they have been there and how happy they are in their jobs.
- Does the staff seem friendly and caring?
- How does staff respond to residents? Do they treat them with dignity, humor, and affection or do they talk down to them, bully them, or ignore them?
- Does staff treat residents as individuals and know about their backgrounds and interests?

Admission

- What kind of admissions procedure does the home carry out before admitting residents?
- Do they offer to compile a detailed list of the person's habits and preferences?
- Will there be a member of staff who is particularly responsible for the person?
- Does each resident have a personal care plan? Each resident should have his or her care plan reviewed annually, and it is good practice to review it 4 to 6 weeks after admission.
- How does the home welcome new residents and help them settle in?

Table 9–2.	INFORMATION THAT NURSING HOME STAFF REQUIRE ON OR SOON AFTER ADMISSION

- Medical history
- Current medications
- Allergies to food and medications
- Family names and contact details
- Personal history and life story, including interests and hobbies
- Religion and practices
- Names and contact details of enduring power of attorney and enduring guardianship
- Details of health funds, Medicare, or pension arrangement
- Names and phone numbers of general practitioner; community nurse; social worker; and vision, hearing, and dental professionals
- Special dietary requirements
- Likes and dislikes
- Preferences for showering and bathing
- Continence (urinary and bowel problems)
- Mobility: Need for lifting equipment, walkers, wheelchairs, or other mobility devices
- Funeral arrangements and end-of-life options and advance directives
- Choice of doctor

a major obstacle to adjustment. Four stages of adaptation to the nursing home have been characterized:

1. Orienting: Getting to know the physical neighborhood and neighbors
2. Normalizing: Adapting to institutional rules such as meal times and times to get up and go to bed
3. Rationalizing: Coming to terms with the need to be in the nursing home and accepting the environment
4. Stabilizing: Settling into the rhythm of daily life in the nursing home

Table 9–3.	COMMON BEHAVIORS SEEN DURING ADJUSTMENT OF NEW RESIDENTS TO A NURSING HOME

Grief

Anger

Dysphoria

Depression

Apathy

Sleep disruption

Disorientation

Withdrawal

Attempts to "escape"

Stopping eating

Falls

Table 9–4.	FACTORS ASSOCIATED WITH POSITIVE ADJUSTMENT TO LIVING IN A NURSING HOME

Preconception of nursing homes

Self-efficacy

Social support (staff, other residents)

Family relationship or support

Self-reported health

Satisfaction with the facility

Family caregivers have a variety of responses to admission of a loved one to a nursing home (Table 9–5). The roles of family caregivers in the nursing home are to contribute to the nursing home community, monitor the quality of care and special needs of their family member, and maintain the continuity of the resident's life. The latter includes maintaining their loving relationship with their relative and teaching the staff, other residents, and other family members about their loved one's life history (i.e., who the resident was and is). A number of factors have been shown to allow the family caregiver to adapt in a minimally stressful way to the placement of his or her loved one in a nursing home (Table 9–6). Nursing home–sponsored support groups for family and social events for family and residents represent important approaches the nursing home can implement to increase family satisfaction.

SETTLING IN

Admission into a nursing home evokes many emotions. The first day can often be taken up with practical matters that leave the family feeling exhausted and emotional. A review of resettlement literature examining psychosocial factors affecting the health of older people after admission to long-term care concluded that death after relocation is influenced by a number of factors, including the preparation and processes of transfer and settling in. The more that individuals felt involved and in control of what was happening to them, the better their outcome and long-term survival. This is obviously a complex area, and the health status and overall condition of the person are major

Table 9–5.	REASONS GIVEN BY CAREGIVERS FOR NURSING HOME PLACEMENT

No choice

Relief

Guilt

Justification

Ambiguity

Physical relief

Emotional relief

Table 9–6.   FACTORS THAT ENHANCE SATISFACTION OF FAMILY CAREGIVERS WHEN A LOVED ONE IS IN A NURSING HOME

Caregivers have positive interactions with loved ones

Positive interactions with other nursing home residents

Strong family and friends aid

Positive relationships with nursing and other staff

Nursing home–sponsored support group

Incorporation as full partners in the care process

factors. However, evidence is accumulating suggesting that the first few days of being a nursing home resident are critical to the development of trust between the care for person and staff as well as the resident's subsequent quality of life and satisfaction with care. Registered nurses and the wider nursing team need to recognize the importance of proactive "settling in" strategies to support the adaptation process and how they can help the new resident deal with the inevitable turmoil of emotions, grief, and loss. Arrival in a new environment can be bewildering for anyone, but arrival in a nursing home for people with and without cognitive impairment, particularly for those with sensory impairment, can be an overwhelming and disorientating experience.

Preadmission nursing assessments that include identification of personal preferences, likes, and dislikes are to be recommended so that early interactions with staff are focused on getting to know each other in ways that will feel personalized. If possible, the family can bring personal belongings and arrange them in the room before the arrival of the resident. If the person is accompanied, then the staff member will need to explain where things are to be stored and orientate the person to his or her new home. Arranging the room together and figuring out where everything is can be helpful. It is important to show the new resident and his or her family members how to get nursing assistance if required. Make sure the call bell is in an easy-to-reach place and encourage a family member to try it before they leave. Written information that can be kept for reference by the resident and copies for family members with frequently asked questions about the nursing home are particularly useful along with instructions and contact details if the family wishes to telephone to enquire about the progress of their relative.

A member of the staff should be responsible for welcoming the person, showing him or her to the room, and providing refreshments. Offering assistance with the toilet may be appreciated after the emotional journey to the home. It is also important to establish which medications the person has been prescribed, what medications have been taken immediately before admission, and what medications the person has brought along. It is sensible to check the condition of medications and ensure that supplies have not expired, assuming that they are in their original containers! Although medications need to be properly reviewed (see later discussion) as part of the clinical management, the registered nurse may wish to seek urgent advice from a physician or prescribing advanced nurse practitioner if the medication regimen seems unusual or there are safety concerns.

Although it is sensible not to overwhelm the person with assessments of his or her condition, which can be completed within a given time period, according to local policy, it is important to make some immediate and initial assessments (e.g., of pain, assistance required for mobilization, cognitive function, continence). The exact list depends on the person's reason for admission and comorbidities, and it is important that a registered healthcare professional (physician or nurse) is involved in these decisions. Transfer information from hospitals is notorious for being incomplete, and accompanying family members can provide helpful details, although these details require confirmation.

THE INITIAL ASSESSMENT: PREADMISSION OR ADMISSION

In the ideal world, a full geriatric assessment would be performed on all persons before admission to a nursing home. This allows the recognition of persons who can be cared for in the community when appropriate resources are available. The preadmission assessment also can identify treatable problems that can obviate the need for nursing home admission. A preadmission assessment can ensure that the person is admitted to the appropriate level of care. Unfortunately, in the United States and Europe, most admissions are hurried, either from home or a hospital, in response to a critical event, either involving the future resident or the caregiver. In countries such as Holland, a system is in place to theoretically provide an adequate geriatric assessment. Similarly, in the Toulouse area in France, general practitioners have a simple checklist that can alert them to the need for a geriatric assessment. The Toulouse Gérontopole have opened a day clinic to help families and primary care physicians (PCPs) decide if nursing home entry is needed. This clinic offers comprehensive geriatrics and social assessment to help with decision making. It is important that patient, families, and PCPs to consider that it is better to anticipate nursing entry than do it too late after an emergency hospitalization.

The most common reasons for a person being admitted to a nursing home are outlined in Table 9–7. In many cases, the preadmission assessment is done by an administrator or social worker or case manager. They determine whether there is adequate payment available, if the facility has adequate resources for the persons medical and rehabilitation needs, if there are behavioral issues that will increase the complexity of the care of the person, and whether the individual has the capacity to make their own healthcare decisions. When the person comes directly from the hospital, many of these decisions are made by the hospital social worker, rehabilitation therapists, nurses, and physicians – the focus is on whether the person can live alone or with the available support or whether the required level of rehabilitation can be delivered at home.

Table 9–7.   COMMON REASONS FOR A PERSON NEEDING TO BE ADMITTED TO A NURSING HOME

In the United States[a]	
Need for intensive short-term rehabilitation before returning home	

In All Countries	
Individual characteristics	Extreme age
	Incontinence: Fecal or urinary
	Severe dementia
	Wandering
	Abusive behaviors by the individual to family members
	Inability to perform basic activities of daily living
	Multiple falls
	Severe frailty
Support characteristics	No caregiver
	Frail caregiver
	Employment of caregiver
	Personality disputes with caregiver
Community characteristics	Lack of formal community resources, including adequate housing, home care, home rehabilitation services, home help, and transportation
	Presence and prestige of long-term care institutions
	Lack of an informal support system (e.g., church, friends)

[a]In most countries, this occurs in hospitals, rehabilitation units, or "community" (cottage) hospitals.

Table 9–8.   AREAS COVERED BY MINIMUM DATA SET 3.0 FOR INITIAL ASSESSMENT

	Section	Discipline(S) Responsible for Completing Data
A	Select demographic items	Medical records staff / Nursing staff
B	Hearing, speech, and vision	Nursing / Optometry, audiology, speech therapy, physician
C	Cognitive patterns (brief interview of mental status, delirium)	Social work, nursing
D	Mood (Patient Health Questionnaire 9)	Social work, nursing
E	Behavior (psychosis, behavior symptoms [physical or verbal, rejection of care], wandering, effect on others)	Nursing, physician, social work, psychology
F	Preferences for customary routine, activities, community setting	Social work, recreation therapy nursing
G	Functional status (activities of daily living, mobility, gait, rehabilitation potential)	Physical therapy, nursing, occupational therapy
H	Bladder and bowel	Nursing
I	Active disease diagnosis	Physician, nursing
J	Health conditions (pain, dyspnea, cough, angina, tobacco use, falls assessment)	Nursing, physical therapy, physician
K	Swallowing and nutritional status	Dietitian, speech therapist, nursing
L	Oral and dental status	Nursing, dentist
M	Skin conditions	Nursing, physician
N	Medication	Physician, pharmacist, nursing
O	Special treatments or procedures	Nursing, physical therapy, occupational therapy
P	Restraints	Nursing
Q	Participation (goal setting)	Social work or nursing

On admission, a full assessment needs to be completed within 72 hours (14 days if using Minimum Data Set [MDS] 3.0). Ideally, this includes a physician assessment (mandated in the United States). Others involved are nurses, social workers, rehabilitation therapists, and clerical personnel. Some information is obtained from old records, but much requires a geriatric assessment for the first time. The new MDS 3.0 (see next section) is an excellent assessment tool covering most necessary domains (Table 9–8). An important component is assessing the capacity of the new resident to make decisions and what level of resuscitation he or she would prefer. To determine the resident's decision-making capacity, a formal mental status examination, which also determines if the person has mild cognitive impairment (e.g., SLUMS or Montreal Cognitive Assessment [MoCA]; see Chapter on dementia) should be administered. The person determining decision-making capacity should then determine whether the resident can comprehend relevant information, manipulate information in a rational way, and communicate his or her choices. If he or she cannot, there is a need to determine who will make the person's choices.

It is essential to determine at admission the resident's advance directive wishes. This is helped if the resident has a living will or a durable power of attorney for health.

However, in the nursing home, a relatively simple schema for rapid, easily understandable decision making in emergencies needs to be available. This is best done by the ABC code status method:

A. Resident wants everything done.
B. Resident will go to a hospital but does not want to be resuscitated or ventilated or have blood transfusion or tube feeding or dialysis.
C. Resident does not want to be transferred to a hospital. This can only be done when essential for resident's comfort.

All nursing homes need to have a clear policy regarding resuscitation, and this should be used on admission to the nursing home to establish the therapeutic level of care for each resident based on the resident's wishes and that of his or her power of attorney if the resident cannot express his or her wishes.

After the admission or preadmission assessment, a comprehensive care plan should be developed for the resident. This should focus on the resident's social and psychosocial needs as well as his or her medical needs. A pharmacy review of potential drug–drug interactions should be included in this review. The resident and family member should be given an opportunity to understand and comment on the care plan.

MINIMUM DATA SETS

The Resident Assessment Instrument and the Minimum Data Set

The Omnibus Budget Reconciliation Act of 1987 (OBRA '87) legislated a number of nursing home reforms. One of these required comprehensive functional assessment of nursing home residents. In 1991, the Resident Assessment Instrument (RAI) was mandated for use in nursing homes. The RAI consisted of an MDS and 18 condition-focused resident assessment protocols. Although the original MDS was shown to be relatively valid (but with questionable reliability) and to improve comprehensiveness and accuracy of care plans, it was anything but *minimum*. This led to limited uptake by healthcare staff providing direct patient care. The contrast to this is the Geronte (Figure 9–1). This simple figure of a person allows all staff members to rapidly recognize all the problems that a resident may have. All members of the interdisciplinary team can complete it, making it an ideal interdisciplinary communication tool. It was highly successfully used in LifeCare of St. Louis when it was acting as a subacute care facility.

The RAI was not shown to alter mortality rates or home discharge. Although the RAI did show a number of areas of improvement, it was also associated with negative effects such as increases in pain. The true effects of the RAI are difficult to assess because there major regulatory changes occurred over the same period. The MDS has been translated into multiple languages and implemented in many countries. However, only a few countries (Sweden, Italy, Denmark, Japan, Iceland, and Canada) carried out reliability testing of their version.

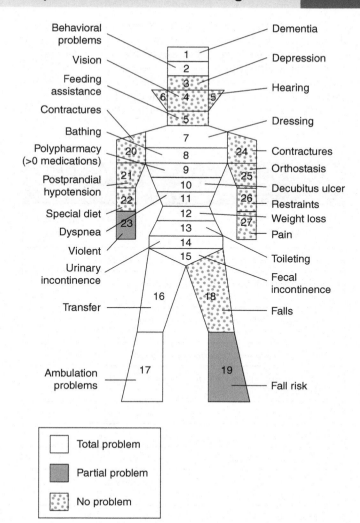

Figure 9–1. Geronte.

Even though the MDS is administratively useful, its clinical usefulness has been questioned. In response to these criticisms, MDS 3.0 was developed. The MDS 3.0 is more clinically useful as perceived by nurses in facilities who have used and, in particular, gave a voice to residents. It is reliable and performed better than the MDS 2.0. It takes approximately half the time to complete (about 60 minutes) compared with the MDS 2.0.

Residents are directly asked about cognition, mood, pain, and their preferences. This makes the MDS 3.0 an excellent geriatric assessment tool. The addition of items based on the Confusion Assessment Methodology heightens the ability to diagnose delirium. ADL questions allow separation of upper and lower body dressing and recognition of the differences between toileting and transfer to the toilet. Pressure ulcers are now categorized using the National Pressure Ulcer's Advisory Panel PUSH toolkit. In developmental testing of the MDS 3.0, more than 80% of nurses said the tool allowed identification of new problems, was more clinically useful, was easier to use, and accurately described the resident. The MDS 3.0 is provided in the Toolkit.

The vast majority of residents want to have their family involved in discussion of their care. More than 70% wanted the choice to go to bed after 8 PM. The most important activities identified by residents were the ability to go outside, keep abreast of the news, have access to religious services, and listen to music that they preferred.

Table 9–9 provides the U.S. national data for the first quarter of using MDS 3.0.

Table 9–9.	U.S. NATIONAL DATA FOR FIRST QUARTER MINIMUM DATA SET 3.0 USE

Long-Stay Residents	National Average
Note: For the following measures, higher percentages are better.	
% of residents given influenza vaccination during the flu season	95
% of residents who were assessed and given pneumococcal vaccination	94
Note: For the following measures, lower percentages are better.	
% of residents experiencing one or more falls with major injury	2
% of residents who have moderate to severe pain	13
% of residents who have pressure sores	8
% of residents who had a urinary tract infection	8
% of low-risk residents who lose control of their bowels or bladder	40
% of residents who have or had a catheter inserted and left in their bladder	4
% of residents who were physically restrained	3
% of residents whose need for help with daily activities has increased	18
% of residents who lose too much weight	8
% of residents who are more depressed or anxious	7
Short-Stay Residents	
Note: For the following measures, higher percentages are better.	
% of residents with a decrease in pain	50
% of residents given influenza vaccination during the flu season	82
% of residents who were assessed and given pneumococcal vaccination	83
Note: For the following measures, lower percentages are better.	
% of residents who had moderate to severe pain	24
% of residents with pressure ulcers that are new or worsened	3

Table 9–10.	THE INTERNATIONAL ASSOCIATION OF NUTRITION AND AGING'S FRAILTY DEFINITION: "FRAIL"[a]

Fatigued
Resistance: Cannot walk up a flight of stairs
Aerobic: Cannot walk 1 block
Illnesses: More than five
Loss of 5% weight in 6 months

[a]More than two positives designates the person as frail.

ASSESSMENT OF CLINICAL NEED AND MEDICATIONS

In the United States, the basic assessment of clinical need is now done by the MDS 3.0, which needs to be completed within 14 days of admission (Table 9–10). In many other countries, the assessment is still based on the inter-RAI (MDS 2.0). The MDS 3.0 provides an excellent, validated assessment that is completed by the interprofessional team working together with the resident and, when necessary, the social workers.

Another important step on admission is to assess the advance directives together with the resident and family members. It is particularly important to determine if the resident would prefer not to go back to the hospital. Medical treatments and acceptable forms of resuscitation need to be documented.

Ideally, the physician should see the resident within 48 hours of admission. At this time, medical diagnoses should be verified; a basic history and physical examination completed; and functional problems, pressure ulcers, and cognitive or behavioral issues documented. The physician should determine if the resident is expecting to return home. Potentially remediable conditions should be recognized, and appropriate referrals should be made to therapists in the nursing home. Medications should be reviewed in detail and potentially inappropriate or unnecessary medicines discontinued. The physician should understand the needs of the resident and, when possible, family members. Advanced directives should be reviewed and documented. Short- and long-term goals for the resident should be documented. A thorough medical treatment plan should be outlined. The Toolkit contains an example of a form for initial medical evaluation.

As soon as possible, the pharmacist should review the medication list and note any drug interactions or inappropriate dosing for older persons. Potentially inappropriate drugs based on recommendations such as the Beers list should be noted. Appropriate monitoring for different drugs should be outlined. This information should be provided to the nursing staff and physician as soon as possible.

Therapy staff should see the resident as requested by the physicians. They should develop and document an appropriate therapy plan. Other specialists such as old age psychiatry (geriatric psychiatry), audiology, podiatry, optometry, and psychology should see the resident as appropriate. When necessary, the need for the resident to

Table 9–11.	ACTIVITIES OF DAILY LIVING (ADL)
Bathing	
Dressing	
Toileting	
Transfers	
Continence	
Feeding	
ADL score: ___/6	

Table 9–13.	ITEMS TESTED BY THE BARTHEL INDEX
Help with bathing	
Help climbing stairs	
Help with dressing	
Help with walking	
Help with transfers	
Help with feeding	
Help with toilet use	
Help with grooming	
Urinary incontinence	
Fecal incontinence	

see other specialists or to go out of the facility for procedures (e.g., dialysis) should be noted and arrangements made to get the resident to these appointments.

Assessing Frailty

Frailty is defined as a state of vulnerability in which a further insult to the person will result in a high potential of the person's becoming disabled. Persons with severe frailty have a 20% increased chance of dying within the year if they are nursing home residents. In 2004 using the Cardiovascular Health Study (CHS), an objective definition for frailty was developed. The five criteria were weight loss, exhaustion, low energy expenditure, slowness (walking time), and weakness or grip strength. Another frailty model was developed from the Study of Osteoporosis Fractures using weight loss, fatigue, and arising from a chair five times. The SHARE-frailty index was developed in Europe and is similar to the CHS frailty index. Another frailty scale was developed from the Canadian Study of Health and Aging (CSHA). This measures the cumulative burden of a variety of deficits. All of these scales are difficult to use clinically. For this reason, the International Association of Nutrition and Aging (IANA) developed the FRAIL Scale (Table 9–10). This is a simple scale that includes components of the CHS and CSHA scale. It takes less than 30 seconds to be administered.

Assessing Function

Most persons residing in a nursing home have poor function in one or more areas. The most basic measurement

of function is the Katz ADL scale. This measures six areas of function, namely bathing, dressing, toileting, transferring, feeding, and continence (Table 9–11). Many authorities believe that continence should be excluded. Failure in any of the other areas means the person cannot live at home alone. An older person who is lacking one or more ADLs has a 30% of dying and a 50% chance of being admitted to a nursing home over the next 6 months.

The Lawton instrumental ADL (IADL) scale measures a higher level of ADLs than the Katz scale (Table 9–12). It takes about 12 minutes to administer and has eight items. It determines the amount of need an older person has to live at home.

The Barthel Index was developed at Johns Hopkins Hospital in 1965. This is a reliable scale with reasonable test–retest reliability. There are 10 items that are tested (Table 9–13).

The modified Rankin Scale is a simple scale used to determine the level of disability in persons with stroke (Table 9–14).

The Functional Index Measure (FIM) is an excellent measure of the burden of care. It consists of 18 items using a 7-point Likert scale for each item with a total score of 126 (Table 9–15). It measures both physical and cognitive

Table 9–12.	INSTRUMENTAL ACTIVITIES OF DAILY LIVING (IADL)
Using the telephone	
Shopping	
Food preparation	
Housekeeping	
Laundry	
Transportation	
Taking medicine	
Managing money	
IADL score: ___/8	

Table 9–14.	MODIFIED RANKIN SCALE
0	No symptoms
1	Comes out for activities despite some symptoms
2	Looks after own affairs but cannot do all previous activities
3	Requires help but can walk unassisted
4	Cannot attend to own bodily needs or walk without assistance
5	Requires full-time nursing care; is bedridden and incontinent
6	Dead

Table 9–15.	ITEMS MEASURED BY THE FUNCTIONAL INDEX MEASURE	
Physical Items		
Bladder management	Toileting	Bowel management
Toilet transfer	Bathing transfer	Mobility
Stair climbing	Bathing	Eating
Grooming	Upper body dressing	Lower body dressing
Bed-to-chair transfers		
Cognitive Items		
Social interaction	Memory	Problem solving
Comprehension	Expression	

domains. An increase of 22 points determines significant clinical improvement. It requires training of persons who are to administer it. It is highly reliable and valid. It appears to be the best score to measure effectiveness of rehabilitation. A number of shorter modified FIM scores exist.

FUNCTIONAL REHABILITATION

In some countries such as the United States, skilled nursing facilities provide functional rehabilitation for persons discharged from hospitals who are expected to return home. However, there is also a need for functional rehabilitation for long-term residents. A systematic review of long-term residents demonstrated that relatively simple exercise programs aimed at walking, endurance, and ADLs improved function, mobility, strength, and ADLs. These programs also improved balance, reduced fear of falling, and decreased agitated behavior. Programs that included resistance exercise and balance training had even better outcomes. A year-long study of adding resistance exercise therapy two times a week dramatically improved outcomes in persons who had sustained a hip fracture. When types of therapy intensity were reviewed, 88% of persons receiving high-intensity therapy improved; improvement was only observed in 33% of persons receiving usual therapy.

The World Health Organization (WHO) introduced the International Classification of Impairment, Disabilities and Handicaps in 1980. An impairment is any pathologic process in the body that can lead to disability. Disability is the loss of function. A handicap is a disability that leads to a loss of an individual's role in society. In addition, the WHO classification examines continual factors such as environment and personal factors that interact with an impairment to produce a handicap.

The principles of rehabilitation are to start intervention as early as possible but recognize that maintenance and late rehabilitation also are important components for an optimal outcome. Rehabilitation should aim at the highest intensity that can be tolerated. Psychological motivation of the person ongoing rehabilitation is a key component. Persons should be set achievable but movable goals. A variety of exercise apparatus, aids, and adaptive devices should be available to enhance function. Obtaining the best outcomes for rehabilitation requires a high-quality team approach.

Outcomes of rehabilitation depend on the type and severity of the impairment, comorbidities, and physiological reserve. This is coupled with the attitude, personality, and ability to adjust of the person undergoing rehabilitation. Although treatment is focused on the primary disability to enhance residual function, the therapists need to also focus on preventing secondary disabilities.

Although the rehabilitation team has multiple members, the key members are the physical (physio) therapist and occupational therapist. Physical therapists focus on reversing impairments by predominantly using a variety of specialized exercises. Enhancing movement potential is their key specialty. They can be assisted by physical therapy assistants (physical rehabilitation therapists). Occupational therapists focus on improving health and well-being through engagement in occupations that lead to an enhancement in the person's ability to carry out basic and IADLs. Occupational therapists also adapt the individual's environment to make it easier to perform specific activities and undertake home visits with the resident to help identify and fix problems in the home environment.

The speech therapist deals with dysphagia, speech problems, and improving communication in residents with dementia. Nursing plays a central role in motivating residents to use their skills outside of therapy and providing maintenance therapy. The recreation therapist provides both physical and mental exercises to maintain gains. Psychologists and social workers provide psychotherapy and motivation and help work with families. The physician is responsible for identifying the problem that requires therapy and working with the therapist to develop a treatment plan. In the United States, for acute rehabilitation, a number of Medicare regulations limit who can get therapy (Table 9–16), and the physician is responsible for certifying that these are met. Although it is recognized that these criteria limit true rehabilitation potential, the physician needs to legally abide by them. Finally, the dietitian needs to provide adequate high-quality protein (1–1.5 g/kg/day) to allow enhancement of muscle strength.

Table 9–16.	THERAPY SITUATIONS NOT COVERED BY MEDICARE

- Therapy performed repetitively to maintain level of function
- Restorative potential is insignificant in relation to therapy required to achieve such potential
- It has been determined that treatment goals will not materialize
- The therapy performed is considered to be a general exercise program

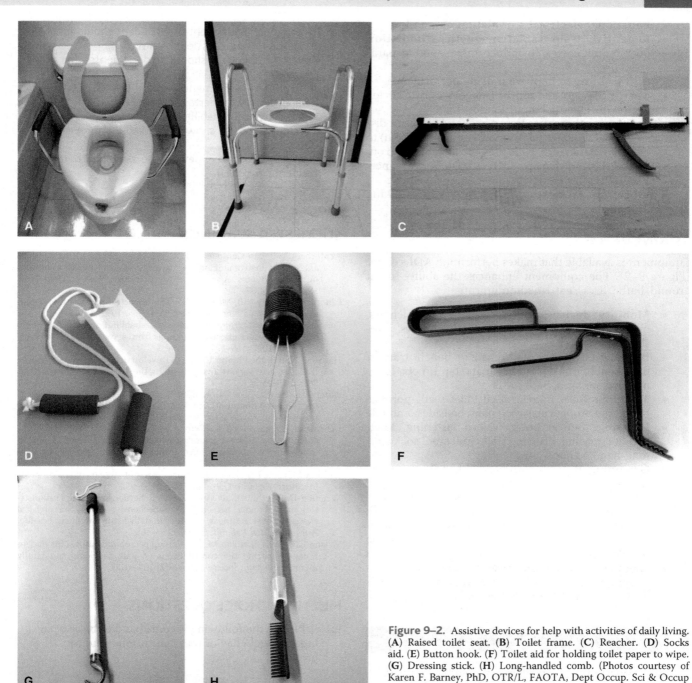

Figure 9–2. Assistive devices for help with activities of daily living. (**A**) Raised toilet seat. (**B**) Toilet frame. (**C**) Reacher. (**D**) Socks aid. (**E**) Button hook. (**F**) Toilet aid for holding toilet paper to wipe. (**G**) Dressing stick. (**H**) Long-handled comb. (Photos courtesy of Karen F. Barney, PhD, OTR/L, FAOTA, Dept Occup. Sci & Occup Therapy, Saint Louis University, St. Louis, Missouri.)

Specific Physical Rehabilitation Techniques

- **Aerobic exercise:** Increasing walking distance and speed aiming at 1 m/s for men and 0.8 m/s for women. The aim should be to be able to walk for 6 minutes with or without an assistive device
- **Resistance exercise:** Progressive training intensity at 40% to 80% of RM (repetition maximum) with one set of 8 repetitions for each limb to three sets of 8 repetitions three times a week

- **Body weight–supported treadmill activity:** Useful for person with strokes but no better than outcomes with a physical therapist
- **Balance exercises:** Standing with the feet together, standing on one leg with the eyes closed, movement training on an obstacle course
- **Biofeedback** to allow visualization of effort and muscle function
- **Constraint-induced movement therapy:** Limits function on the working arm with a sling or mitten

- **Functional electrical stimulation** of muscle
- **Repetitive transcranial magnetic stimulation** over motor cortex to induce movement in paralyzed limb
- **Gait training** to improve walking performance
- **Mirror therapy** and **motor imagery** to help cortex to provide essential input to movement
- **Positioning therapy** to train persons with specific diseases (e.g., shoulder subluxation, contralateral pain) to prevent contractures, pain, pressure ulcers, and so on
- **Task-oriented therapy** such as ADL performance
- **Virtual reality games** to encourage movement
- **Vibration exercises** for persons with walking limitations

Assistive Devices

Equipment is available that makes performing ADLs easier (Figure 9–2). The equipment enhances the ability to get around, bathe, dress, eat, or communicate.

- **Mobility devices:** Canes, walkers, wheelchairs, motorized walkers, motorized wheelchairs, exoskeletons, crutches
- **Bathing:** Grab bars, bath chair or bench, transfer bath bench, nonslip rubber mats, tap timers, long-handled sponges, bath mitts
- **Toileting:** Toilet frame, raised toilet seats, portable bidet, spill proof urinals, bed pans, bedside commode
- **Dressing:** Button hook, Velcro fastening, long-handled reacher, dressing stick, foot stool sock aids, long-handled shoe horn
- **Grooming:** Brushes with padded handle or universal cuff; long-handled comb
- **Eating:** Rocker knife (cut food with one hand), heavy-handled spoon, combined utensil (e.g., fork and knife), adhesive placemats, plate guards, built-up handle, cups with T-shaped handles, attachable handle to add to glass or soft drink can, universal cuff
- **Augmentative communication devices** such as communication boards or electronic devices
- **Low vision and hearing devices**

KEY POINTS

1. Admission to the nursing home should be discussed by all involved, and a choice that is most suitable for the person entering the nursing home should be made.
2. A number of factors play a role in adjustment to the nursing home, and a smooth adjustment requires effort by the resident, family, and nursing staff.
3. Many residents struggle to adapt to the nursing home and may show a variety of behaviors such as anger, dysphoria, apathy, sleep disruption, disorientation, anorexia, falls, and attempts to "escape."
4. The MDS 3.0 is an excellent initial assessment tool.
5. The Geronte is an ideal communication tool for an interprofessional team.

6. The original assessment of a resident should involve the entire interprofessional team.
7. Advanced directives should be documented for all residents.
8. A number of assessments beyond the MDS 3.0 may be appropriate for certain residents.
9. Newer physical rehabilitation techniques are being developed and are showing markedly improved outcomes.
10. A variety of assistive devices are available to improve residents' function.

SUGGESTED READINGS

Achterberg WP, can Campen C, Pot AM, et al. Effects of the resident assessment instrument on the care process and health outcomes in nursing homes. A review of the literature. *Scan J Rehab Med.* 1999;31:131-137.

Chiodo LK, Gerety MB, Mulrow CD. The impact of physical therapy on nursing home patient outcomes. *Phys Ther.* 1992;72:168-173.

Forster A, Lambley R, Young JB. Is physical rehabilitation for older people in long-term care effective? Findings from a systematic review. *Age Ageing.* 2010;39:169-175.

Hawes C, Morris JN, Phillips CD, et al. Development of the nursing home Resident Assessment Instrument in the USA. *Age Ageing.* 1997; 26(S2):19-25.

Hutchinson AM, Milke DL, Maisey S, et al. The Resident Assessment Instrument-Minimum Data Set 2.0 quality indicators: a systematic review. *MBC Health Serv Res.* 2010;10:166-170.

Matusik P, Tomaszewski K, Chmielowska K, et al. Severe frailty and cognitive impairment are related to higher mortality in 12-month follow-up of nursing home residents. *Arch Gerontol Geriatr.* 2012;55(1):22-24.

Smith AE, Crome P. Relocation mosaic: review of 40 years of resettlement literature. *Rev Clin Gerontol.* 2000;10:81-95.

Weening-Dijksterhuis E, de Greef MHG, Scherder EJA, et al. Frail institutionalized older persons: a comprehensive review on physical exercise, physical fitness, activities of daily living and quality-of-life. *Am J Phys Med Rehabil.* 2011;90:156-168.

Wilson CB, Davis S, Nolan M. Developing personal relationships in care homes: realizing the contributions of staff, residents and family members. *Ageing Society.* 2009;29(7):1041-1063.

MULTIPLE CHOICE QUESTIONS

9.1 Which of the following is considered to be a social breakdown behavior that institutions tend to promote?

a. Attempts to "escape"
b. Falls
c. Apathy and submissiveness
d. Disorientation
e. Dysphoria

9.2 Which of the following does not enhance satisfaction of family caregivers when a loved one is in a nursing home?

a. Aid from family and friends
b. Poor self-reported health
c. Nursing home–sponsored support group
d. Incorporation as partners in care process
e. Positive interactions with other residents

9.3 Which of the following items is not covered in the Minimum Data Set (MDS) 3.0?

    a. Payment details
    b. Medications
    c. Patient Health Questionnaire 9.0
    d. Pain
    e. Mobility

9.4 Which rarely used but simple picture of a person is an excellent rapid communication tool in nursing homes?

    a. MDS 2.0
    b. MDS 3.0
    c. Stick figure
    d. Geronte
    e. MoCA

9.5 Which of the following is a component of the FRAIL tool for screening for frailty?

    a. Dyspnea
    b. Pain
    c. Bathing
    d. Fatigue
    e. Continence

Chapter 10

EDUCATION AND RESEARCH

To advance nursing home practice and raise standards of care, it is essential that there is investment in both nursing home education and research. We also need to challenge two deep-rooted assumptions. The first assumption is that practitioners who are unfamiliar with nursing home culture and practice are automatically equipped with the skills and competences they require to work safely and effectively with older vulnerable nursing home residents. The second assumption is that the evidence base required to inform nursing home practice is adequate and can be generalized from studies of non–nursing home resident populations.

We also need to challenge the myth that nursing homes are unsuitable training areas and recognize those that provide excellent care that cannot be observed or understood in other care settings. In the United States, the vast majority of care for complex, vulnerable older people is provided outside of acute care hospitals. Yet much of the training in medical schools and residency programs still occurs in acute care hospitals. The nursing home provides an opportunity for multiple critical learning experiences, including (1) the management of complex, vulnerable older patients with multiple comorbidities and psychosocial as well as medical conditions; (2) understanding what happens to patients when they are discharged from the hospital to a postacute care environment; (3) appreciating the strengths and limitations of care provided in nursing homes, including the critical role of the interdisciplinary team; (4) and gaining a perspective on the regulatory and legal liability issues that are a critical aspect of practicing medicine outside the acute care setting. In many regions with robust quality assurance and regulatory systems, nursing homes are becoming a major resource for education of physicians, nurses, and other health and social care professionals. Nursing homes also represent an ideal situation to introduce students to the complexity and rewards of working with older persons. A great opportunity exists to get to know nursing home residents and their families as individuals and develop a better appreciation of the benefits of person-centered care. In many nursing homes, the complexity of clinical and psychosocial care needs provides a rich set of learning experiences for students and those wishing to advance their geriatric and gerontologic practice skills and competences. From a resident's perspective, meeting students can be a pleasant interlude to relieve the "boredom" of living in a nursing home. As in other care settings, students can provide "extra hands" in providing care. Although preparing for students to come to the nursing home takes commitment, the benefits are plentiful.

Ensuring that the nursing home provides a suitable learning environment for student placement helps to maintain a positive work culture, with quality improvement benefits. Involvement of nursing homes in education is an opportunity for the nursing home to improve its image in the community and increase the awareness of the role nursing homes play in providing high-quality care for older persons. Accreditation to act as a practice placement usually requires the educational institution to assess the quality of the practice and to identify practice mentors who will ensure that the students' learning objectives are satisfied.

An International Association of Gerontology and Geriatrics (IAGG)/World Health Organization (WHO) position paper has strongly advocated a need to increase research in nursing homes. There is recognition that management of diseases and geriatric syndromes in persons with disabilities and dementia requires different approaches, as has been outlined in this book. However, there is a paucity of good-quality research on which care approaches produce the best outcomes. There is also a need to better understand who is admitted to nursing homes and what community services would allow a person to "age in place" in a more cost-effective manner. There is a desperate need for research on how to replace the use of dangerous, ineffective drugs for difficult behaviors with appropriate, feasible behavioral programs and demonstrate their effectiveness. The IAGG/WHO Taskforce paper points out that although many new drugs are used in the nursing home population, they have been rarely tested in this older, vulnerable population. As such, the Taskforce called for a need for controlled drug studies in nursing homes before these drugs are approved for use in older persons.

RESEARCH

Research is essential to improving the quality of nursing home care, the quality of life of nursing home residents, and staff satisfaction with their jobs through evidence-informed changes. In most chapters within this book, we identify gaps in current knowledge and highlight research opportunities and priorities. Nursing home research can take many forms from explorations of culture and resident

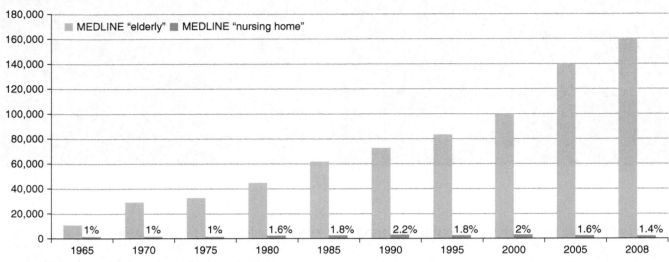

Figure 10–1. Research in nursing home is scarce in 2009.

experiences to the testing of new healthcare technologies, medications, and nonpharmacologic interventions. In general, there is a scarcity of nursing home research (Figure 10–1). Figure 10–2 provides a graphic description of key issues that have been addressed in nursing home research. The most highly cited articles in nursing home research in the *Journal* of *American Medical Directors Association* (*JAMDA*) are given in Table 10–1. A myriad of other issues also warrant investigation in the nursing home setting.

Although a number of small studies (usually focused on a single nursing home) have shown that certain best-care practices will improve care, there is a paucity of multisite randomized controlled trials (RCTs) that have demonstrated that specific interventions will improve care (Figure 10–3). Epidemiologic studies have focused on describing trends in nursing home populations, and a plethora of small-scale studies have qualitatively examined a range of nursing strategies and resident experiences, but few robust trials have been attempted that increase knowledge about resident outcomes and nursing-sensitive

indicators. There is also a dearth of major implementation studies that demonstrate how research-based interventions can be translated into practice within nursing homes. Furthermore, there is limited evidence about the impacts of new nursing home roles and the most effective methods to educate and prepare practitioners to work in and to lead nursing homes.

At present, most studies reported from nursing homes are observational studies that may include case control or cross-sectional studies. Very few RCTs have been conducted in nursing homes (see Figure 10–3), yet these are the gold standard for producing evidence-based medicine. Even when these trials have been conducted, most are of 3 months or less duration. For a true evidence base to exist, there should be at least two RCTs examining the same intervention. At present, there are inadequate data to produce a true meta-analysis to allow the development of high-quality evidence-based recommendations for nursing home care. Many studies that have provided information on quality care are of the "quality improvement" type. Within a facility, high-quality "continuous quality improvement" studies often have become the publications on which we are presently basing our care practices.

There are numerous challenges to overcome for high-quality research to occur in nursing homes (Table 10–2). Although some of these challenges are more in perception than reality, many of them represent clear barriers to research in nursing homes. In addition, many institutional review boards (IRBs; ethics approval committees) have little insight into nursing homes and the challenges involved in undertaking research in nursing homes. A major positive is the Minimum Data Set (MDS) 3.0, which will greatly improve the quality of outcome data in nursing homes. For research to be successful in nursing homes, there is a need for the development of networks of researchers and nursing homes to allow multisite, high-quality studies to be undertaken. The American Medical Directors Association (AMDA) Foundation has put a large amount of time into identifying and training physicians to

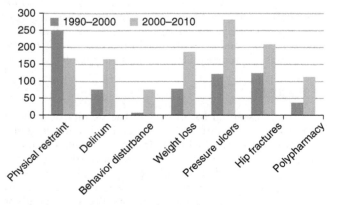

Figure 10–2. Key issues in nursing homes and research.

Table 10–1. ALL TIME TOP 10 *JOURNAL OF AMERICAN MEDICAL DIRECTORS ASSOCIATION* ARTICLES BASED ON GOOGLE SCHOLAR

No.	Year	Authors	Subject	Citations (*n*)
1	2003	Warden et al.	Develop pain assessment scale	304
2	2005	Vu et al.	Falls in the nursing home	126
3	2006	Bostick et al.	Review of staffing and quality in nursing home	104
4	2003	Villaneuva et al.	Pain assessment ... dementing elderly	97
5	2005	Oliver et al.	End-of-life care U.S. nursing homes	87
6	2008	Rolland et al.	Physical activity or Alzheimer's disease	86
7	2008	Abellan van Kan et al.	Frailty: Toward a clinical definition	80
8	2003	Baum et al.	Effectiveness of a group exercise program	74
9	2004	Mitchell et al.	Tube feeding versus hand feeding	71
10	2007	Rockwood et al.	How should we grade frailty?	71

Source: Statistics from Google Scholar. Accessed July 14, 2012.

undertake multicenter nursing home research. The AMDA has had some success in doing a series of smaller studies but has also recognized the difficulties in successfully carrying out research in nursing homes. A highly successful development of a nursing home research network is the *Reseau de Recherche en Etablissement d'Hebergement pour Persones Agees* (REHPA). REHPA is a research network of 240 nursing homes and the department of geriatrics of Toulouse University Hospital. Its purpose is to compensate for the lack of evidence-based research in nursing homes. The investigators have found that this research program has been successful because it has targeted areas that are perceived to be clinically relevant.

It is important to recognize that there are many costs to the nursing home when research is conducted in the facility. The potential costs of research in nursing homes are listed in Table 10–3. These costs need to

be discussed with the nursing home administration and agreed upon before the research budget is prepared. It is becoming less realistic for the nursing homes in multisite studies to bear these costs, and there needs to be a mechanism to reimburse their costs. Some advantages of funded research in the nursing home include extra help to perform comprehensive geriatric assessments and to organize specific interventions. Nursing homes in which research is being undertaken may be more attractive to high-quality geriatricians and nursing staff.

Table 10–2. CHALLENGES FACED IN DEVELOPING HIGH QUALITY RESEARCH IN NURSING HOMES

- Ethical issues in obtaining informed consent from cognitively impaired individuals
- Lack of enthusiasm by administrators, directors of nursing, staff, family, and residents about research
- Belief that researchers are using a vulnerable population for their own benefit
- High dropout level because of hospitalizations, transfer to another facility or home, acute illnesses, or death
- Questionable quality of nursing home records
- Lack of availability of specialized equipment such as a dual-energy X-ray absorptiometry for bone or sarcopenic studies or cardiac ultrasonography for cardiovascular studies
- Need for multiple sites to obtain a large enough sample size
- Assessment of nursing home residents is time consuming compared with other persons
- Costs to the facility that need to be reimbursed
- Inadequate research support from funding agencies and the pharmaceutical industry

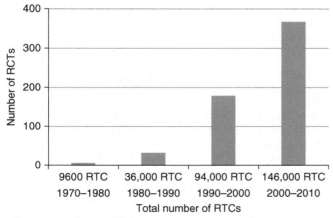

Figure 10–3. High quality research in nursing homes.

Table 10–3.	COST OF RESEARCH TO THE NURSING HOME

- Administrative time in discussing and developing the protocol
- Disruption of usual care routines
- Preparing and transporting residents to research activities
- Identifying surrogates and witnessing informed consent
- Providing information on functional status
- Answering questions of residents and families
- Minor supplies, space, and telephones used by research staff
- Assisting in administering treatment protocols
- Assisting in assessing outcomes

Adapted from *Medical Care in the Nursing Home.*

An important issue in research in nursing homes is the maintenance of fidelity between sites. This requires making certain that the intervention has been implemented as intended. This requires a motivational intervention and high-quality training of the involved staff before the study is initiated. In addition, there needs to be continuous monitoring of the fidelity of the intervention during the study. Finally, all studies need to have a measurements of fidelity included in the final assessment of the intervention.

Similar to many areas of medicine and nursing, most nursing homes implement only a few of the best-care practices that are available via research and organizational practice guidelines. The reasons for this are many. Many research interventions and guidelines are not considered to be useful by nursing home staff. A number of other reasons for failed dissemination have also been suggested (Table 10–4). There is a need for research into the best methods of successful dissemination (see education section of this chapter). Dissemination can be further helped by advocacy organizations, such as the National Coalition on Advancing Excellence in American's Nursing Homes (http://www.nhqualitycampaign.org).

Many persons working in nursing homes have little experience in doing research and even when they complete

Table 10–4.	REASONS WHY BEST-CARE PRACTICES BASED ON RESEARCH ARE NOT IMPLEMENTED

- Not perceived as an improvement
- Incompatible with existing practices
- Difficult to understand and use
- Increase workload without adequate resources
- Do not demonstrate easily visible results
- Can be introduced on a limited trial basis
- Difficult to implement
- Require a change in staff beliefs
- Lack of organizational support
- Poor communication of new research findings
- Payers slow to reward best practices

Table 10–5.	KEYS TO CONDUCTING SUCCESSFUL RESEARCH IN THE NURSING HOME

- Make sure the research is supported by the administrator and staff.
- Hold a family and resident meeting to enlist their support.
- Design a project that is scientifically sound with limited risk that is clinically useful.
- Consider conducting quality improvement research as opposed to traditional controlled trials.
- Train the staff to perform the tasks necessary.
- Reward the staff involved in the study (e.g., thank them, have a pizza party, give fiscal reimbursement).
- Try out the protocol before starting the study.
- Use clear criteria for informed consent. (The decision for which residents can make their own decisions without use of a surrogate should be based on objective criteria.)
- Make sure all costs to the facility are covered or the facility agreed to assume them.
- Provide feedback on the outcomes of the study to administration, staff, family, and residents.

a laudable project become blocked at writing a publishable article. *JAMDA* now has the highest impact factor of all clinical geriatric journals. The editorial staff prides itself on working with junior authors to develop publishable studies. They have published guidelines for writing an article for *JAMDA*.

Table 10–5 provides an approach to performing successful research in nursing homes. Make sure that all research is approved by the appropriate IRB (ethics committee) even if it is conducted as quality improvement research and informed consent has been waived. Data collection strategies should be pilot tested in a nursing home to ensure that data you wish to collect are available. Explain to the staff, family, and residents the potential benefit of the project to those involved. Projects should have limited risks to residents, and if major risks are possible, an independent data review board needs to be created. A written memorandum of understanding between the administration and the investigator should be created. This should delineate what indirect costs to the facility will be reimbursed. At the end of the study, the results should be provided to the staff, residents, and family.

QUALITY IMPROVEMENT PROJECTS VERSUS HUMAN RESEARCH

Many important research questions in the nursing home setting relate to improving the quality of care and costs. These studies may be conducted as quality improvement projects rather than research requiring informed consent. Although there are advantages to this approach and it is recognized that high-quality improvement projects can provide useful information, it also has disadvantages. In general, these studies lack the rigorous design of high-quality research and the lack of a control group means these studies fail to prove true effectiveness or necessarily identify the key reasons that were responsible for the interventions being effective. The SQUIRE (Standards for Quality Improvement Reporting Excellence; http://squire-statement.org) guidelines provide an approach to developing and reporting quality improvement research. Consultation with an IRB should be undertaken to determine the need for informed consent.

SERVICE USER INVOLVEMENT IN NURSING HOME RESEARCH

The drive for public and patient involvement in research is gaining momentum in some countries, and as nursing home research is developed, it is important that attention is given to resident and family participation. Involvement of residents, family members, and staff in designing the research can foster new ways of framing research questions that address the fundamental concerns of nursing home residents and those who care for them. If we buy into resident-centered philosophies for care, then it follows that resident involvement in research should be embraced. In the 1980s, emerging ideas about user-led and user-controlled research generated some interesting and heated discussion among medical and healthcare scientific communities. Although there are understandably few examples of nursing home resident–led research, there is no reason why family members and staff cannot pursue and direct research if given the opportunity and support to do so. In the 1990s, many Westernized nations promoted active citizenship, and the concept of expert patients emerged. In the United Kingdom, advances in service user involvement in research have led researchers to factor in user engagement strategies within funding applications. Indeed, user involvement in research as part of the overall research metrics is a growing international trend. In the United States, "community-based participatory research" is being encouraged and funded by the federal government. Although underdeveloped in nursing home research, numerous accounts suggest that the use of experiential service user knowledge enhances the quality of research.

In theory, at least nursing home residents and family members can be involved at all stages of the research process as noted below:

- Suggesting topics for research
- Selective contributions to the development of research proposals
- Advising on methods and the best ways to approach data collection
- Preparing accessible participants information sheets and consent forms
- Advocating for studies and promoting recruitment
- Assisting selectively with data analysis and interpretation of findings
- Dissemination activities to nursing home communities and the public

Involvement can take many forms, and when inviting people to serve on stakeholder reference groups or as part of a research team, it is important to equip these participants with the necessary skills and confidence to make a meaningful contribution.

EDUCATION

Education in the nursing home industry comes in two forms, macro and micro. As was pointed out in the research section of this chapter, the ability to disseminate new research and incorporate it into care in the nursing home is a complex and difficult task (Table 10–6). Macro education is the processes necessary to efficiently carry out this dissemination at a national level (see Table 10–6).

Macro education begins with the publication of a study in a major geriatric journal (Table 10–7). This knowledge is then disseminated at major meetings and through newsletters, review articles, and the Internet. The AMDA provides further dissemination through its Certified American Directors course. Numerous local continuing education meetings further disseminate the information. Textbooks such as this one represent another method of providing consolidated data. The IAGG has piloted a certificate course for nursing home professionals in China and Hong Kong and in a mini form in India. An online version of this certificate is available in conjunction with this book. Online courses with individual topic-based modules that are endorsed or accredited by national organizations can facilitate rapid and consistent dissemination of educational interventions. Many nursing home chains hold meetings for their nursing, medical, and administrative leadership, which can serve as an additional strategy for regional and national dissemination. A second component of macro education is the universities and colleges that train the professionals who will work in nursing homes. This represents a "bottom-up" educational approach in which the recently qualified students bring new information with them. A final form of macro education is detailing of new medications, devices, and other technologies by well-trained and experienced sales representatives from industry.

Table 10–6.	PROCESS NECESSARY TO CHANGE NURSING HOME PRACTICE ON A NATIONAL LEVEL

- Obtain support from major national organizations
- Have organizations endorse a best practice and publicize it
- Mass media: Journal articles and newsletters, conferences, webinars, newspapers, and television
- Internet as an interactive process
- Development of national leaders to carry the interpersonal messages and act as change agents
- Obtain support from the owners or administrators of nursing home chains
- Obtain change in regulations or nursing home inspection process
- Consider innovative dissemination methods such as the Community of Practice
- Alter payment systems to make the innovation cost effective

Table 10–7.   EXAMPLES OF JOURNALS AND MEETINGS THAT PROVIDE DISSEMINATION OF NEW NURSING HOME KNOWLEDGE

Journals	Meetings
Journal of the American Medical Directors Association	American Medical Directors Association Annual Meeting
Journal of the American Geriatrics Society	American Geriatrics Society Annual Meeting
Journal of Nutrition, Health, and Aging	International Association of Nutrition and Aging Meetings
Age and Ageing	International Association of Gerontology and Geriatrics Meeting
International Journal of Geriatric Psychiatry	British Geriatrics Society
BMC Geriatrics	European Geriatric Medicine Society Meeting
American Journal of Geriatric Psychiatry	National Gerontological Society
Journal of Gerontological Nursing	Gerontological Advanced Practice Nurses Association
Geriatric Nursing	Canadian Geriatrics Society
McKnight's Long Term Care	NADONALTC Annual
News and Assisted Living	
International Journal of Nursing Older People	

Because of the difficulties in disseminating knowledge in nursing homes, innovative approaches are needed. One such approach is the Community of Practice (CoP) model, which has been adapted from industry and was recommended by the IAGG/WHO position paper.

In its simplest form, a CoP is a group of people who share a common concern or area of practice and who deepen their knowledge and expertise in this area by interacting on an ongoing basis. Group maturity is achieved through four processes: identity building, social interaction, knowledge sharing, and knowledge creation. Knowledge creation includes developing new approaches to practice and practice-based problem solving that are highly relevant to nursing home teams striving to introduce evidence-informed changes to practice. As the CoP matures, it builds its capability for improvement and innovation through sharing knowledge, finding and sharing solutions and developing resources (toolkits for practice) that embody the *accumulated* group knowledge. In general, this requires both face-to-face meetings and an online platform to be successful.

CoPs can form organically or can be cultivated, and they may have clarity of purpose or their goals might evolve overtime. A recent systematic review that endorsed the potential of CoPs for driving practice change in health and social care cautioned that it is not enough to simply form a group and call it a CoP. To derive the benefits for deliverable practice-based change, the group must behave as a CoP, as exemplified in the four processes noted above.

When the CoP behaves as a CoP, it can provide a new form of practice leadership, creating a transformational change dynamic that most teams find energizing.

An improvement model using CoP as a vehicle for learning about and delivering best practice within nursing homes has been developed through a decade of research in the United Kingdom. The so-called Caledonian improvement model includes three core elements, which provide the dimensions and mechanisms to support practice improvement and culture change: (1) infrastructure and communication mechanisms, (2) knowledge conversion processes, and (3) learning and development processes. A facilitator steers the transformational learning journey, beginning with confidence building activities and cultivating CoP behaviors. Values reconciliation focuses application of an agreed value base to daily work situations in relation to the aspect of practice targeted for improvement (e.g., oral healthcare or falls prevention), as well as to interactions with residents and family members. CoP members benchmark current practice against evidence-based best practice protocols and action plans and are guided through their choice of change strategies. Implementation solutions are rehearsed and compared across the CoP to efficiently identify the best ways to improve and change the behaviors of colleagues. Outcome data are collected appropriate to the change project, including resident-centered case studies, which are shared and critically reflected upon as a group. CoP members share and collaboratively develop their change and practice leadership skills as they learn from one another to overcome barriers to change. Nursing home CoPs can function as real—face-to-face communities or virtually via Internet-based collaborative workplaces—or in blended models that combine both approaches. Many homes may not have adequate numbers of computers to support online education, which presents a barrier to this strategy.

In the United States, the CoP approach has been successfully piloted by St. Louis University with the Veterans Administration and the NHC nursing home chain.

At the micro level, the focus is on education within a single nursing home. A key is training nurses' aides (healthcare assistants). These individuals often have minimal educational background and may also face language barriers. As Nolan and Keady state: "Training should be integrated with, and embedded within, an overall philosophy of care from which aims, objectives and procedures are derived."

Basic needs of a training course for nurses' aides are outlined in Table 10–8. There is a need for development of high-quality online courses for nurses' aides, as well as onsite bedside case-based teaching. Education in improving clinical skills can be given by advanced nurse practitioners and physicians. One example of an educational and clinical practice tool that can be used by nurses' aides is the "Stop

Table 10–8.   CORE KNOWLEDGE AND SKILLS FOR NURSES' AIDES (ASSISTANTS)

- Core values of caring for vulnerable residents
- Basic nursing care
  - Dressing
  - Feeding
  - Washing
  - Transferring
- Basic nursing assessment
- Care planning
- Understanding of the individual's history and its contribution to their present self
- Promotion of independence in activity
- Understanding of meaningful activities
- Skin care
- Communication skills with older persons
- Understanding and recognizing dementia, delirium, and depression
- Management of confusion and difficult behaviors
- Incontinence
- Constipation
- Falls risk identification and interventions
- Recognition of early illness
- Working with families
- Elder abuse
- Recognition of lines of authority and resources for help

care also provides an opportunity for students to understand what happens to patients discharged from the hospital and all of the complexities of transitions in care. A study from the Netherlands pointed out the strength of a nursing home experience in building emotional learning for medical students. A survey of medical students in the United States found that 38% felt uneasy about caring for older persons in nursing homes. Although teaching students in nursing homes is generally well accepted, a number of barriers have been identified:

- Nursing home often at a distance from academic center
- Lack of acceptance or respect for geriatrics
- Lack of adequately trained teachers or mentors
- Ability to provide one-on-one supervision
- Conflicting priorities with curricula needs for other specialties

Similarly, there are a number of advantages for including nursing homes in the medical resident (registrar) training. In the United States, a survey of internal medicine residency programs found that 67% had a required nursing home component and 97% in family medicine (general practitioner) training programs. There is much disagreement regarding whether block or longitudinal experience produce a better outcome. Block rotations in geriatrics have been shown to improve geriatric knowledge, skills, and attitudes as have longitudinal rotations. Table 10–9 compares block versus longitudinal rotations. A number of educational domains that are now required for medical

and Watch" Early Warning Tool that is a fundamental component of the INTERACT quality improvement program (http://interact2.net). This tool is designed for use by nurses' aides (as well as other direct care staff) to recognize early changes in condition and communicate them effectively to the licensed nurses. Research into best methods to educate and motivate nursing assistants is a major need.

The education of other health professionals (e.g., social workers, rehabilitation therapists, pharmacists, dietitians, administrators) comes in part by involvement in interdisciplinary rounds and continuous quality improvement meetings. However, the majority of their education comes from their professional organizations.

Nursing homes are from many perspectives an ideal environment to teach physicians and medical students at all levels of their training. Nursing homes provide an excellent opportunity to teach medical students the basics of history taking and examination. Time is usually not of the essence for nursing home residents, allowing the student to do a full history and examination. Residents in nursing homes usually have not only interesting symptoms but also a variety of signs. There is ample opportunity for students to learn to communicate with individuals with visual, hearing, and cognitive impairments. More formal rotations either in block form or as a longitudinal experience give the student ample opportunity to learn how to carry out a comprehensive geriatric assessment, as well as to manage a variety of conditions that occur in older persons. Postacute

Table 10–9.   COMPARISON BETWEEN BLOCK AND LONGITUDINAL ROTATIONS IN NURSING HOMES FOR EDUCATING MEDICAL RESIDENTS (REGISTRARS)

Block	Longitudinal
Repeated exposures in short time (4 weeks)	Intermittent exposures over 1–3 years
Intensive exposure	Less intensive
More didactics	Less didactics
No primary care role	Primary care role
Management of acute problems	Often miss acute problems
No opportunity to observe changes over time	Opportunity to follow time course of diseases
Faculty readily available	Variable availability of faculty
Rounds part of rotation	Difficult to find set time for rounds
More observation of interdisciplinary and administrative issues	May miss interdisciplinary and administrative issues

Table 10–10.	EDUCATIONAL DOMAINS EASILY TAUGHT IN LONG-TERM CARE

- Quality improvement
- Interprofessional teamwork
- Group dynamics
- Health systems
- Transitions of care

resident (registrar) training are often more easily taught in a nursing home setting (Table 10–10).

Nursing home rotations are a component of the training for advanced geriatric trainees in the United States. In 2011, there were 301 trainees in the 148 programs. Sixty percent of the trainees were international medical graduates. There were 187 positions that were unfilled. Thus, there is a major need to increase the number of geriatric trainees in the United States. In most other countries, the requirement for a nursing home experience is variable. In Holland, trainees can train especially to be nursing home physicians. Table 10–11 lists the educational and attitudinal objectives of a nursing home rotation for trainees in geriatric medicine.

Table 10–11.	EDUCATIONAL AND ATTITUDINAL OBJECTIVES OF A NURSING HOME ROTATION FOR TRAINEES IN GERIATRIC MEDICINE

- Improve the ability to care for nursing home residents.
- Understand how to evaluate and manage common problems in nursing home residents.
- Learn rehabilitation techniques.
- Learn to work in interprofessional teams.
- Recognize the importance of care transitions.
- Develop competence in the continuous quality improvement process.
- Understand the role of inter-RAI and MDS 3.0.
- Be able to help train other health professionals in the nursing home.
- Understand administrative issues, including the role of nursing home inspections.
- Recognize that illness and disability are not inevitable consequences of aging.
- Goals of nursing home care can differ from other settings.
- Caring rather than curing is the most appropriate goal.
- Small changes in function can make large changes in quality of life.
- An interprofessional approach is essential for effective care.
- Recognize common ethical and legal issues in the nursing home.

MDS, minimum data set; RAI, resident assessment instrument.
Adapted from *Medical Care in the Nursing Home.*

SUGGESTED READINGS

Abellan van Kan G, Rolland YM, Morley JE, Vellas B. Frailty: toward a clinical definition. *J Am Med Dir Assoc.* 2008;9:71-72.

Baum EE, Jarjoura D, Polen AE, et al. Effectiveness of a group exercise program in a long-term care facility: a randomized pilot trial. *J Am Med Dir Assoc.* 2003;4:74-80.

Baum EE, Nelson KM. The effect of a 12-month longitudinal long-term care rotation on knowledge and attitudes of internal medicine residents about geriatrics. *J Am Med Dir Assoc.* 2007;8:105-109.

Bostick JE, Rantz MJ, Flesner MK, Riggs CT. Systematic review of studies of staffing and quality in nursing homes. *J Am Med Dir Assoc.* 2006;7:366-376.

Buhr GT, Paniagua MA. Update on teaching in the long-term care setting. *Clin Geriatr Med.* 2011;27:199-211.

Fitzpatrick JM, Roberts JD. Challenges for care homes: education and training of healthcare assistants. *Br J Nurs.* 2004;13:1258.

Grady MJ, Earll JM. Teaching physical diagnosis in the nursing home. *Am J Med.* 1990;88:519-521.

Helmich E, Bolhuis S, Prins J, et al. Emotional learning of undergraduate medical students in an early nursing attachment in a hospital or nursing home. *Med Teach* 2011;33:e594-e601.

Google Scholar. http://scholar.google.com/scholar?q=JAMDA+most+cited+articles&hl=en&as_sdt=1%2C26. Accessed July 14, 2012.

Karlawish JH, Hougham GW, Stocking CB, Sachs GA. What is the quality of the reporting of research ethics in publications of nursing home research? *J Am Geriatr Soc.* 1999;47:76-81.

Li LC, Grimshaw JM, Nielsen C, et al. Use of communities of practice in business and health care sectors: a systematic review. *Implement Sci.* 2009;4:27.

Mayo-Smith MF, Gordon V, Gillie E, Brett A. Teaching physical diagnosis in the nursing home: a prospective, controlled trial. *J Am Geriatr Soc.* 1991;39:1085-1088.

Messinger-Rapport BJ, Gammack J, Thomas DR. Writing an article for a geriatrics journal: guidelines from the Journal of the American Medical Directors Association. *J Am Med Dir Assoc.* 2008;9:4-8.

Mitchell SL, Buchanan JL, Littlehale S, Hamel MB. Tube-feeding versus hand-feeding nursing home residents with advanced dementia: a cost comparison. *J Am Med Dir Assoc.* 2004;5(2 suppl):S22-S29.

Nolan MR, Keady J. Training in long-term care: the road to better quality. *Rev Clin Gerontol.* 1996;6:333-342.

Oliver DP, Porock D, Zweig S. End of life care in U.S. nursing homes: a review of the evidence. *J Am Med Dir Assoc.* 2005;6(3 suppl): S21-S30.

Rahman AN, Applebaum RA, Schnelle JF, Simmons SF. Translating research into practice in nursing homes: can we close the gap? *Gerontologist.* 2012;52(5):597-606.

Resnick B, Cayo J, Galik E, Pretzer-Aboff I. Implementation of the 6-week educational component in the Res-Care intervention: process and outcomes. *J Contin Educ Nurs.* 2009;40:353-360.

Resnick B, Gruber-Baldini AL, Zimmerman S, et al. Nursing home resident outcomes from the Res-Care intervention. *J Am Geriatr Soc.* 2009;57:1156-1165.

Resnick B, Simpson M, Bercovitz A, et al. Testing of the Res-Care pilot intervention: impact of nursing assistants. *Geriatri Nurs.* 2004;25: 292-297.

Rockwood K, Abeysundera MJ, Mitnitski A. How should we grade frailty in nursing home patients? *J Am Med Dir Assoc.* 2007;8:595-603.

Rolland YM, Abellan van Kan G, Vellas B. Physical activity and Alzheimer's disease: from prevention to therapeutic perspective. *J Am Med Dir Assoc.* 2008;9:390-405.

Staley K. *Exploring Impact; Public Involvement in NHS, Public Health and Social Care Research.* Eastleigh, UK: INVOLVE; 2009.

Tolson D, Lowndes A, Booth J, et al. The potential of Communities of Practice to promote evidence informed practice within nursing homes. *J Am Med Dir Assoc.* 2001;12(3):161-242.

Turner M, Beresford P. *User Controlled Research: Its Meanings and Potential. Final Report. INVOLVE, Shaping Our Lives and the Centre for Citizen Participation.* Easleigh, UK: Brunel University, INVOLVE; 2005.

Villaneuva MR, Smith L, Erickson JS, et al. Pain assessment for the dementing elderly (PADE): reliability and validity of a new measure. *J Am Med Dir Assoc.* 2003;4:1-8.

Vu MQ, Weintraub N, Rubenstein LZ. Falls in the nursing home: are they preventable? *J Am Med Dir Assoc.* 2005;6(3 suppl):S82-S87.

Warden V, Hurley AC, Volicer L. Development and psychometric evaluation of Pain Assessment in Advanced Dementia (PAINAD) scale. *J Am Med Dir Assoc.* 2003;4:9-15.

White HK. The nursing home in long-term care education. *J Am Med Dir Assoc.* 2008;9:75-81.

Wiener M, Shamaskin A. The nursing home as a site for teaching medical students. *Acad Med.* 1990;65:412-414.

MULTIPLE CHOICE QUESTIONS

10.1 Which of the following was *not* a key issue in nursing home research between 2001 and 2010?

   a. Pressure ulcers
   b. Weight loss
   c. Hip fractures
   d. Chronic obstructive pulmonary disease
   e. Delirium

10.2 Nursing homes tend to implement most of the best-care practices that exist.

   a. True
   b. False

10.3 Which of the following is true concerning randomized controlled trials in nursing homes?

   a. Many such trials have been conducted.
   b. Most trials are of 3 months or less duration.
   c. It is easy to do a meta-analysis to support best practices in nursing homes.
   d. Many trials concern testing new drugs before they are released.

10.4 Which of the following is true concerning the Community of Practice approach?

   a. It requires little infrastructure.
   b. It is not evidence based.
   c. It involves distance learning.
   d. It is not a culture change process.

10.5 Almost all medical students are comfortable caring for older persons in nursing homes.

   a. True
   b. False

Part 3
MANAGING AGE-RELATED SYNDROMES AND CHANGES

Chapter 11

ACHES AND PAINS: MANAGING PAIN IN THE NURSING HOME

Pain is what the person says it is and exists wherever he or she says it does.

—Margo McCaffey

The experience of pain at whatever stage of life has far-reaching consequences for the individual in terms of function, ability to fully participate in activities, and quality of life. There is increasing recognition that access to pain management is a fundamental human right, and some have described pain as the fifth vital sign (in addition to pulse, respiration, blood pressure, and temperature).

Pain is often thought of as a sensation but is more accurately conceived of as a perception (similar to vision, hearing, smell, or touch) and as such is subject to the same kind of influences (e.g., memory, mood, context, culture). It is well known that some people can experience pain (and display all the physiologic responses associated with pain) in the absence of tissue damage, and others have evident major tissue damage and yet report no pain. Acute pain is relatively short lived and is often associated with tissue damage resulting from injury, some diseases, and transient conditions common in later life such as constipation. For these reasons, acute pain is said to be a biologic alert system that something is wrong, prompting the individual to take corrective action. In contrast, chronic and enduring pain serves no such simple biologic alert function but does have severe emotional and physical consequences for the individual. Realizing that a resident may be in pain is straightforward if the person can tell you, or if his or her visitors or staff recognizes their distress. However, not all pain is reported or recognized among nursing home residents for a variety of reasons.

Pain is extremely common in nursing homes. However, the reported prevalence of pain varies widely throughout the world from 7.8% to 72% (Table 11–1). This is accounted for by both cultural attitudes to pain and varying quality of assessment methods. In most parts of the world, pain is underestimated. Many older persons tolerate pain because it is seen as a normal part of aging.

Persons with pain are more likely to be dysphoric or frankly depressed. Pain limits nursing home residents' mobility, ability to carry out activities of daily living, and involvement in other activities. Pain has also been associated with a loss of cognitive ability. The Institute of Medicine in the United States has enunciated a series of principles for managing pain (Table 11–2).

A number of different types of pain have been identified (Table 11–3). It is important that the cause of pain is identified to allow appropriate management. In addition, numerous factors modulate the central perception of pain (Figure 11–1). These factors need to be taken into account when developing a pain management system. In older persons joint aches are the most common form of pain, followed by back ache, headache, and muscle pains.

PAIN ASSESSMENT

It is now clearly demonstrated that the use of faces, verbal , and visual analog scales is essential to fully document pain in cognitively intact older persons (Figure 11–2). Just asking about pain or documenting a nursing or physician opinion is inadequate. In persons with cognitive impairment, nonverbal pain signs need to be carefully observed and recorded (Table 11–4).

Evaluation of pain requires accepting the resident's view of the severity of the pain. Pain needs to be asked about regularly (at least once a shift). It needs to be recognized that when a resident is isolated, addressing psychological and social problems will reduce both physical and intrapsychic pain. Nonverbal pain signs need to be noticed. Several scales have been developed for this purpose, and the Minimum Data Set (MDS) 3.0 contains resident- and staff-based assessments of pain. Pain characteristics (including type, radiation, and associated symptoms such as sweating) need to be evaluated. Finally whether or not the pain impairs function needs to be recorded. The PAINED mnemonic is a useful tool to remember the steps in evaluating pain (Table 11–5).

PAIN MANAGEMENT

Management of pain should use the modified World Health Organization's (WHO's) analgesic pyramid (Figure 11–3). Factors that have been found to improve pain management in nursing homes are models that use a systematic implementation of this approach, algorithms that lead to clinical decision making, interprofessional involvement including the resident as a member of the care team, continuous evaluation of the program, and onsite consultation with a pain specialist. Numerous nonpharmacologic pain management strategies have been used. Although there is a variable

Table 11–1.   THE REPORTED PREVALENCE OF PAIN AMONG NURSING HOME RESIDENTS IN DIFFERENT PARTS OF THE WORLD

Country	Prevalence (%)
Iran	72
Holland	69
Taiwan	59
Finland	57
Norway	55
United States	15–50
Canada	49
England	37
Sweden	33
Italy	32
Scotland	32
Ireland	27
Singapore	14
Germany	7

Table 11–3.   DIFFERENT TYPES OF PAIN

Psychological
- Dysphoric
- Anxiety
- Somatization

Nonspecific
- Tension headaches
- Brain headaches

Vascular
- Migraines
- Ischemia
- Angina

Neuropathic
- Peripheral
- Central
  - Thalamic
  - Radiculopathies

Nociceptive
- Trauma
- Pressure
- Inflammation
- Ischemia

evidence base for these approaches, many seem to produce an excellent placebo response (Table 11–6). For example, many bitemporal headaches in older persons are attributable to cervical osteophytes causing neck muscle spasm. These headaches can be alleviated by hard neck massage. It is important to recognize that placebo has been shown to have an effect on reducing pain through the endogenous opioid system. As such, whenever an analgesic is given, the nurse should tell the resident that it will improve his or her pain. This is particularly important in cognitively impaired residents.

For many older persons, regular (as opposed to as needed) use of acetaminophen (paracetamol) is more effective for chronic pain relief. Acetaminophen is safe in doses from 2000 to 3000 mg/day. Persons with liver disease should not use acetaminophen. Acetaminophen can interact with

Table 11–2.   PRINCIPLES FOR MANAGING PAIN AS ENUNCIATED BY THE INSTITUTE OF MEDICINE

- Pain management is a professional responsibility and the duty of all persons in the health professions.
- Chronic pain should be considered a disease entity on its own.
- Interprofessional approaches produce the best outcomes to treating chronic pain.
- Chronic pain is disruptive of an individual's life.
- Present knowledge concerning pain management is not always used effectively, resulting in many persons suffering needlessly.
- Opiates, when prescribed and appropriately monitored, can be safe and effective. Fear of diversion and abuse should not limit their use.
- Clinician–person relationships play an important role in the effectiveness of pain management programs.

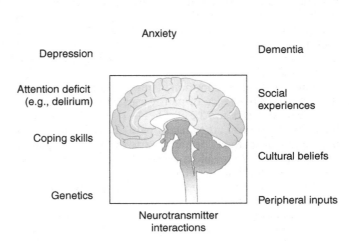

Figure 11–1. Modalities that modulate the perception of pain in the nursing home. (Morley JE. Pain—God's megaphone. *J Am Med Dir Assoc.* 2012;13:316-318. Copyright 2012, with permission from Elsevier.)

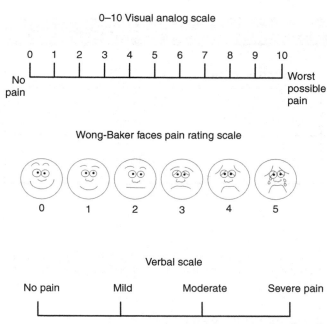

Figure 11–2. Pain rating scales. (Reprinted with permission from Hockenberry MJ, Wilson D, Winkelstein ML. *Wong's Essentials of Pediatric Nursing.* 8th ed. St. Louis; 2009. Used with permission. Copyright Mosby.)

Table 11–4. NONVERBAL SIGNS OF PAIN	
Behavior	**Responses**
Altered activity	More or less sleep or rest
	Reduced social interaction
	Insomnia
	Decreased activities of daily living
	Decreased mobility
	Limited movement of a limb
Facial expressions	Tears
	Frowns
	Grimaces
	Shutting eyes
	Staring
Aggression	Verbal
	Biting
	Hitting
Vocal behaviors	Screaming
	Crying
Body movements	Rocking
	Pulling legs to chest
	Holding one part of body
	Head movements
	Rigidity
Others	Withdrawal
	Irritability
	Delirium

Table 11–5. THE "PAINED" MNEMONIC EVALUATION OF PAIN
Pain is real (believe the resident)
Ask about pain regularly
Isolation (social and psychological problems)
Notice nonverbal pain signs
Evaluate pain characteristics
Does pain impair function?

warfarin and increase the international normalized ratio. Nonsteroidal antiinflammatory drugs (NSAIDs) have many potential serious adverse effects among nursing home residents. They increase the risk of gastrointestinal bleeding, myocardial infarction, and stroke. NSAIDs also cause salt and water retention and increase blood pressure. They can cause interstitial nephritis and acute renal failure. They decrease the efficacy of warfarin and selective serotonin reuptake inhibitor antidepressants. Although an older paper suggested that NSAID use is one of the most common causes of hospitalizations in older persons, a newer one did not find this association. The American Geriatrics Society recommends that NSAIDs should only rarely be used only if other treatments have failed. They should not be used concurrently with aspirin. If used, they should be used with a proton pump inhibitor. Topical NSAIDs (diclofenac or salicylates) can be used safely and effectively for up to 4 weeks.

Tramadol is a drug with μ opioid activity combined with weak inhibition of norepinephrine and serotonin uptake. Major side effects include dizziness, orthostasis, anorexia, and delirium. Tramadol can also precipitate epileptic seizures. Tapentadol is a combined μ opioid agonist with an inhibitor of norepinephrine uptake. Side effects include nausea, constipation, pruritus, and somnolence.

Weak-acting opiates are codeine, hydrocodone, and oxycodone. Their major side effects are constipation and sedation. In Europe, an oral combination of oxycodone and naloxone is available to reduce the constipation produced by oxycodone. These agents also cause

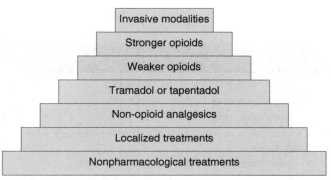

Figure 11–3. A modified approach to the World Health Organization pain pyramid.

Table 11–6.   NONPHARMACOLOGIC PAIN MANAGEMENT STRATEGIES

Distraction Therapy	Behavioral Modification	Physical Therapy	Neurostimulation	Other
Movies	Imagery or meditation	Massage	Transcutaneous nerve stimulation (TENS)	Chiropractic manipulation
Laughter	Relaxation techniques	Ultrasound		
Art therapy	Hypnosis	Hot–cold therapies	Acupuncture	Prototherapy (counter irritation)
Music therapy	Biofeedback	Exercise		

nausea, vomiting, itching, problems concentrating, and poor quality of sleep. Both physicians and persons taking these drugs often prefer to have less pain relief in return for fewer side effects. Buprenorphine patches (20 μg/day equivalent to 240 mg/day of codeine) is approved for chronic pain in Europe. Table 11–7 provides a reminder that persons with severe pain benefit from opiates, and opiates rarely cause unacceptable side effects in this population. A careful inventory of opioid stocks needs to be kept in the nursing home, and they need to be kept in a locked cupboard because theft is not rare. In the United States, a number of nursing homes have seen fentanyl removed from the patches with a syringe after being placed on residents. Dose equivalents of different opiates are given in Table 11–8.

Chronic pain is associated with increased N-methyl-D-aspartate (NMDA) activity. Ketamine, methadone, and propoxyphene (no longer available in many countries because of low efficacy to toxicity ratio) all block NMDA and thus may be effective in blocking the chronic pain cycle. Memantine has anti-NMDA effects, and its ability to decrease agitated behavior in some residents with dementia may be attributable to its NMDA antagonism.

Cannabinoids can relieve pain in some persons with persistent pain. They may be particularly useful in end-of-life care (see section on hospice in Chapter 6). In older persons, lower doses should be used. The major side effects are confusion and delirium. Available cannabinoids are nabilone and dronabinol.

Table 11–9 and Figure 11–4 provide straightforward approaches to pain management that summarize this discussion.

NEUROPATHIC PAIN

Neuropathic pain results from damage to the nervous system. Symptoms include hyperalgesia, sensory neuropathy, burning pain, and hypersensitivity to stimuli. A number of screening questionnaires, such as the pain-DETECT and the self-administered Leeds Assessment of Neuropathic Symptoms and Signs (S-LANSS) Questionnaire have been developed (http://www.geriatricpain.org/Content/Assessment/Intact/Pages/default.aspx) (Accessed February 17, 2012). Typical causes of neuropathic pain are herpes zoster pain, diabetic neuropathy, phantom limb pain, and ischemic neuropathy.

Treatment for neuropathic pain starts with monotherapy and then moves to combination therapy. The tricyclics with low anticholinergic activity (desipramine and

Table 11–7.   DISPELLING MYTHS ABOUT OPIATES

- Opiates can be given orally and sublingually.
- Opiates rarely cause respiratory depression.
- Opiates rarely cause death.
- Opiates are unlikely to be severely addictive when used to treat major pain.
- Opiates rarely are the cause of nausea and vomiting.
- Opiate tolerance is less common than expected when treating pain.

Table 11–8.   DOSE EQUIVALENTS OF DIFFERENT OPIATES

Drug	Delivery Route	Equivalent Dose
Morphine	IM, SC, IV	60 mg
Morphine	PO	180 mg
Methadone	PO	10–40 mg
Hydromorphone	PO	45–60 mg
Oxycodone	PO	120 mg (90 mg in France)
Codeine	PO	1200 mg
Fentanyl	Patch	50–100 mcg/hr (change every 72 hours)

IM, intramuscular; IV, intravenous; PO, oral.

Table 11–9.	FACTORS TO CONSIDER IN DEVELOPING A PAIN MANAGEMENT PROGRAM

- Choose a simple pain assessment tool for cognitively intact residents.
- Educate staff about nonverbal pain signs.
- Be aware of cultural differences in dealing with pain.
- Document the effects of pain on function.
- Train staff in nonpharmacologic approaches to pain management (e.g., relaxation, imagery distraction, music, conversation, appropriate positioning, massage).
- Provide analgesics on a routine basis not "as needed," for chronic pain.
- Always evaluate the effectiveness of analgesics.
- Evaluate for complications of pain and its treatment.
- Document response to allow an informed decision-making process to changing medications.

neuropathy reported relief. Forty percent of persons with fibromyalgia, and one third of persons with postherpetic neuralgia were substantially improved. Carbamazepine is the drug of choice for trigeminal neuralgia. A topical lidocaine patch applied for 12 hours a day is an excellent treatment for localized pain (e.g., herpetic neuralgia). Capsaicin cream can also be useful for some regional pain syndromes but with limited evidence for effectiveness. Topiramate together with α lipoic acid has been shown to reverse diabetic neuropathy over 3 to 6 months in persons who can tolerate high doses of topiramate.

LOW BACK PAIN

At least 80% of persons will have trouble with low back pain sometime in their life. Low back pain is very common among nurses' aides in a variety of countries with a prevalence of 40% to 50%. Approximately half of these persons have sought medical care for their low back pain. The Cochrane Systematic Review could find no evidence supporting training or the provision of assistive devices in preventing low back pain.

In nursing home residents, back pain is also common. It is important in this population to identify serious underlying conditions (Table 11–10). There is no evidence that routine radiographs for persons with low

nortriptyline) are cheap and have the best efficacy for pain relief. Other first-line treatments include duloxetine, venlafaxine, pregabalin, and gabapentin. A study on pregabalin showed that by themselves, these drugs have poor pain relief. Only half of patients with diabetes with peripheral

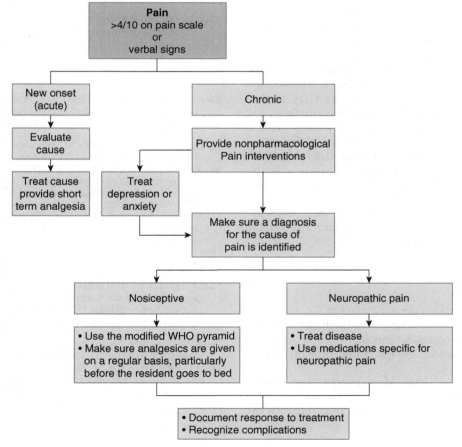

Figure 11–4. Algorithm for pain management in nursing homes.

Table 11–10.	FEATURES OF SERIOUS CONDITIONS CAUSING LOW BACK PAIN	
Condition	**Signs and Symptoms**
Spinal infection	Fever, localized tenderness, source of infection
Disk disease with herniation	Sciatic pain, lower limb sensory loss or weakness
Cancer	Localized tenderness, known cancer diagnosis, weight loss, no relief with bed rest
Compression fracture	Pain is nonspecific with localized tenderness. Evidence of osteoporosis
Spinal stenosis	Leg pain on walking relieved when standing, sitting down, or bending forward; gait is wide based; lumbar extension for 30 to 60 seconds causes thigh pain

back pain improve diagnosis. Magnetic resonance imaging should be considered with persistent low back pain and symptoms or signs of spinal stenosis or radiculopathy are present.

The treatment of choice for low back pain is to remain active, and supervised exercise programs, especially involving stretching, may improve outcomes. Spinal manipulation and massage appear to have a small effect. Superficial heat or cold is helpful for acute low back pain. First-line analgesics (acetaminophen [paracetamol]) are the treatment of choice for pain relief. NSAIDs need to be used with caution. Muscle relaxants (e.g., baclofen and cyclobenzaprine) may reduce spasm. Cyclobenzaprine is structurally related to amitriptyline and has high rates of drowsiness and dizziness, making it potentially unsuitable for older persons. Opiates are, in general, no more effective than first-line analgesics. There is little evidence to support use of antidepressants, anticonvulsants, or corticosteroids. Although commonly recommended and used, evidence for use of steroid or local anesthetic injections is poor in improving long-term outcomes.

USEFUL WEBSITES

Geriatric Pain: http://www.geriatricpain.org
Oxford Pain Internet Site: http://www.medicine.ox.ac.uk/gandolier/booth/painpag/#chronic
International Association for the Study of Pain: http://www.iasp-pain.org
American Academy of Pain Management: http://www.aapainmanage.org
American Academy of Pain Medicine: http://www.painmed.org

KEY POINTS

1. Pain perception is complex and multidimensional, requiring the health professional to accept the subjective viewpoint of the resident.
2. Pain assessment scales are available for both cognitively intact and cognitively impaired nursing home residents and should be used regularly.
3. In cognitively impaired residents, the diagnosis of pain requires noticing nonverbal pain signs.
4. Depression commonly coexists with pain and needs to be treated to obtain adequate pain relief.
5. Pain management requires starting with nonpharmacologic treatments and using the WHO's pain pyramid.
6. Chronic pain requires scheduled medicines.
7. Neuropathic pain should be treated differently and almost always requires at least two medications.

TOOLKITS

1. MDS 3.0
2. Comprehensive Pain Assessment
3. PAINAD
4. LANSS Pain Scale

Toolkits for Practice: What you will see, what you should say, what you should do?
Toolkits for Practice: Knowing when specialist referral is indicated.

SUGGESTED READINGS

American Geriatrics Society Panel on the Pharmacological Management of Persistent Pain in Older Persons. Pharmacological management of persistent pain in older persons. *J Am Geriatr Soc.* 2009;57:1331-1346.
Brennan F, Carr DB, Cousins M. Pain management: a fundamental human right. *Anesth Analg.* 2007;105:205-221.
Burgess G, Williams D. The discovery and development of analgesics: New mechanisms, new modalities. *J Clin Invest.* 2010;120(11):3753-3759.
Dumas LG, Ramadurai M. Pain management in the nursing home. *Nurs Clin North Am.* 2009;44:197-208.
Freynhagen R, Baron R, Gockel U, Tolle TR. painDETECT: A new screening questionnaire to identify neuropathic components in patients with back pain. *Curr Med Res Opin.* 2006;22:1911-1920.
Herr K, Bursch H, Ersek M, Miller LL, Swafford K. Use of pain-behavioral assessments tools in the nursing home: expert consensus recommendations for practice. *J Gerontol Nurs.* 2010;36:18-29.
Kamel HK, Phlavan M, Malekgoudarzi B, et al. Utilizing pain assessment scales increases the frequency of diagnosing pain among elderly nursing home residents. *J Pain Symptom Manage.* 2001;21:450-455.
Morley JE. Pain—"God's megaphone." *J Am Med Dir Assoc.* 2012;13:316-318.
Pizzo PA, Clark NM. Alleviating suffering 101—Pain relief in the United States. *N Engl J Med.* 2012;366(3):197-198.
Snow L, Rapp MP, Kunik M. Pain management in persons with dementia. BODIES mnemonic helps caregivers relay pain-related signs, symptoms to physicians and nursing staff. *Geriatrics.* 2005;60:22-25.
Swafford KL, Lachmann Miller L, Tsai P-F, et al. Improving the process of pain care in nursing homes: a literature synthesis. *J Am Geriatr Soc.* 2009;57:1080-1087.

MULTIPLE CHOICE QUESTIONS

11.1   Which of the following drugs is most likely to lead to severe adverse effects, leading to hospitalization?

    a. Acetaminophen (paracetamol)
    b. NSAIDs
    c. Codeine
    d. Pregabalin
    e. Morphine

11.2   What is the most common side effect of opiates?

    a. Respiratory depression
    b. Nausea
    c. Pruritus
    d. Constipation
    e. Vomiting

11.3   Which of these drugs can precipitate seizures and thus should not be given to a person with seizures?

    a. Tramadol
    b. Acetaminophen (paracetamol)
    c. Topiramate
    d. Morphine
    e. Pregabalin

11.4   Which cause of low back pain leads to pain on walking, which is relieved by sitting down or bending forward?

    a. Herniated disc
    b. Cancer
    c. Compression fracture
    d. Spinal stenosis
    e. Spinal infection

11.5   Which of these analgesics increases the efficacy of warfarin?

    a. Acetaminophen (paracetamol)
    b. Morphine
    c. NSAIDs
    d. Tramadol
    e. Fentanyl

11.6   Which of the following is *not* true about pain management?

    a. Present knowledge about pain management is not always effectively used.
    b. Clinician–person relationships play a minor role in the effectiveness of pain management.
    c. Analgesics should be given on a routine basis.
    d. Analgesics should be provided before activity.

11.7   Which factor has been shown *not* to improve pain management in the nursing home?

    a. A systematic implementation approach
    b. Use of algorithms
    c. Interprofessional involvement
    d. Onsite consultation with a pain specialist
    e. Acupuncture

Chapter 12

LOW MOOD, ANXIETY, AND DEPRESSION

In recent years, there has been a shift in how depression is conceptualized. Depression is now considered to exist on a continuum from normal sadness to pathologically severe depression. In nursing homes, staff must recognize the difference between low mood that is reactive and a normal consequence of the experiences and challenges faced by the resident that may come and go compared with depressive disorders that may be enduring manifestations of mild to major depressive disorders. Members of the care team who spend the most time with residents and know them as individuals are well placed to see subtle behavioral changes as well as more extreme changes. At all ages, the prevalence of subthreshold depression significantly exceeds that of major depression. For older nursing home residents, there may be many reasons to feel sad because of the multiple experiences of loss, including the admission to the nursing home, and these may be compounded by a lack of interest, motivation, or opportunity to participate in meaningful activities before and during their stay in the nursing home. Whereas apathy may be resolved through provision of resident-centered activities and behavioral interventions, depression is more likely to respond to psychological treatments and medications.

It is helpful if team members can distinguish between apathy, lack of stimulation, and depression because this is necessary in order to plan appropriate care and treatments. Hypoactive delirium may also be mistaken as apathy (see Chapter 13), and residents may sit with their closed eyes and appear apathetic as they try to get relief from uncomfortable dry eyes (see Chapter 22).

Loneliness is also a factor in low mood, and time spent with residents early in their admission or preadmission identifying the people who are important in their lives and planning ways to maintain contact can assist in deflecting feelings of social isolation that compound low mood and the sense of isolation.

It is also important that all staff appreciate the different ways that older people may minimize obvious displays of sadness through stoicism and a desire not to bother the doctor or nurse. Others may report multiple trivia to seek attention in ways that can obscure the underlying problem. Table 12–1 provides an overview of what nursing staff need to know based on the Scottish Best Practice Guidance *Working with Older People Towards Prevention and Early Detection of Depression.*

DEPRESSION

In a review of depression prevalence in nursing homes from around the world, 15.5% had major depression, and 25% had minor depression (dysphoria). More than 40% had some depressive symptoms. About 20% to 40% of persons with dementia have been reported to have coexistent depression. Depressive symptoms are particularly high on admission to the nursing home, but close to 40% no longer show depressive symptoms after 1 year.

The Minimum Data Set (MDS) 2.0 used 15 indicators of low mood. It has been shown to have poor sensitivity for identifying major or minor depression and has been considered an inadequate tool by experts in geriatrics. The MDS 3.0 uses the nine-item Patient Health Questionnaire-9 (PHQ-9), which has been validated in frail populations and is responsive to changes over time (Figure 12–1). Major depression is defined as five or more symptoms and minor depression two to four symptoms present more than half of the days in the last week. To be a positive result, one of the positives needs to be either "Little or no interest in doing things" or "Feeling or appearing down, depressed or hopeless." This scoring showed an 18% incidence of minor depression and a 17% incidence of major depression in the MDS 3.0 validation study. The Geriatric Depression Scale had less of an agreement with the modified Schedule for Affective Disorders and Schizophrenia, and the Cornell Scale for Depression in Dementia, which were used as the "gold standard" for diagnosis of depression.

The Cornell Depression Scale was developed to diagnose depression in persons with dementia (Mini-Mental Status score of 15 of 30 or less). It requires direct observation, a resident interview and interviews with caregivers. In the MDS 3.0 validation, the observed PHQ-9 performed at least as well.

The *Diagnostic and Statistical Manual*, edition four, text revision (*DSM-IV-TR*) is the gold standard to diagnose depression (www.behavenet.com/diagnostic-and-statistical-mental-disorders-fourth-edition-text-revision). These criteria can be remembered using the SIG-E-CAPS mnemonic (Table 12–2). The *DSM-5* criteria are expected to be available in May 2013 (www.dsm5.org).

The definitive diagnosis for depression in a person with dementia uses the Provisional Diagnostic Criteria for Depression in Alzheimer Disease (PDC-dAD).

Table 12–1.   NURSING CARE ESSENTIALS IN THE EARLY DETECTION AND PREVENTION OF DEPRESSION

Nursing Care Essentials: Low Mood and Depressions	Rationale
Nursing staff are aware of the impact of life changes on the emotional well-being of residents.	Move to a nursing home is major life stress. Multiple losses increase the risk of low mood and depression. Bereavement, including the loss of spouse and pets, can be intense, and normal grieving may be extended.
Nursing staff are aware that psychological, spiritual, and social support can improve a resident's quality of life and sense of well-being.	With appropriate and timely support, transient causes of low mood can be alleviated.
Nursing staff are knowledgeable about the early signs and symptoms of depression and its causes and complete formal assessments and repeat assessments at appropriate intervals.	Prompt intervention and preventive strategies can prevent major deterioration; an objective measure of depression risk or severity is essential. Assessment is a prerequisite to appropriate referral to specialists.
Resident-centered approaches are adopted, and the resident is fully involved in decisions about his or her care and treatment.	Strategies that preserve the unique identity and interests of individuals are affirming, and involvement of older people (with or without the family) in planning care is central to the achievement of person-centered approaches.
Nursing staff recognize and appropriately manage sensory disabilities, including vision and hearing impairments.	Communication is key to resident-centered approaches, including shared decision making.
Nursing staff ensures residents have opportunities to participate in meaningful activities and maintain friendships.	Lack of stimulation and loneliness lead to boredom, social isolation, and low mood and can exacerbate cognitive problems.

In older people, a number of atypical symptoms of depression are not rare (Table 12–3). Depression should always be considered to be a cause of new or worsening cognitive function. Because depression can lead to severe anorexia in older persons, it is the most common cause of weight loss in this population. The risk for suicide should always be recognized and assessed. In persons who express suicidal thoughts, a careful history should be obtained. Some residents display "subintentional suicide," which presents as withdrawn behavior with rejection of food, fluids, and medical care.

Residents who articulate specific plans for suicide should be seen by a geriatric psychiatrist or other qualified mental health professional as soon as possible, transferred to a geriatric psychiatry unit, or both.

A number of medical disorders can cause depression, and these should be considered when a diagnosis of depression is made. These include hypothyroidism, hyperthyroidism, hypoadrenalism, vitamin B_{12} deficiency, pancreatic cancer, medication effects, hypercalcemia, stroke, vascular dementia, and Alzheimer's disease.

Psychotic depression can present with hallucinations, paranoia, delusions, or other unusual symptoms. Bipolar disorders that include symptoms of hypomania should be excluded because these conditions are treated differently (Table 12–4). Persons with suicidal thoughts, psychotic depression, or bipolar disorder should be treated by a geriatric (old age) psychiatrist.

MANAGEMENT OF DEPRESSION

For persons with minor depression (dysphoria or dysthymia), a supportive environment may be sufficient to reverse the symptoms. Placebo has been shown to reverse depression in up to 40% of older persons. In Hong Kong, the introduction of Mah Jong playing in the nursing home reduced depressive symptoms. There are limited data suggesting that physical activity programs, especially resistance exercise, can reduce depressive symptoms and improve quality of life. Table 12–5 provides components of a supportive program to reduce depressive symptoms in nursing home residents.

Psychotherapies ("talk therapies") have been found to be as effective as medications in curing depression. Cognitive behavioral therapy has the best evidence for its effectiveness in treating older persons but is not feasible in residents with dementia. Because psychotherapy has fewer side effects, the use of psychotherapists (psychologists, social workers, or trained therapy aides) in the nursing home represents a reasonable approach to the management of depression in nursing homes. A combination of individual and group therapy appears to be the most cost-effective approach.

Numerous medications exist for the treatment of depression (Table 12–6). These drugs are more effective for severe depression than for dysphoria. For optimal response, these drugs need to be coupled with some form of supportive therapy. Recent studies have suggested that antidepressants are minimally effective in persons with dementia.

Both tricyclic antidepressants (TCAs) and selective serotonin reuptake inhibitors (SSRIs) have a variety of side effects (Table 12–7). Originally, SSRIs were thought to be safer than TCAs. However, a community study found that SSRIs are more likely to cause hip fractures and death than amitriptyline, a drug not considered safe for older persons.

PHQ-9 Patient Questionnaire
Nine symptom checklist

Patient Name: _____   Date: _____

Dear Patient,

In an effort to provide the highest standard of care and meet the requirements of your insurance company, we ask that you fill out the form below. This form is used as both a screening tool and a diagnostic tool for depression. Your provider will discuss the form with you during your visit. Thank you for your cooperation and the opportunity to care for you.

1. Over the *last 2 weeks*, how often have you been bothered by any of the following problems?

	Not at all 0	Several days 1	More than half the days 2	Nearly every day 3
a. Little interest or pleasure in doing things.	☐	☐	☐	☐
b. Feeling down, depressed, or hopeless.	☐	☐	☐	☐
c. Trouble falling/staying asleep, sleeping too much.	☐	☐	☐	☐
d. Feeling tired or having little energy.	☐	☐	☐	☐
e. Poor appetite or overeating.	☐	☐	☐	☐
f. Feeling bad about yourself – or that you are a failure or have let yourself or your family down.	☐	☐	☐	☐
g. Trouble concentrating on things, such as reading the newspaper or watching television.	☐	☐	☐	☐
h. Moving or speaking so slowly that other people could have noticed. Or the opposite – being so fidgety or restless that you have been moving around a lot more than usual.	☐	☐	☐	☐
i. Thoughts that you would be better off dead or of hurting yourself in some way.	☐	☐	☐	☐

2. If you checked off any problem on this questionnaire so far, how difficult have these problems made it for you to do your work, take care of things at home, or get along with other people?

Not difficult at all	Somewhat difficult	Very difficult	Extremely difficult
☐	☐	☐	☐

Figure 12–1. Patient Health Questionnaire-9 (PHQ-9).

An early side effect of TCAs is orthostasis, so all persons taking these drugs should have their blood pressure measured while standing. Blood levels for TCAs should be monitored. The demonstration that long-term treatment with SSRIs leads to osteoporosis makes long-term treatment questionable in older persons. Methylphenidate has been used as an activating agent in older persons with severe apathy and depression. There is limited evidence in controlled trials for the effectiveness of methylphenidate.

Electroconvulsive therapy (ECT) is the most effective treatment for depression in older persons with an 80% response rate. ECT is safe in the majority of older persons. ECT should be strongly considered for residents with severe depression that is causing weight loss and who

Table 12–2.   CRITERIA FOR MAJOR DEPRESSION
Sad (depressed mood)
Insomnia with awakening between 2 and 4 AM
Guilt
Energy decreased
Concentration difficulties
Anorexia or weight loss
Psychomotor agitation or retardation
Suicidal thoughts

Table 12–4.   SYMPTOMS OF HYPOMANIA
Talk incessantly
Abnormally excited
Do not sleep
Irritable
Rapid thinking process
Problems with judgment
Inappropriate social behavior

have comorbidities that make drug or behavioral therapies impractical or unsafe.

Vagal nerve stimulation and repetitive transmagnetic stimulus have a possible use in some persons, but there is no strong evidence for their effectiveness. High-lux (2000-lux) light may decrease depression in nursing home residents.

ANXIETY

Generalized anxiety disorder (GAD) occurs in about 6% of nursing home residents. In addition, about one in five residents with depression have an anxiety component. Anxiety is especially common when persons first enter a nursing home and have to deal with new situations. The diagnostic criteria for GAD are pervasive anxiety for at least 6 months together with at least three of six of the following symptoms:

- Irritability
- Fatigue
- Insomnia
- Restlessness
- Muscle tension
- Concentration problems

Anxiety-like symptoms can occur in response to pulmonary embolism, myocardial infarction, unresolved pain, chronic obstructive pulmonary disorders, atrial fibrillation or other arrhythmias, repeated falls (fear of falling), and medications that result in tachycardia or hypotension (dizziness).

Table 12–3.   ATYPICAL SYMPTOMS OF DEPRESSION IN OLDER PERSONS
Cognitive impairment
Anorexia or weight loss
Pain syndromes
Fatigue
Constipation
Excessive sleepiness
Apathy

In general, an acute anxiety attack can be treated with a short-acting benzodiazepine such as lorazepam and reassurance. Long-acting benzodiazepines such as benzodiazepam and chlordiazepoxide should not be used. Recurrent or continuous anxiety requires medication coupled with cognitive behavioral therapy, relaxation techniques, or both. Cognitive behavioral therapy alone produces a response in fewer than half of the persons treated. Citalopram and other SSRIs have been shown to be effective in treating GAD. Buspirone has a slower onset but can be particularly effective at treating anxious persons in the nursing home who have accompanying personality disorders ("the angry old man syndrome"). Table 12–8 provides the drugs that can be used to treat anxiety in the nursing home.

PSYCHOTIC DISORDERS

Psychotic disorders commonly accompany dementia and depression in older nursing home residents. The new onset of schizophrenia is rare in this population, but many nursing home residents may have a longstanding history of this condition.

Table 12–5.   COMPONENTS OF A SUPPORTIVE THERAPY PROGRAM FOR DEPRESSIVE SYMPTOMS IN A NURSING HOME
• Diagnose depression and make sure that staff know who is depressed.
• Have active recreation therapy programs.
• Provide an exercise program at least 3 days a week.
• Encourage regular visiting by family and volunteers.
• Provide outings from nursing home when possible.
• Develop trust with resident.
• Interact to build self-esteem and sense of personal power.
• Ascertain need for spiritual support and provide religious counseling and access to worship services when appropriate.
• Provide supportive "active" listening ("being with" the resident) and encouragement.
• Encourage positive reminiscences.
• Reinforce positive behaviors and personal strengths.
• Monitor for suicidal tendencies.
• Assess effects on one's own feelings and reactions and recognize times when another person should be assigned to a resident.

Table 12–6. SOME ANTIDEPRESSANT DRUGS USED FOR OLDER PERSONS

Class	Drug	Starting Dose (mg)	Maximal Dose in Older Persons (mg)
Selective serotonin reuptake inhibitors[a]	Paroxetine	10	20
	Sertraline	25	100
	Citalopram	10	40
	Escitalopram	10	20
Serotonin–norepinephrine reuptake inhibitors	Duloxetine	20	30
	Venlafaxine XR	37.5	150
Tricyclics[b]	Desipramine	25	150
	Nortriptyline	10	75
Tetracyclics	Trazodone	25	100
	Mirtazapine	7.5	30
Monoamine oxidase inhibitors	Phenelzine	15	60
	Tranylcypromine	10	40
	Moclobemide	150	300
Aminoketone	Bupropion	75	300

[a]Fluoxetine should be avoided because of long half-life and potential to cause severe weight loss.

[b]Amitriptyline and imipramine are very anticholinergic and should not be used in older persons.

Table 12–7. SIDE EFFECTS OF TRICYCLIC AND SELECTIVE SEROTONIN REUPTAKE INHIBITOR ANTIDEPRESSANTS

Tricyclic Antidepressants	Selective Serotonin Reuptake Inhibitors
Dry mouth	Serotonin syndrome
Blurred vision	Tinnitus
Constipation	Severe weight loss
Urinary retention	Anorexia
Postural hypotension	Akathisia
Drowsiness	Suicidal ideation
Confusion	Nightmares
Dizziness	Falls
Sweating	Osteoporosis
Apathy	Hip fracture
Muscle twitching	Hyponatremia
Arrhythmias	Delirium
Falls	Gastrointestinal bleeding
	Myocardial infarction
	Stroke

Table 12–8. DRUGS USED TO TREAT ANXIETY

Treatment	Comments
Benzodiazepines	Useful for a single attack Side effects include falls, cognitive impairment, drowsiness, delirium, and withdrawal syndrome
Azaspirones (e.g., buspirone)	Slow onset of action Variable efficacy
SSRIs/SNRIs	First line of treatment Major side effects include falls, hip fracture, hyponatremia, and delirium
α2 δ ligand of voltage-dependent calcium channel (e.g., pregabalin)	Effective in trials Side effects include blurred vision, diplopia, drowsiness, tremors, cognitive impairment, falls, delirium, and ataxia

SNRI, serotonin–norepinephrine reuptake inhibitor; SSRI, selective serotonin reuptake inhibitor.

Schizophrenia is the prototypical psychotic disorder. Positive symptoms include delusions, hallucinations, illusions, and paranoia. These symptoms respond well to antipsychotic drugs. Negative symptoms (e.g., being asocial, the inability to experience pleasure, poor dress and hygiene, lack of motivation, poor judgment, disorganized speech) respond poorly to antipsychotics.

Antipsychotics are predominately antidopaminergic drugs, but they also have anticholinergic and antiserotonergic effects. It can take 7 to 14 days for the drugs to be effective. There is little evidence that the newer atypical antipsychotics, which are more expensive, are more effective or have fewer side effects than the older drugs. Major side effects are dystonia, tardive dyskinesia, confusion, hip fracture, aspiration pneumonia, stroke, and neuroleptic malignant syndrome. These drugs are ineffective in one in five persons and only partially effective in 40% of persons. In older persons, the lowest possible dose should be used to control symptoms, (e.g., haloperidol or risperidone 0.5–1 mg/day). Atypical antipsychotics can cause hyperglycemia and weight gain and are associated with an increased incidence of stroke and death in older people. For these reasons, the U.S. Food and Drug Administration has placed

Table 12–9.	NURSING CARE FOR PERSONS WITH PSYCHOSES

- Avoid physical contact because it may be seen as threatening. Always inform the resident before touching him or her to carry out care.
- Remain calm.
- To decrease paranoia, do not talk to other staff in a soft voice.
- Encourage verbalization of feelings.
- Do not argue with resident.
- Promote trust.
- Avoid competitive activities.
- Watch for resident pocketing medications in mouth and do mouth checks when necessary.
- Encourage physical exercise.
- Keep your distance when the resident is angry.
- Do not use physical restraints.
- When possible, use the same nurses' aides who the resident recognizes and trusts.
- Allow resident to choose own food to decrease belief that he or she is being poisoned.

a "black box warning" on their use. In addition, the Centers for Medicare and Medicaid have recently begun a major campaign to reduce the inappropriate use of these drugs for behavioral symptoms of dementia that are not true psychoses.

From the nursing perspective, it is essential to take an existential approach to these residents' wild ideas and not to disagree with their reality whenever possible. Remaining calm in their presence is also difficult but important (Table 12–9).

KEY POINTS

1. Both residents and their family caregivers need support after admission to a nursing home.
2. Help new residents become oriented and use volunteer resident to help them form friendships.
3. Depression is underdiagnosed.
4. The MDS 3.0 (but not 2.0) provides a suitable screen for depression.
5. Depression should always be considered in a resident with weight loss.
6. A supportive environment, innovative activities, adequate lighting, and physical exercise are often sufficient to treat dysphoria.
7. Cognitive behavioral therapy is as effective and has fewer side effects compared with medications to treat depression.
8. All antidepressants have potentially severe side effects and have a poor therapeutic window for dysphoric residents.
9. ECT is very effective for treatment of major depression.

10. Anxiety alone or in combination with depression occurs in up to 20% of residents.
11. SSRIs are the first line of therapy for chronic anxiety.
12. Antipsychotic drug treatment should be reserved for residents with true psychosis because they have many severe side effects. They should not be used for behavioral disturbances associated with dementia in the absence of psychosis.

SUGGESTED READINGS

American Psychological Association. *Diagnostic and Statistical Manual.* 4th edition , text revision. Washington, DC: Author; 1994.

Arroll B, Elley CR, Fishman T, et al. Antidepressants versus placebo for depression in primary care. *Cochrane Database Syst Rev.* 2009; (3):CD007954.

Bergh S, Selbaek G, Engedal K. Discontinuation of antidepressants in people with dementia and neuropsychiatric symptoms (DESEP study): Double blind, randomised, parallel group, placebo controlled trial. *Br Med J.* 2012;344:e1566.

Candy M, Jones L, Williams R, et al. Psychostimulants for depression. *Cochrane Database Syst Rev.* 2008;(2):CD006722.

Chalder M, Wiles NJ, Campbell J, et al. Facilitated physical activity as a treatment for depressed adults: Randomised controlled trial. *Br Med J.* 2012;344:e2758.

Chen F, Hahn TJ, Weintraub NT. Do SSRIs play a role in decreasing bone mineral density? *J Am Med Dir Assoc.* 2012;13:413-417.

Cipriani A, La Ferla T, Furukawa TA, et al. Sertraline versus other antidepressive agents for depression. *Cochrane Database Syst Rev.* 2010;(4):CD006117.

Coupland C, Chiman P, Morriss R, et al. Antidepressant use and risk of adverse outcomes in older people: population based cohort study. *Br Med J.* 2011;343:d4551.

Daley A, Jolly K. Exercise to treat depression. *Br Med J.* 2012;344:e3181.

Frenchman IB. Atypical antipsychotics for nursing home patients: a retrospective chart review. *Drugs Aging.* 2005;22:257-264.

Goncalves DC, Byrne GJ. Interventions for generalized anxiety disorder in older adults: systematic review and meta-analysis. *J Anxiety Disord.* 2012;26:1-11.

Harvey PD, Bowie CR. Late-life schizophrenia. What providers need to know. *Director.* 2005;13:90, 93-94.

Karakaya MG, Bilgin SC, Ekici G, et al. Functional mobility, depressive symptoms, level of independence, and quality of life of the elderly living at home and in the nursing home. *J Am Med Dir Assoc.* 2009;10:662-666.

Mead GE, Morley W, Campbell P, et al. Exercise for depression. *Cochrane Database Syst Rev.* 2009;(3):CD004366.

Morley JE. Depression in nursing home residents. *J Am Med Dir Assoc.* 2010;11:301-303.

NHS Quality Improvement Scotland. *Best Practice Statement Working with Older People Towards Prevention and Early Detection of Depression.* Edinburgh: Author; 2004.

Olin JT, Schneider LS, Katz IR, et al. Provisional diagnostic criteria for depression of Alzheimer disease. *Am J Geriatr Psychiatry.* 2002;10(2):125-128.

Reinhold JA, Mandos LA, Rickels K, Lohoff FW. Pharmacological treatment of generalized anxiety disorder. *Expert Opin Pharmacother.* 2011;12:2457-2467.

Rodda J, Walker Z, Carter J. Depression in older adults. *Br Med J.* 2011;343:d5219.

Royer M, Ballentine NH, Eslinger PJ, et al. Light therapy for seniors in long term care. *J Am Med Dir Assoc.* 2012;13:100-102.

Strome TM. Schizophrenia in the elderly: what nurses need to know. *Arch Psychiatr Nurs.* 1989;3:47-52.

Thakur M, Blazer DG. Depression in long-term care. *J Am Med Dir Assoc.* 2008;9:82-87.

Watanabe N, Omori IM, Nakagawa A, et al. Mirtazapine versus other antidepressive agents for depression. *Cochrane Database Syst Rev.* 2011;(12):CD006528.

Wilson KC, Mottram PG, Vassilas CA. Psychotherapeutic treatments for older depressed people. *Cochrane Database Syst Rev.* 2008;(1):CD004853.

MULTIPLE CHOICE QUESTIONS

12.1   Which of the following has been shown to be important for adjustment to the nursing home?

a. Family attitude
b. Having a roommate
c. Promoting conformity
d. Ability to have choice and control over one's environment
e. Institutional design of building

12.2   Which scale is used in the MDS 3.0 to screen for depression?

a. Patient Health Questionnaire-9 (PHQ-9)
b. Patient Depression Questionnaire-9 (PDQ-9)
c. Geriatric Depression Scale
d. Cornell Depression Scale
e. Hamilton Depression Scale

12.3   Which of the following has been shown to be most effective in treating depression?

a. Cognitive behavioral therapy
b. Antidepressant drugs
c. Exercise
d. Light therapy (200 lux)
e. A combination of a and b

12.4   Which of the following symptoms is *not* a component of general anxiety disorder?

a. Irritability
b. Insomnia
c. Muscle tension
d. Dysphoria
e. Concentration problems

12.5   Which of the following is a side effect of selective serotonin reuptake inhibitors (SSRIs) used to treat depression?

a. Blurred vision
b. Urinary retention
c. Arrhythmias
d. Osteoporosis
e. Orthostasis

12.6   Which of the following is *not* a positive symptom of schizophrenia that is responsive to antipsychotics?

a. Illusions
b. Disorganized sleep
c. Paranoia
d. Delusions
e. Hallucinations

Chapter 13

CONFUSION, AGITATION, AND OTHER BEHAVIORAL DISTURBANCES

The term *confusion* is not in itself a diagnosis but a popular term to describe a syndrome characterized by disorientation in time, place, and person and degrees of difficulty with memory, attention, and cognitive abilities. When a person is said to be confused, he or she is thinking or behaving in ways that are not considered normal; thus, the term is associated with stigma and negative connotations. In thinking about older nursing home residents, it is important to make differential diagnosis to ensure appropriate management of chronic and acute manifestations of confusion, depression, and other disorders. Acute confusion is a common presentation of physical illness in older people, and sometimes it is the only visible sign of infection or physical and mental stress. Therefore, it is important for nurses to be aware of delirium and to regard its development as a signal to act quickly and in collaboration with the physician identify the causative factors and begin treatment. This chapter also covers dementia and behavioral disturbances often seen in persons with dementia.

DELIRIUM

The presence of delirium is common in nursing home residents, ranging from 8.9% in Dutch nursing homes to 24.9% in Finnish nursing homes. Studies in Switzerland and the United States suggested that in new admissions, subsyndromal delirium (one or two delirium symptoms) was present in 40% of residents. Delirium is associated with a doubling of rehospitalization and five times the chance of dying. Persons with delirium have less functional improvement and are half as likely to be discharged home.

Dementia is the main predisposing and therefore main risk factor for delirium; up to two thirds of cases of delirium occur in patients with dementia. Studies indicate that age older than 65 years, dementia, severe illness defined as a clinical condition that is deteriorating or is at risk of deterioration, anticholinergic medications, and current hip fracture are consistent risk factors. Delirium may be understood as a reaction of the brain to metabolic disturbances, infections, stress, malnutrition, or medications. A new underlying mechanism has recently been proposed, that of overreacting responses of the brain to psychological and illness stress. Research shows a clear systemic inflammation-induced exacerbation of neurodegenerative disease, with the likelihood that every episode of delirium will speed up the progression of dementia.

Delirium is a clinical syndrome consisting of attentional deficits, change in cognition, and generalized disorganized behavior that is of acute onset and fluctuating during the day. Three distinctive clinical presentations of delirium have been described: hyperactive, hypoactive, and mixed. In the hyperactive form, the person is hyper alert, visibly restless, excitable, and vigilant. A nursing home resident with hyperactive delirium may be continuously on the move, searching, shouting, combative, and resistive when staff members attempt to calm them. Although not recommended practice, this may result in staff members' opting to physically restrain the resident in the belief that this will protect the individual and other residents.

An individual with hyperactive delirium can experience frightening and vivid hallucinations, leading to outbursts of intense fear and rage. Persons with new-onset falls in a nursing home should be considered to have delirium until proven otherwise.

A resident with hypoactive delirium is less easy to recognize because apathetic or withdrawn behaviors are more accepted and stand out less than the physicality of hyperactive delirium. Staff members who know the resident are more likely to identify abnormally lower levels of activity and alertness and be concerned about residents who are quiet, fail to respond to simple greetings, appear listless, and easily drift off to sleep during hygiene activities and other interventions. Residents who lie with their eyes open but are indifferent to what is going on around them may be experiencing hypoactive delirium.

Mixed forms of delirium in which the resident alternates between the two forms are common, and fluctuations in behavior and altered sleep–wake cycles may occur over several hours or days; in some cases, changing behaviors may falsely suggest spontaneous recovery. Although for some residents delirium may be transient and a relatively brief episode, growing evidence suggests that delirious episodes may recur for several weeks or months, especially at night, and that outcomes may be poor.

The care of residents with delirium is an interdisciplinary endeavor between nursing and medical interventions commencing with prevention or diagnosis of delirium followed by supportive nursing care and simultaneous medical treatment of the underlying cause.

Delirium is often underdiagnosed. For this reason, a number of screening tools have been developed. Of these, the gold standard is the Confusion Assessment Method (CAM)

Table 13–1. THE CONFUSION ASSESSMENT METHOD DIAGNOSTIC ALGORITHM

Consider the diagnosis of delirium if 1 and 2, AND either 3a or 3b are positive:

1. **Acute Onset and Fluctuating Course**

   Is there evidence of an acute change in mental status from the patient's baseline?

   Did the (abnormal) behavior fluctuate during the day (tend to come and go, or increase and decrease in severity)?

2. **Inattention**

   Did the patient have difficulty focusing attention (e.g., being easily distractible) or have difficulty keeping track of what was being said?

3a. **Disorganized Thinking**

   Was the patient's thinking disorganized or incoherent: such as rambling or irrelevant conversation, unclear or illogical flow of ideas, or unpredictable switching from subject to subject?

3b. **Altered Level of Consciousness**

   Overall, how would you rate this patient's level of consciousness? (alert [normal], vigilant [hyper-alert], lethargic [drowsy, easily aroused], stupor [difficult to arouse], or coma [un-arousable]). Positive for any answer other than "alert."

Table 13–2. NURSING HOME CONFUSION ASSESSMENT METHOD BASED ON MDS 3.0

1. Mental function varies over the course of the day (B5f)

   OR

   Mood decline over last 90 days (E3)

   AND

2. Easily distracted (B5a)

   AND EITHER

3. Periods of altered perception or

   Awareness of surroundings (B5b) or
   Episodes of disorganized speech (B5c) or
   Cognitive decline over last 90 days (B6)

   OR

4. Periods of restlessness (B5d) or
   Periods of lethargy (B5e) or
   Behavior decline over the last 90 days

(Table 13–1). The Minimum Data Set (MDS) 3.0 uses the CAM for diagnosis of delirium. Observing the person while saying the days of the week backward or by asking the person to lift his or her hand when hearing a vowel in between a number of consonants can detect more subtle versions of delirium. The Nursing Home Confusion Assessment Method was developed for the MDS 3.0 (Table 13–2). The Veterans Administration Delirium Group has developed a set of "faces" to be used as a vital sign to help in the identification of delirium (Figure 13–1).

There are multiple causes of delirium (Table 13–3), and many persons with delirium have more than one cause. Anticholinergic drugs play a major role in precipitating delirium. Most persons with delirium have increased serum anticholinergic activity. Hyponatremia caused by selective serotonin receptor uptake inhibitors is another common cause. Partial complex seizures can take up to nearly 2 years before the diagnosis is made and should be considered in all persons with delirium without a cause. Infection is the most common cause of delirium, but it should be remembered that fever and leukocytosis can occur with myocardial infarction and pulmonary embolism. Pain can also precipitate delirium.

A number of approaches to prevent delirium are available (Table 13–4). Remember that untreated delirium or subsyndromal delirium can last for months. The treatment for delirium involves early recognition, diagnosing and treating the causes, and providing support (including removing illusionary objects, good lighting, and care in approaching and addressing the resident). Physical restraints should *never* be used. Low-dose lorazepam (0.5 mg) may be necessary but should be avoided. There is no evidence that antipsychotics (e.g., haloperidol, risperidone, olanzapine) have a beneficial effect in persons with delirium.

The European Delirium Association has developed an excellent toolkit for recognizing preventing and treating delirium. The STOP DELIRIUM! Intervention has been shown to reduce delirium in nursing homes (http://www.europeandeliriumassociation.com/delirium-information).

The care of nursing home residents with delirium can be highly challenging and stressful for nursing staff, other residents, and visitors, and in some cases, the severity of underlying problems necessitates transfer to hospital. In all cases, it should be recognized as a serious condition. All forms of delirium put the individual at risk of negative outcomes, including dehydration; incontinence and urinary tract infection; increased risk for accidental injury and falls; acceleration of dementia progression; and not least, loss of dignity. Restraint of delirious individuals should never be used.

Unarousable	Difficult to arouse	Drowsy	Lethargic	Can't pay attention	Alert and calm	Restless or anxious	Vigilant or hyperalert	Agitated	Very agitated	Combative
−5	−4	−3	−2	−1	0	+1	+2	+3	+4	+5

Figure 13–1. The "faces" mental status vital sign.

Table 13–3. CAUSES OF DELIRIUM	
Drugs (any drug with anticholinergic activity)	
Emotional (depression or acute psychosis)	
Low PO$_2$	Pulmonary embolus
	Myocardial infarction
	Anemia
	Stroke
Infection	
Retention of urine and feces	
Ictal (especially partial complex seizures and absence seizures)	
Undernutrition (especially dehydration)	
Metabolic	Thyroid disorder
	Hyperglycemia
	Vitamin B$_{12}$ deficiency
	Hyponatremia
	Liver or renal failure
Subdural hematoma	

DEMENTIA

Memory is a passion no less powerful or pervasive than love.
     —Elie Wesel, *All Rivers Run to the Sea*

The ability to learn and remember things peaks between 25 and 28 years of age. After that, there is a slow decline in our cognitive abilities. Harvard physicians were shown to have an 18% cognitive decline between 40 to 70 years, although the rate of decline varied tremendously among individuals.

Between normal age-related cognitive impairment and dementia is a twilight zone condition known as mild cognitive impairment (MCI). The definition of MCI includes the following elements:

- Complaints and objective evidence of memory problems
- No functional impairment
- Abnormal memory for age
- The person is not depressed or demented.

Table 13–4.   PREVENTION OF DELIRIUM
• Reduce disorientation (e.g., clocks, calendars).
• Correct sensory impairment (lighting, glasses, hearing aides).
• Reduce dehydration.
• Reduce constipation (use osmotic laxatives).
• Reduce risk of infections (use vaccines, avoid bladder catheters).
• Avoid polypharmacy and utilization of anticholinergic drugs.
• Control pain.

The condition is not benign. Persons with MCI have poor functional recovery after major events such as myocardial infarction, pneumonia, or prolonged surgery. One third develop Alzheimer's disease, and one third are dead within 5 years. This form of MCI is designated amnestic MCI (aMCI). People with nonamnestic MCI have mild declines in attention, language use, or visuospatial skills. Nonamnestic MCI may be a precursor to some forms of non-Alzheimer's dementia.

Assessment for amnestic MCI can be done using the St. Louis University Mental Status Examination (SLUMS), Montreal Cognitive Assessment (MoCA)(http://www.mocatest.org/pdf_files/test/MoCA-Test-English_7_1.pdf), or Short Test of Mental Status (STMS). All perform at approximately the same level for diagnosing MCI. The diagnosis depends on educational status and needs to be corrected for whether or not the person completed high school. See the Toolkit for the tests. Amnestic MCI is often reversible, and depression, medication effect, vitamin B$_{12}$ deficiency, and hypothyroidism should be excluded. Exercise is the only known treatment.

At present, 42.3 million people are living with dementia worldwide with about 60% of these persons residing in developing countries. By 2040, there will be 81.1 million persons with dementia, with more than 20% living in developing countries. Alzheimer's disease is the third most costly disease after heart disease and cancer. Eighty percent of persons with Alzheimer's disease live at home. Caregivers of people with dementia often have psychological problems and ill health. Being a caregiver can markedly alter a person's ability to maintain his or her job.

Both family and physicians fail to recognize when a person has dementia. This requires the use of formal screening tests such as the Mini-Mental Status Examination (MMSE). The MMSE has been highly successfully used worldwide as a screening tool. It is educationally dependent, has both false-positive and false-negative results, and has minimal testing of visuospatial testing. It is a poor tool for diagnosing MCI. It is copyrighted and costs approximately $1 each time it is used.

The VAMC-SLUMS (Figure 13–2) performs better than the MMSE at diagnosing dementia and can be used to screen for MCI. It has better visuospatial and executive function components. The copyright belongs to the United States government and as such its usage is free. It has been translated into 13 languages (http://aging.slu.edu/index.php?page=saint-louis-university-mental-status-slums-exam). The MoCA has similar specificity and sensitivity to the VAMC-SLUMS test for MCI and dementia. A number of computerized tests for examining residents with dementia have been developed (Figure 13–3).

There are a number of reversible causes of dementia (Table 13–5). These should be considered in all persons with dementia.

There are more than 100 different forms of dementia. The most common dementia is Alzheimer's disease. Vascular disease is the next most common disorder and often coexists with Alzheimer's disease. When dementias are associated with tremor, Lewy body damage, pure tauopathy, Parkinson's dementia with Alzheimer's disease, and fragile X syndrome should be considered. Abnormal behaviors similar to delirium occur with Lewy

VAMC
SLUMS EXAMINATION

Questions about this assessment tool? E-mail aging@slu.edu

Name_____ Age_____

Is the patient alert?_____ Level of education_____

__/1 **1. What day of the week is it?**

__/1 **2. What is the year?**

__/1 **3. What state are we in?**

4. Please remember these five objects. I will ask you what they are later.

    Apple   Pen   Tie   House   Car

5. You have $100 and you go to the store and buy a dozen apples for $3 and a tricycle for $20.

    How much did you spend?

__/3   **How much do you have left?**

6. Please name as many animals as you can in one minute.

__/3   **0** 0-4 animals   **1** 5-9 animals   **2** 10-14 animals   **3** 15+ animals

__/5 **7. What were the five objects I asked you to remember? 1 point for each one correct.**

8. I am going to give you a series of numbers and I would like you to give them to me backwards. For example, if I say 42, you would say 24.

__/2   **0** 87   **1** 649   **1** 8537

9. This is a clock face. Please put in the hour markers and the time at ten minutes to eleven o'clock.

    2 Hour markers okay

__/4   **2** Time correct

1 10. Please place an X in the triangle.

__/2   **1** Which of the above figures is largest?

11. I am going to tell you a story. Please listen carefully because afterwards, I'm going to ask you some questions about it.

Jill was a very successful stockbroker. She made a lot of money on the stock market. She then met Jack, a devastatingly handsome man. She married him and had three children. They lived in Chicago. She then stopped work and stayed at home to bring up her children. When they were teenagers, she went back to work. She and Jack lived happily ever after.

    2 What was the female's name?   **2** What work did she do?

__/8   **2** When did she go back to work?   **2** What state did she live in?

_____ **TOTAL SCORE**

SCORING		
HIGH SCHOOL EDUCATION		**LESS THAN HIGH SCHOOL EDUCATION**
27-30	NORMAL	25-30
21-26	MILD NEUROCOGNITIVE DISORDER	20-24
1-20	DEMENTIA	1-19

_____   _____   _____
CLINICIAN'S SIGNATURE   DATE   TIME

SH Tariq, N Tumosa, JT Chibnall, HM Perry III, and JE Morley. The Saint Louis University Mental Status (SLUMS) Examination for detecting mild cognitive impairment and dementia is more sensitive than the Mini-Mental Status Examination (MMSE) - A pilot study. *Am J Geriatr Psych* 14:900-10, 2006.

Figure 13–2. The VAMC-SLUMS (Veterans Administration Medical Center-St. Louis University Mental Status Examination).

body dementia and apathy with Pick's disease (frontotemporal dementia). The different forms of common dementia are compared in Table 13–6.

Alzheimer's disease pathologically is characterized by amyloid-β plaques and neurofibrillary tangles caused by hyperphosphorylation of tau. The course of the disease usually is over 10 years, and it takes 2 to 3 years for family members to notice problems. Between 4 and 7 years, the resident needs full-time care. At this time, the persons are usually incontinent and cannot dress and groom themselves adequately. Toward the end of life, they become aphasic, rigid, and bedridden. The stages of Alzheimer's dementia

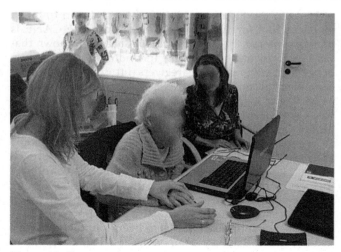

Figure 13–3. Typical computerized test conditions for a resident with Alzheimer's disease in a nursing home.

Table 13–5.   REVERSIBLE CAUSES OF DEMENTIA
Drugs (all anticholinergic)
Emotional (depression)
Metabolic (hypothyroid)
Eyes and ears (sensory isolation)
Normal-pressure hydrocephalus (ataxia, incontinence, dementia)
Tumor or other space occupying lesions
Infection (syphilis, AIDS, Lyme disease, chronic infections)
Anemia (vitamin B_{12} deficiency)

are delineated in Figure 13–3. A simple approach to the diagnosis of the causes of dementia is given in Table 13–7.

A number of drugs have been approved by the U.S. Food and Drug Administration for Dementia (Table 13–8). Both the cholinesterase inhibitors and memantine have effects that are statistically significant but whose clinical significance has been questioned. Occasional persons have a dramatic response to the drugs.

These drugs may preserve function for longer than placebo, but again, the effect is small. Memantine is an

N-methyl-D-aspartate (NMDA) antagonist approved for moderate to severe dementia. It decreased agitation in 12% of persons compared with 8% receiving placebo. Its effect on agitated behavior may be secondary to decreasing pain by blocking NMDA activity. Overall these drugs perform at about the same level as the older nootropics (i.e., piracetam and Hydergine).

Numerous botanicals and nutraceuticals have been said to improve cognition (Table 13–9). The efficacy of any of these agents is at the best borderline. A variety of drugs acting on different systems, mainly β-amyloid production and aggregation or oxidative metabolism, are under development (Table 13–10). Cerebrolysin, a peptide preparation that provides nerve growth factor effects and is given intravenously, has been shown to have short-term cognitive improvement.

Table 13–6.	COMPARISON OF DIFFERENT KINDS OF DEMENTIA				
	Alzheimer's Disease	**Lewy Body**	**Vascular Dementia**	**Depression**	**Pick's Disease**
Onset	Slow	Slow	Abrupt	Insidious	Slow
Progression	Progresses slowly with fluctuations over months	Progressive with fluctuations within a single day	Stepwise	Progressive	Progressive
Clinical features	Deficits in at least two areas of cognition Consciousness intact Hyperphagia early followed by anorexia Loss of ADLs Loss of executive function Agitation (midway) Depression (midway) Paranoia (midway) Wandering (midway) Loss of speech (late) Loss of mobility (late) Increased muscle tone (late) Seizures (late) Illusions, hallucinations (late)	Poor social function Attention deficits Visuospatial deficits Altered alertness Agitation Falls Inappropriate sexual behavior Visual hallucinations Systemized delusions Parkinsonism Syncope	Focal neurologic disease Cognitive defects are patchy Often depressed Other vascular disease	Sad Does not try to answer mental status testing Poor motivation Subjective complaints prominent and much greater than objective findings Tearful	Apathy fluctuations

ADL, activity of daily living.

Table 13–7.   SIMPLIFIED APPROACH TO DIAGNOSIS OF DEMENTIA

1. SAD = Depression
2. Exclude other reversible dementias
3. No loss of function = Mild cognitive impairment
4. Abrupt onset, stepwise progression, other vascular disease = Vascular dementia
5. Behavioral disturbance early (socially inappropriate or apathy) = Frontotemporal or Lewy body dementia
6. All others = Alzheimer's disease

Physical exercise has been shown to slow hippocampal shrinkage, improve cognition, decrease depression, and slow the rate of loss of activities of daily living. Overall, at present, exercise appears to be the most potent therapy for slowing the ravages of dementia.

High-quality ongoing dementia care requires adherence to a number of steps (Table 13–11). The needs of residents with dementia and their likes and dislikes are often poorly identified in nursing homes. The Camberwell Assessment of Need in the Elderly (CANE) has been shown to be an excellent tool for identifying these needs. The CANE is person centered with good validity. It has been shown that the CANE identifies needs for individuals with dementia better than either staff or caregivers (http://www.ucl.ac.uk/cane/#background). The CANE performs better than the MDS 2.0 at identifying individual needs. The MDS 3.0 has a similar resident-centered approach to determining unmet needs of residents.

In the United Kingdom, cognitive stimulation therapy (CST) has been developed as an evidence-based approach to treating dementia. CST has been found to improve memory, orientation, visuospatial skills, and a variety of language skills (e.g., naming, comprehension, word finding). It appears to be as effective as a number of drugs used for dementia. CST has also been found to improve quality of life. The key components of CST are given in Table 13–12. Nineteen separate sessions have been developed. The content of these include, for example, physical games, using money, art discussion, being creative, and household treasures. Each session has a series of consistent warm-up activities to maintain continuity. The CST website is http://www.cstdementia.com, and a manual and CD can be purchased.

Table 13–8.   COMPARISON OF COMMONLY USED AGENTS FOR THE TREATMENT OF ALZHEIMER'S DISEASE

	Donepezil	**Galantamine**[a]	**Rivastigmine**[a,b]	**Memantine**
Dementia stage	All	Mild to moderate	Mild to moderate	Moderate to severe
Action	AChEI	AChEI	AChEI	NMDA receptor antagonist
Dose range	5–23 mg/day	4 mg twice a day ER 8 mg/day	1.5–6 mg twice a day TD 4.6 mg every 24 hr	5 mg/day 10 mg twice a day
Side effects	Nausea Vomiting Diarrhea	GI side effects more common	GI side effects more common	Dizziness Hypotension Nausea Confusion Headache Incontinence Nightmares

Prolongation of QT_c interval

Increased tremor

Ataxia

Syncope

Delusions

Insomnia

Muscle cramps

Fatigue

Anorexia or weight loss

Aggression

AChEI, acetyl cholinesterase inhibitor; BuCHEI, butryl choleresterase inhibitor; ER, extended release; GI, gastrointestinal; NMDA, N-methyl-D-aspartate; TD, transdermal.

[a]Available in liquid formulations.

[b]Available as a patch.

Table 13–9.	NUTRACEUTICALS USED TO TREAT COGNITIVE DECLINE

Huperzine A

Polyphenols (curcumin)

Gingko biloba

Panax ginseng

Withaniasomnifera

Coenzyme Q10

Melatonin

Dehydroepiandrosterone

Pregnenolone

Phosphatidylserine

Acetyl-L-carnitine

Vitamins and minerals

Omega-3 fatty acids (Docosahexanoic acid)

α-Lipoic acid

Souvenaid (uridine monophosphate, choline, N-3 fatty acids)

Lutein + docosahexaenoic acid

Table 13–11.	KEY POINTS IN HIGH-QUALITY DEMENTIA CARE

1. Ongoing assessment that involves the individual and relatives with a focus on care that is acceptable to the individual
2. A focus on improving verbal and nonverbal communication with recognition of barriers to communication (including hearing and visual problems and understanding of language and cultural differences)
3. Recognition of appropriateness or not of pharmacotherapy
4. Maintaining the individual's nutritional needs
5. Providing appropriate recreation therapy to stimulate the individual while maintaining a calming environment
6. Enabling the individual to maintain and develop relationships and for the individual to recognize that his or her personhood is respected
7. Maximizing independence and sense of individuality
8. Providing a regular exercise program and encourage the individual to participate as much as he or she can
9. Providing a safe, homey environment with easily understandable signs posted and access to garden space
10. Educating staff members to be aware of innovative dementia care programs (e.g., cognitive stimulus therapy) and encouraging them to develop their own approaches to meet the individual needs of each resident

Cognitive therapy has been advocated as an alternative treatment modality to antidepressant medications or pharmacotherapy. Some studies show that cognitive therapies such as reminiscence have some short-term beneficial effect on mood and behavior for persons with dementia. The basic principle underpinning cognitive therapies is that low mood is triggered by thoughts related to the individual's interaction with his or her environment and his or her physiologic and emotional responses to that environment.

One type of cognitive therapy popular within dementia care is reminiscence. Initially, interest in reminiscence arose from the potential to tap into intact memories rather than with a view to the alleviation of low mood, the emphasis being on enabling people with dementia to review their lives, bringing unresolved conflicts into conscious awareness. More recently, however, the emphasis has shifted toward giving voice to people with mild to moderate dementia who can share well-rehearsed memories with others and engage in cognitively stimulating activities associated with personal interests that promote a sense of well-being. The potential to improve family interaction through

reminiscence work may likewise help to sustain caring relationships. It is widely recognized that structured reminiscence around a person's life experiences can be beneficial in terms of stimulating interest and enjoyment and maintaining identity and self-esteem. Many nursing home practitioners and family intuitively engage in informal reminiscence work to stimulate older residents to talk about topics of personal interest. Despite its popularity and the existence of some evidence to suggest that improvements in quality of life, behavior, and communication can be gained through reminiscence for people with mild to moderate dementia, the evidence of sustained therapeutic benefit is not strong.

Nonetheless, the international nursing home development agenda advocates the provision of meaningful activities that are both stimulating and enjoying. In theory, any topic might form a useful basis upon which to plan reminiscence activities, and knowing the interests of the

Table 13–10.	DRUGS UNDER DEVELOPMENT TO TREAT ALZHEIMER'S DISEASE		
Immunotherapy	Active		γ-Secretase inhibitor
	Passive		β-Secretase inhibitors
			α-Secretase activators
Antisenses	Antiamyloid precursor protein		Amyloid aggregate inhibitors
	Antipresenilin		Tau phosphorylation inhibitors
	Anti-GSK-β		Inhibitors of oxidative metabolism

Table 13–12.	PRINCIPLES OF COGNITIVE STIMULATION THERAPY

- Providing orientation in a sensitive manner
- Using implicit learning in which opinion is more important than learned facts
- Using multiple forms of sensory stimulation
- Having a variety of flexible activities available to maintain stimulation
- Using reminiscence to help maintain older memories
- Creating new relationships and strengthening old relationships
- Sing supportive groups to increase mood and concentration

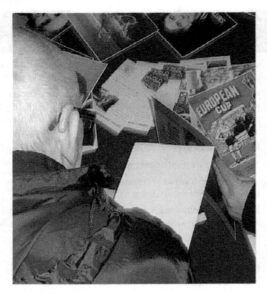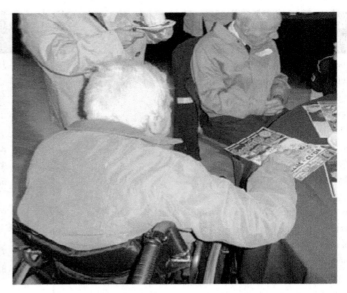

Figure 13–4. Nursing home residents visiting the National Scottish Football Museum.

resident is key to planning appropriate activities. In the United Kingdom, an ongoing program of collaborative research has identified concern among male nursing home residents and community-dwelling men with dementia about the feminization of the activities that are provided for them. This lack of meaningful activity stimulated the development of soccer-focused reminiscence projects (http://www.facebook.com/MemoriesFC). Promising early results suggests that this is a popular and particularly powerful anchor subject with therapeutic potential (Figure 13–4).

Although the mechanisms that make soccer reminiscence potentially powerful are not fully understood, a possible explanation might lie in the combination or the place of this national sport in the United Kingdom in personal and shared identities and in the symbolism of the soccer stadium as home and the comforting effect of this strong emotional attachment. Sports-based reminiscence therapy can be applied in a personalized way, thus stimulating both personal and cultural identity and providing much needed social interaction. The potential of other sports-based reminiscence activities tailored to local interests could be explored by nursing home staff as this may offer new ways to engage local communities in nursing home life. A project at St. Louis University, for example, is developing a program of baseball reminiscence for nursing home residents, and similar to the Scottish project, it is proving popular.

Another dementia program that has been successful is the STAR (Staff Training for Assisted living Residences) program. This program reduced both behavioral and affective distress. This program deals with training staff and family to have realistic expectations, enhance communication, and increase pleasant events using visual and activity aids (http://www.depts.washington.edu/adrcweb/STAR.shtml).

BEHAVIORAL DISTURBANCES

Altered behaviors occur commonly in nursing home residents with dementia. Apathy is present in 27%, depression in 24%, and agitation with or without aggression in 24%. In addition, delusions occur in 19% and hallucinations in 25%. The classic course as dementia worsens is that the residents go from social withdrawal to depression to paranoia. The most common inappropriate behaviors in dementia are resistance to care and vocal behaviors. In addition, more than half of residents with dementia have restlessness and times when they are physically aggressive (Table 13–13).

The management of inappropriate behaviors whenever possible should be a psychosocial intervention. Drugs should be avoided whenever possible; antipsychotics are greatly overused for behavioral problems associated with dementia. Table 13–14 demonstrates a way to highlight for nursing home staff why antipsychotics should be avoided.

In the classical study in the *New England Journal of Medicine*, antipsychotics failed to statistically improve behavior. Placebo improved behavior in 21%, and olanzapine, quetiapine, and risperidone all improved behavior by 55 to 10% compared with placebo but insufficiently to produce statistical significance. Antipsychotics clearly can reduce hallucinations, illusions, delusions, and paranoia and should be used when their symptoms are bothersome to residents. Reasons why antipsychotics are commonly used but are clearly ineffective are listed in Table 13–15. Antipsychotics have been shown to accelerate the production of neurofibrillary tangles and thus accelerate the dementia process. The side effects of neuroleptics are listed in Table 13–16. In the United Kingdom, 180,000 people with dementia are receiving antipsychotics, leading to an excess of 1800 deaths. When used, neuroleptics should be used in the lowest possible dose (e.g., 0.5 mg for haloperidol or 1 mg for risperidone). There is little evidence to support that at these low doses the newer antipsychotics are safer. In nursing homes, antipsychotic use should be limited to residents with schizophrenia; some patients with severe bipolar disorder; and persons with hallucinations, illusions, delusions, or paranoia that is troublesome to the resident. Always remember that sensory deprivation caused by auditory or visual loss can

Table 13–13.	INAPPROPRIATE BEHAVIORS SEEN IN NURSING HOME RESIDENTS WITH DEMENTIA	
Behavior	**Prevalence (%)**	
Resistance to care	>70	
Vocal behaviors	>60	
Restlessness	>50	
Physical regression	>50	
Rummaging	25–50	
Hallucinations	25–50	
Pacing	10–20	
Spitting	1–5	
Sexual behaviors	1–5	

Table 13–15.   BEHAVIORS FOR WHICH ANTIPSYCHOTICS SHOULD NOT BE USED

- Wandering
- Restlessness
- Unsociability, including physical and verbal aggression
- Poor self-care
- Impaired memory
- Anxiety
- Insomnia
- Fidgeting
- Indifference to surroundings
- Nervousness
- Uncooperativeness
- Depression (without psychotic features)
- Distressed behaviors that are not a danger to the resident or others

Based on F329 tag used by nursing home surveyors in the United States.

be the cause of illusions or hallucinations, as can tinnitus. Residents taking neuroleptics should have a dose reduction tried after 3 months and at least yearly thereafter. Possible side effects should be recorded on a weekly basis, and a monthly review of their necessity and possible side effects should be done by a registered nurse, pharmacist, and physician.

Dextromethorphan–quinidine (marketed as Nuedexta in the United States) has been shown to have a small positive effect on pseudobulbar symptoms (inappropriate laughing and crying) in persons with amyotrophic lateral sclerosis and multiple sclerosis. It is an NMDA receptor antagonist and a σ-1 receptor agonist. This drug combination increases the QT_c interval, and as such, increases the propensity for arrhythmias. It can produce dissociative hallucinations. It can cause histamine release, leading to itching, dizziness, and hypotension. When used with monoamine oxidase inhibitors or serotonin reuptake inhibitors, it can cause serotonin syndrome. It has been suggested that it can be used for some behaviors in dementia, but at present, no data support this.

There is no place for physical restraints to treat behavioral symptoms. Mittens produce sensory deprivation and increase inappropriate behaviors.

When nursing home residents become agitated, the possibility that they have delirium or untreated pain should

be the first approach. Regular use of pain medications rather than as needed is a key because persons with dementia often do not ask for pain medicines. Physical violence often occurs when a resident is startled by a caregiver approaching too rapidly or from behind or trying to get the resident to do a task that he or she does not want to do. Regular exercise has been shown to markedly decrease aggressive behavior. Namaste therapy can be successful in some agitated residents (Table 13–17). Caregivers need to be taught to deal with or ignore agitation because this is often the best approach. The caregiver should keep his or her distance; walk alongside an aggressive individual; and talk to the person in a quiet, nonagitated voice. Time-outs either in the resident's room or in a "Snoezelen" room, if available, are

Table 13–14.   WOULD YOU GIVE YOUR MOTHER A DRUG THAT...

- Caused aspiration?
- Made her think less well?
- Could make her feel more agitated?
- Increased falling and hip fractures?
- Caused aspiration pneumonia?
- Increased her chance of dying by 10?
- Did not work?

Table 13–16.   SIDE EFFECTS OF NEUROLEPTICS

- Tardive dyskinesia
- Parkinson's disease
- Dystonia
- Sedation
- Falls
- Osteoporosis
- Hip fractures
- Diabetes mellitus
- Hypotension
- Anticholinergic symptoms such as dry mouth, urinary problems, constipation
- Cognitive decline
- Increased neurofibrillary tangles
- Q-T prolongation
- Stroke
- Myocardial infarction
- Neuroleptic syndrome (hyperthermia, rigidity)
- Increased mortality

Table 13–17.   NAMASTE THERAPY[a]

Concept: From Sanskrit

Nam = bow

Aham = false ego

Te = you

"Greeting you while giving up false ego."

Recognition of one's existence by another person

Components

Seven days a week

Dedicated room for programs

Touch (e.g., hand and foot massage, brushing or combing hair with slow movements)

Moisturizing face with cold cream

Providing different scents

Using shaving cream

Blowing bubbles

Moving limbs to music

Food and drink 24 hours a day

Talking to in a gentle voice

Music in background

Comfortable chairs and quilts

Pictures of the past and mementos

Bird sounds

[a]The concept of Namaste Therapy was created by Joyce Simard.

Table 13–18.   MUSIC THERAPY PROGRAMS

Intervention	Notes
Background music	Decreases agitation
Active listening groups	Attention and socialization
Therapeutic singing	Cognition and socialization
Movement to music	Exercise and range of motion
Gait training with music	Uses music to improve cadence and velocity of gait
Reminiscence with music	Cues recall for life review
Playing an instrument	Self-expression; improves attention and short-term memory
Imagery with music	Relaxation; reduces pain and anxiety
Iso-principle	Matching music cadence to resident's voice and movements and then changing volume and cadence to a less agitated mode

very useful. Low dose of a benzodiazepam, such as the short-acting lorazepam (0.5 mg), can be used in difficult cases.

Both formal or informal music therapy programs have been used to reduce behavioral disturbances in residents. Dancing and playing a musical instrument are recreational activities that have been associated with a slowing of cognitive decline. Music reminiscence groups can improve recall of past events and help maintain cognitive function. Music therapy produces active engagement, enhancing attention and participation. Music therapy can be used to reduce disruptive behaviors, and in an informal setting, background music can have a calming effect on residents. Music therapy can increase socialization within groups. Finally, music therapy can be helpful for staff and caregivers in enhancing positive interactions with the residents. Table 13–18 provides examples of different approaches to music therapy.

SUNDOWNING: TWILIGHT AGITATION

"Sundowning" is agitated behavior that occurs in the evening. There are multiple causes of "sundowning." Persons with dementia have a phased advancement in their circadian rhythm, making them more active at dinnertime and at the time they would normally go to bed. Use of high-lux light (2000 lux) has been shown to decrease agitation, and the concurrent use of melatonin may be more effective. Shadows occurring at sunset can lead to illusions, especially in persons with cataracts or age-related macular degeneration. Many persons had a fear of darkness as a child, and

this can return in persons with dementia, leading to altered behaviors. Both relative hypo- or hyperglycemia around suppertime can result in altered behavior as can postprandial hypotension. Hunger while waiting for dinner is a trigger for agitation. Making snacks available while waiting for dinner can reduce residents' conflicts around dinner time. Stress thresholds tend to be lowered as residents become tired at the end of the day.

SCREAMING

Uncontrollable, continuous screaming by a resident can be very disturbing in the nursing home ambience. Pain or other reasons for the resident's being uncomfortable should be the first area to be addressed. Use of activities, exercise, reading, and a relaxing environment can all help reduce screaming. If these approaches fail, using a pocket talker (hearing amplifier) with the volume turned high can allow the resident to hear his or her own voice and reduce the screaming. Screaming may be caused by intrapsychic stress and in many cases responds to electroconvulsive therapy.

APPROACH TO MANAGEMENT OF BEHAVIORAL PROBLEMS

A simple method of behavioral management is the ACE approach:

A = Assess behavior. Is the cause the environment, the staff, or the patient?

C = Care planning

E = Exercise

Special care units isolate problematic patients. To be successful, they require increased staffing. Staff needs to be carefully chosen and rotated regularly to avoid burnout.

Table 13–19.	MANAGEMENT OF NONCOGNITIVE BEHAVIORAL SYMPTOMS

Caregiver support and education. The ability to deal with agitation is often more important than agitation itself.

Behavioral therapy

- Reality orientation
- Validation therapy
- Reminiscence therapy
- Music and other creative arts therapies
- Namaste therapy

Environmental modifications

- Clear environmental distinctions
- Restraint-free environment
- "Snoezelen" room
- Wander garden
- "Time-out" space

Exercise therapy

Recreation therapy (keeps a high level of activity)

Avoidance of pharmacotherapy

Assess for and treat pain as a cause (regular, not as needed, pain medications)

Exclude delirium as a cause

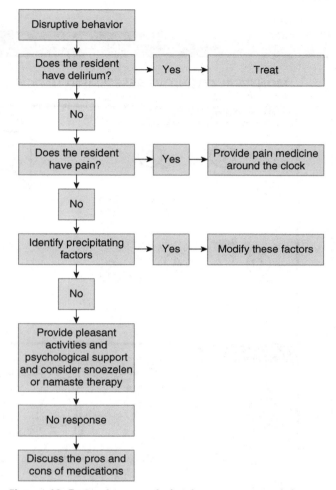

Figure 13–5. Simple approach for the management of disruptive behaviors in a nursing home.

Education for the staff in managing problematic behaviors is essential. Availability of a "Snoezelen" or time-out area is very helpful. A wander garden, an exercise program, and multiple activities are also helpful. Controlled studies have failed to show that special care units are efficacious or cost effective. However, this fails to account for positive effects on other residents who no longer have to deal with difficult residents.

The major principles of management of noncognitive behavioral symptoms are outlined in Table 13–19. A simple approach to managing problematic behaviors is provided in Figure 13–5.

KEY POINTS

1. Delirium and subsyndromal delirium are common in nursing homes and lead to falls, functional decline, and increased mortality rates.
2. There are many treatable causes of delirium. In older persons with delirium, there is often more than one cause.
3. MCI should be identified and treatable causes, such as anticholinergic drugs, identified. There is no evidence that it responds to drugs used to treat dementia.
4. Dementia has a variety of reversible and nonreversible causes. Depression should always be considered as a cause of "pseudo-dementia."
5. CST has been shown to be as effective as drugs as a treatment for dementia.
6. Physical exercise slows cognitive and functional impairment in persons with dementia.
7. A variety of behavioral disturbances occur in persons with dementia.
8. Physical restraints should *not* be used in persons with dementia.
9. Antipsychotics (neuroleptics) should only be used in persons with psychosis or clear hallucinations, illusions, delusions, or paranoia. Antipsychotics increase mortality rates.
10. Treatments such as "Snoezelen" or "Namaste" therapy should be available to help manage agitation.
11. Exercise decreases agitated behaviors.

TOOLKIT

MoCA

MONTREAL COGNITIVE ASSESSMENT (MOCA)
Version 7.1 Original Version

NAME :
Education :   Date of birth :
Sex :   DATE :

VISUOSPATIAL / EXECUTIVE

Copy cube

Draw CLOCK (Ten past eleven)
(3 points)

POINTS

[ ]   [ ]   [ ]   [ ]   [ ]   __/5
                                                              Contour   Numbers   Hands

NAMING

[ ]   [ ]   [ ]   __/3

MEMORY Read list of words, subject must repeat them. Do 2 trials, even if 1st trial is successful. Do a recall after 5 minutes.		FACE	VELVET	CHURCH	DAISY	RED	No points
	1st trial						
	2nd trial						

ATTENTION	Read list of digits (1 digit/ sec.).	Subject has to repeat them in the forward order	[ ] 2 1 8 5 4	__/2
		Subject has to repeat them in the backward order	[ ] 7 4 2	

Read list of letters. The subject must tap with his hand at each letter A. No points if ≥ 2 errors
[ ]   F B A C M N A A J K L B A F A K D E A A A J A M O F A A B   __/1

Serial 7 subtraction starting at 100   [ ] 93   [ ] 86   [ ] 79   [ ] 72   [ ] 65   __/3
4 or 5 correct subtractions: **3 pts**, 2 or 3 correct: **2 pts**, 1 correct: **1 pt**, 0 correct: **0 pt**

LANGUAGE	Repeat : I only know that John is the one to help today. [ ] The cat always hid under the couch when dogs were in the room. [ ]	__/2

Fluency / Name maximum number of words in one minute that begin with the letter F   [ ] _____ (N ≥ 11 words)   __/1

ABSTRACTION	Similarity between e.g. banana - orange = fruit [ ] train – bicycle [ ] watch - ruler	__/2

DELAYED RECALL	Has to recall words **WITH NO CUE**	FACE [ ]	VELVET [ ]	CHURCH [ ]	DAISY [ ]	RED [ ]	Points for UNCUED recall only	__/5
Optional	Category cue							
	Multiple choice cue							

ORIENTATION	[ ] Date [ ] Month [ ] Year [ ] Day [ ] Place [ ] City	__/6

© Z.Nasreddine MD   **www.mocatest.org**   Normal ≥ 26 / 30 | TOTAL   __/30 |

Administered by: _____   Add 1 point if   ≤ 12 yr edu

SUGGESTED READINGS

An Introduction to Cognitive Stimulation Therapy (CST). http://www. cstdementia.com. Accessed April 18, 2013.

Baillon S, Van Diepen E, Prettyman R, et al. A comparison of the effects of Snoezelen and reminiscence therapy on the agitated behaviour of patients with dementia. *Int J Geriatr Psychiatry.* 2004;19:1047-1052.

Charleston S. The English football ground as a representation of home. *J Environ Psychol.* 2009;29:144-150.

Enmarker I, Olsen R, Hellzen O. Management of person with dementia with aggressive and violent behaviour: a systematic literature review. *Int J Older People Nurs.* 2011;6:153-162.

Flaherty JH. The evaluation and management of delirium among older persons. *Med Clin North Am.* 2011;95:555-577.

Flaherty JH, Shay K, Weir C, et al. The development of a mental status vital sign for use across the spectrum of care. *J Am Med Dir Assoc.* 2009; 10:379-380.

Flaherty JH, Steele DK, Chibnall JT, et al. An ACE unit with a delirium room may improve function and equalize length of stay among older delirious medical inpatients. *J Gerontol A Biol Sci Med Sci.* 2010;65: 1387-1392.

Gibson F. *The Past in the Present.* Baltimore: The Health Professions Press; 2004.

Gillette Guyonnet S, Abellan van Kan G, Alix E, et al. International Academy on Nutrition and Aging Expert Group. Weight loss and Alzheimer's disease. *J Nutr Health Aging.* 2007;11:38-48.

Inouye SK. Delirium in older persons. *N Engl J Med.* 2006;354:1157-1165.

Ishii S, Weintraub N, Mervis JR. Apathy: a common psychiatric syndrome in the elderly. *J Am Med Dir Assoc.* 2009;10:381-393.

Lai CK, Yeung JH, Mok V, Chi I. Special care units for dementia individuals with behavioural problems. *Cochrane Database Syst Rev.* 2009;(4):CD006470.

MacLullich A, Ferguson KJ, Miller T, et al. Unravelling the pathophysiology of delirium: a focus on the role of aberrant stress responses. *J Psychosom Res.* 2008;65:229-238.

Mazoteras Muñoz V, Abellan van Kan G, Cantet C, et al. Gait and balance impairments in Alzheimer disease patients. *Alzheimer Dis Assoc Disord.* 2010;24:79-84.

Morley JE. Alzheimer's disease: future treatments. *J Am Med Dir Assoc.* 2011;12:1-7.

Morley JE. Dementia-related agitation. *J Am Med Dir Assoc.* 2011;12: 611-612.e2.

Morley JE. Editorial: Can we improve care for patients with dementia? *J Nutr Health Aging.* 2011;15:523-525.

Morley JE. Managing persons with dementia in the nursing home: high touch trumps high tech. *J Am Med Dir Assoc.* 2008;9:139-146.

National Institute for Clinical Excellence. *Diagnosis, Prevention and Management of Delirium* [draft for consultation]. http://www. nice.org.uk/Nicemedia/Pdf/Delirium_Nice_Guideline.Pdf 2009. Accessed July 24, 2012.

Orrell M, Woods B, Spector A. Should we use individual cognitive stimulation therapy to improve cognitive function in people with dementia? *Br Med J.* 2012;344:e633.

Rolland Y, Abellan van Kan G, Hermabessiere S, et al. Descriptive study of nursing home residents from the REHPA network. *J Nutr Health Aging.* 2009;13:679-683.

Rolland Y, Abellan van Kan G, Vellas B. Physical activity and Alzheimer's disease: from prevention to therapeutic perspectives. *J Am Med Dir Assoc.* 2008;9:390-405.

Rolland Y, Pillard F, Klapouszczak A, et al. Exercise program for nursing home residents with Alzheimer's disease: a 1-year randomized, controlled trial. *J Am Geriatr Soc.* 2007;55:158-165.

Rupke S, Blecke D, Renfrow M. Cognitive therapy for depression. *Am Fam Physician.* 2006;73:83-86.

Schofield I, Tolson D, Fleming V. How nurses understand and care for older people with delirium in the acute hospital: a critical discourse analysis. *Nurse.* 2011;19(2):165-176.

Simard J, Volicer L. Effects of Namaste care on residents who do not benefit from usual activities. *Am J Alzheimers Dis Other Demen.* 2010;25:46-50.

STAR (Staff Training for Assisted living Residences). http://www.depts. washington.edu.adrcweb/STAR.shtml. Accessed April 18, 2013.

Tariq SH, Tumosa N, Chibnall JT, et al. Comparison of the Saint Louis University mental status examination and the mini-mental state examination for detecting dementia and mild neurocognitive disorder—a pilot study. *Am J Geriatr Psychiatry.* 2006;14:900-910.

Teri L, Huda P, Gibbons L, et al. Star: a dementia-specific training program for staff in assisted living residents. *Gerontologist.* 2005;45(5):686.

The Camberwell Assessment of Need in the Elderly (CANE). http://www. ucl.ac.uk/cane#background. Accessed April 18, 2013.

The European Delirium Association. STOP Delirium Project. http:// www.europeandeliriumassociation.com/delirium-information/ healthprofessionals/stop-delirium-project/. Accessed April 18, 2013.

Tolson D, Schofield I. Football reminiscence for men with dementia: Lessons from a realistic evaluation. *Nurse Inquiry.* 2012;19:63-70.

Trzepacz P, van der Mast R. The neuropathophysiology of delirium. In: Lindesay J, Rockwood K, MacDonald A (eds). *Delirium in Old Age.* Oxford, UK: Oxford University Press; 2002.

Villars H, Oustric S, Andrieu S, et al. The primary care physician and Alzheimer's disease: an international position paper. *J Nutr Health Aging.* 2010;14:110-120.

Volicer L. Is your nursing home a battlefield? *J Am Med Dir Assoc.* 2012; 13:195-196.

Volicer L, Hurley AC. Management of behavioral symptoms in progressive degenerative dementias. *J Gerontol A Biol Sci Med Sci.* 2003;58:M837-M845.

Volicer L, McKee A, Hewitt S. Dementia. *Neurol Clin.* 2001;19:867-885.

Wang J-Y. Group reminiscence therapy for cognitive and affective function of demented elderly in Taiwan. *Int J Geriatr Psychiatry.* 2007;22: 1235-1240.

Woods B, Aguirre E, Spector AE, Orrell M. Cognitive stimulation to improve cognitive functioning in people with dementia. *Cochrane Database Syst Rev.* 2012;2:CD005562.

Woods, B, Spector A, Jones C, et al. Reminiscence therapy for dementia. *Cochrane Database Syst Rev.* 2005;(2):CD001120.

Worden A, Challis D, Hancock G, et al. Identifying need in care homes for people with dementia: the relationship between two standard assessment tools. *Aging Mental Health.* 2008;12:719-728.

MULTIPLE CHOICE QUESTIONS

13.1   Which of the following is *not* true of delirium in nursing homes?

    a. Delirium is associated with a doubling of rehospitalization rates.

    b. Delirium does not affect functional improvement.

    c. Delirious patients are more likely to be physically restrained.

    d. Residents with delirium have a higher mortality rate.

    e. Subsyndromal delirium occurs in up to 40% of residents admitted from a hospital.

13.2   Which of the following cannot be used to screen for amnestic mild cognitive impairment?

    a. Mini-Mental Status

    b. VAMC-St. Louis University Mental Status (SLUMS) Examination

    c. Montreal Cognitive Assessment (MoCA)

    d. Short Test of Mental Status

13.3   A 75-year-old woman has had poor recall and executive function. She has had a number of falls, and her gait is ataxic. She has developed incontinence. Which of the following is a possible reversible diagnosis?

    a. Pick's disease

    b. Fragile X syndrome

    c. Hypothyroid

    d. Lewy body dementia

    e. Normal-pressure hydrocephalus

13.4 An 84-year-old man being treated for dementia has a decrease in pain and angry outbursts
but develops nightmares. His blood pressure is
90/60 mm Hg. Which drug for dementia is he
likely to be receiving?

a. Donepezil
b. Piracetam
c. Memantine
d. Rivastigmine
e. α-Lipoic acid

13.5 Cognitive stimulation therapy has been developed
to improve memory and language skills. It has been
demonstrated to be as effective as drug therapy for
dementia.

a. True
b. False

13.6 Which of the following is *not* a side effect of
antipsychotics?

a. Decreased mortality rate
b. Hip fractures
c. Osteoporosis
d. Cognitive decline
e. Stroke

Chapter 14

EATING AND DRINKING

Eating and drinking is a fundamental activity that most healthy adults associate with pleasure. When we have the resources to do so, we select the food and drink that we consume and choose how it is served and when we take nourishment. Understanding the food preferences and eating habits of nursing home residents is important in the quest to deliver resident-centered care. In addition to the pleasurable and social aspects of mealtimes and beverages, it is important that the healthcare team understand the dietary and nutritional status and requirements of individual residents. Attention to provision of an appropriate diet and fluid intake can assist in promotion of resident health and well-being. Age-related changes that may compromise eating and drinking behaviors and intentions include anorexia, changes in the sense of smell and taste, medication side effects, constipation, and dry mouth. Research has shown that what people choose to eat may not always be rational and often depends on the context of eating. Several studies have shown that people tend to eat more when they eat with others; however, this is not always the case in nursing homes, and if a resident is forced to eat in a communal area against his or her wishes, it may have the opposite effect. Undernutrition is common among older people admitted to nursing homes; lower levels of hunger and increased levels of fullness (satiety) are common complaints. The challenges for nursing home teams are to identify those who are malnourished (or at risk of becoming so), know how to monitor nutritional and hydration status, and know how to intervene and when to refer for further specialized intervention.

Nurses and nurse's aides play key roles in providing residents with help in the selection of food and drink and in preparing residents for meals. To enjoy meals, people should feel clean and comfortable; they should also have been offered the opportunity to go to the toilet and wash their hands. Preparation of the resident for mealtimes should not be rushed, and when spillage is anticipated, dignified napkins should be selected to protect clothing. Mealtime independence can be enabled through the provision of suitable adapted utensils recommended by an occupational therapist when possible. Food should arrive plated attractively and served at the correct temperature. For residents who require mealtime assistance, help should be attentive and considerate, and postmealtime hygiene and bathroom time should leave the resident feeling comfortable and confident.

This chapter focuses on nutritional screening, clinical aspects, and nursing strategies known to be useful within nursing homes for common and more complex problems. The chapter also draws attention to the multiplex of factors discussed elsewhere in this book that may alter a resident's appetite and eating and drinking behaviors such as low mood, boredom, dry mouth, cognitive changes, delirium, constipation, and fear of being incontinent to name but a few.

NUTRITIONAL SCREENING AND ASSESSMENT

Malnutrition of a variety of types is common in nursing homes. The British Association for Enteral and Parenteral Nutrition (2008) conducted a nutritional screening survey and audit of more than 9000 people admitted to care homes, hospitals, and mental health units and found that one third of older people admitted to care homes or "care of older adults" hospital wards were classified as malnourished. Protein energy undernutrition is an excellent indicator of quality of care in the nursing home. Vitamin and mineral deficiencies are not rare but are usually linked to poor food intake. Obesity is less of a problem, and persons with body mass indexes (BMIs) up to 35 usually have better outcomes than those with low BMIs (<22). BMIs greater than 40 are associated with poor function and increased burden on caregivers.

NUTRITIONAL ASSESSMENT

A number of nutritional assessment tools have been developed. BMI is a proxy for body fat. It is calculated as:

$$\text{BMI} = \frac{\text{Mass (kg)}}{(\text{Height [m]}^2)} \text{ or } \frac{\text{Mass (lb)} \times 703}{(\text{Height [m]}^2)}$$

Although a normal BMI is defined as 18.5 to 25 for young persons, an ideal BMI may be considered to be 22 to 30 in nursing home residents.

The Simplified Nutrition Assessment Questionnaire (SNAQ) consists of four simple questions that can be answered by the resident or the caregiver (based on observation of the person eating) (Table 14–1). The SNAQ has been validated as an instrument that predicts weight loss in nursing home residents. It can be considered as an early warning detector of persons at high risk of developing protein energy undernutrition.

Table 14–1.   THE SIMPLIFIED NUTRITION ASSESSMENT QUESTIONNAIRE

Instructions: Complete the questionnaire by circling the correct answers and then tally the results based on the following numerical scale: A = 1, B = 2, C = 3, D = 4, and E = 5.

Scoring: If the SNAQ is less than 14, there is a significant risk of weight loss.

1. My appetite is
   A. Very poor
   B. Poor
   C. Average
   D. Good
   E. Very good

2. When I eat
   A. I feel full after eating only a few mouthfuls.
   B. I feel full after eating about a third of a meal.
   C. I feel full after eating over half a meal.
   D. I feel full after eating most of the meal.
   E. I hardly ever feel full.

3. Food tastes
   A. Very bad
   B. Bad
   C. Average
   D. Good
   E. Very good

4. Normally I eat
   A. Less than one meal a day
   B. One meal a day
   C. Two meals a day
   D. Three meals a day
   E. More than 3 meals a day

The Mini Nutritional Assessment (MNA) is a highly validated tool in older persons and in nursing home residents (Figure 14–1). It has been widely used in many countries and has been translated into a variety of languages. It does not require laboratory tests. It is highly prognostic of future declines in function and of mortality. A short form of the MNA exists and can be used for screening. In addition to diagnosing malnutrition, the MNA also identifies persons with frailty.

A variety of blood tests (albumin, prealbumin, and transthyretin, retinal binding protein, insulinlike growth factor-1 [IGF-1], and transferrin) have been used to determine the nutritional status of the individual. Albumin, transthyretin, and retinol binding protein are all decreased with cytokine excess (seen in the presence of inflammation) and as such are poor indicators of protein energy malnutrition in persons with chronic illnesses. Transferrin is associated with iron status and cytokines and as such is also a poor nutritional marker in nursing homes. IGF-1

declines with aging because of the decrease in growth hormone secretion. Thus, laboratory tests are poor proxies for general nutritional status in nursing home residents.

ANOREXIA AND WEIGHT LOSS

Weight loss, even in persons with diabetes mellitus, is highly predictive of mortality. Weight loss also predicts loss of function, hip fracture, and institutionalization. Figure 14–2 demonstrates the effects of weight gain, loss, or maintenance on mortality in nursing home residents. The reasons why weight loss is bad for older persons in nursing homes is multifactorial:

- Weight loss can be a harbinger of occult disease.
- Weight loss is a marker of protein energy undernutrition.
- Weight loss leads to an increase in small dense low-density lipoprotein, which is highly atherogenic.
- Weight loss is associated with fat loss, and fat padding at the hips protects against hip fracture.
- Weight loss leads to release of toxins (Polychlorinated biphenyl [PCBs] and Dichlorodiphenyl ethane [DDEs]) stored in fat—the so-called "poisonous infusion."
- Weight loss alters the effects of drugs bound to albumin and stored in fat, leading to the need for dose reduction.
- Weight loss leads to a loss of stem cells in fatty tissue, which play an essential role in repair of damaged tissues.

The major causes of weight loss are given in Table 14–2. Measurement of vitamin A or β-carotene in serum and fecal chymotrypsin or elastase are useful for the diagnosis of malabsorption.

Independent of weight loss, anorexia has also been shown to independently predict mortality. Thus, in nursing homes, maintenance of weight is a key to survival and good health in the nursing home.

Older persons develop a physiologic anorexia of aging to balance their decrease in physical activity and physiologic loss of muscle mass (Figure 14–3). Numerous factors are involved in developing the physiologic anorexia of aging. These include a decline in taste and more especially olfaction, a decrease in stomach fundal compliance leading to early satiation, and an increase in the satiety hormone cholecystokinin. Increases in leptin levels and circulating cytokines can further increase the anorexia.

One third of weight loss in nursing home residents is caused by depression, and less than 10% is due to cancer. Chronic obstructive pulmonary disease (COPD) is an important cause of weight loss, mainly caused by oxygen utilization as part of the thermic effect of eating, leading to early dyspnea, which inhibits the ability to continue to eat. Eating multiple small meals is the best way to increase caloric intake in persons with COPD. There are numerous treatable causes of weight loss in nursing home residents as illustrated by the MEALS ON WHEELS mnemonic (Table 14–3).

Mini Nutritional Assessment

MNA®

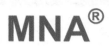

Nestlé
NutritionInstitute

Last name:		First name:	
Sex:	Age:	Weight, kg:	Height, cm:	Date:

Complete the screen by filling in the boxes with the appropriate numbers. Total the numbers for the final screening score.

Screening

A Has food intake declined over the past 3 months due to loss of appetite, digestive problems, chewing or swallowing difficulties?
0 = severe decrease in food intake
1 = moderate decrease in food intake
2 = no decrease in food intake ☐

B Weight loss during the last 3 months
0 = weight loss greater than 3 kg (6.6 lbs)
1 = does not know
2 = weight loss between 1 and 3 kg (2.2 and 6.6 lbs)
3 = no weight loss ☐

C Mobility
0 = bed or chair bound
1 = able to get out of bed / chair but does not go out
2 = goes out ☐

D Has suffered psychological stress or acute disease in the past 3 months?
0 = yes   2 = no ☐

E Neuropsychological problems
0 = severe dementia or depression
1 = mild dementia
2 = no psychological problems ☐

F1 Body Mass Index (BMI) (weight in kg) / (height in m²) ☐
0 = BMI less than 19
1 = BMI 19 to less than 21
2 = BMI 21 to less than 23
3 = BMI 23 or greater ☐

IF BMI IS NOT AVAILABLE, REPLACE QUESTION F1 WITH QUESTION F2.
DO NOT ANSWER QUESTION F2 IF QUESTION F1 IS ALREADY COMPLETED.

F2 Calf circumference (CC) in cm
0 = CC less than 31
3 = CC 31 or greater ☐

Screening score ☐☐
(max. 14 points)

12-14 points: ☐ Normal nutritional status   Save
8-11 points: ☐ At risk of malnutrition   Print
0-7 points: ☐ Malnourished   Reset

Ref.   Vellas B, Villars H, Abellan G, et al. *Overview of the MNA® - Its History and Challenges.* J Nutr Health Aging 2006;10:456-465.

Rubenstein LZ, Harker JO, Salva A, Guigoz Y, Vellas B. *Screening for Undernutrition in Geriatric Practice: Developing the Short-Form Mini Nutritional Assessment (MNA-SF).* J. Geront 2001;56A: M366-377.

Guigoz Y. *The Mini-Nutritional Assessment (MNA®) Review of the Literature - What does it tell us?* J Nutr Health Aging 2006; 10:466-487.

Kaiser MJ, Bauer JM, Ramsch C, et al. *Validation of the Mini Nutritional Assessment Short-Form (MNA®-SF): A practical tool for identification of nutritional status.* J Nutr Health Aging 2009; 13:782-788.

® Société des Produits Nestlé, S.A., Vevey, Switzerland, Trademark Owners

© Nestlé, 1994, Revision 2009. N67200 12/99 10M

For more information: www.mna-elderly.com

Figure 14–1. The Mini Nutritional Assessment.

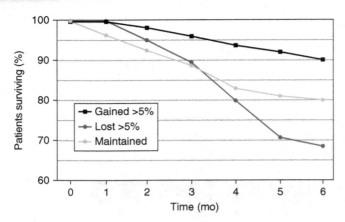

Figure 14–2. The Geriatric Anorexia Nutrition (GAIN) registry survival curve demonstrates that reversal of weight loss increased survival in nursing home.

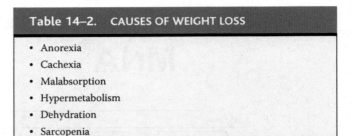

Table 14–2. CAUSES OF WEIGHT LOSS
• Anorexia
• Cachexia
• Malabsorption
• Hypermetabolism
• Dehydration
• Sarcopenia

MANAGING WEIGHT LOSS

Enhancing food intake in the nursing home requires multiple approaches. Since the original studies in Scandinavia, it is now clear that enhancing dining ambience is an important component of improving food intake. This includes nice table settings with tablecloths and food presented in a pleasing style on the plate. The use of buffet dining appears to increase food intake (Figure 14–4). Good conversation at mealtimes increases food intake, thus making it important to ensure the compatibility of the residents sharing a table.

Flavor enhancement of food using substances that activate the unami taste (e.g., glutamate, ribonucleotides [quanylic acid and inosinic acid], glycine, and leucine) may increase food intake. Involving residents in meal preparation has also been successful in Finland. Foods need to be ethnically appropriate as do feeding methods. When foods are mixed together, intake tends to be reduced.

Persons who need help with feeding should ideally be in a separate dining area. Semicircular tables can allow an aide to easily feed five or six residents at the same time. The vast majority of feeding assistance is provided by certified nursing assistants. The better the interaction between the aide and the resident, the longer the time spent feeding and the better the food intake. In addition, trying to maintain as small a number of aides as possible to feed an individual resident improves outcomes. In one study of a large nursing home, residents were exposed to 15 to 20 different nursing assistants to help them eat over a 4-week period.

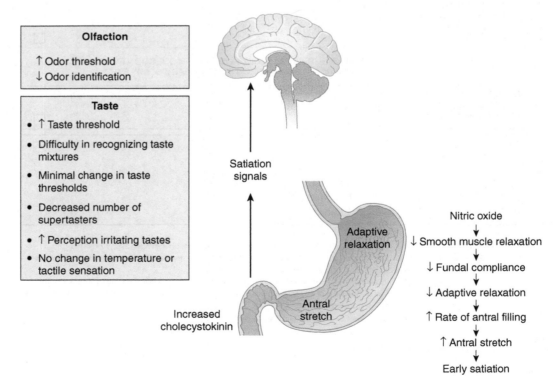

Figure 14–3. Physiologic anorexia of aging.

Table 14–3.	THE "MEALS ON WHEELS" MNEMONIC FOR TREATABLE CAUSES OF WEIGHT LOSS

Medications

Emotional (depression)

Alcoholism, anorexia tardive, abuse (elder)

Late life paranoia

Swallowing problems

Oral problems

Nosocomial infections, no money (poverty)

Wandering or dementia

Hyperthyroidism, hypercalcemia, hypoadrenalism

Enteric problems (malabsorption)

Eating problems (e.g., tremor)

Low-salt, low-cholesterol diet

Shopping and meal preparation problems, stones (cholecystitis)

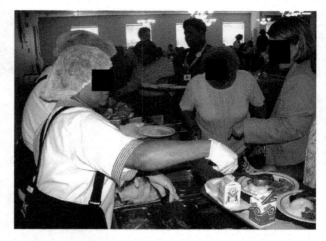

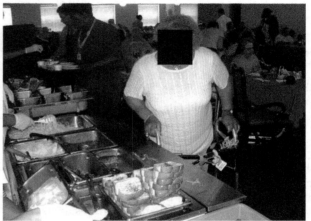

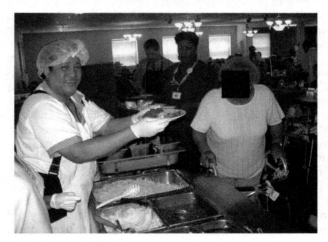

Figure 14–4. Buffet dining.

Families should be encouraged to assist when there are problems with feeding and to bring in food from home or other food favored by the resident. A person needing help with feeding requires approximately 45 minutes of aide time to be appropriately fed. Assessing feeding difficulties in persons with dementia can be carried out with the Edinburgh Feeding Evaluation in Dementia (http://www.nursingcenter.com/prodev/ce_article.asp?tid=807225). The Edinburgh Feeding Evaluation in Dementia Scale and the Mid-Stage Alzheimer's Feeding Behaviors Inventory (http://hdl.handle.net/10755/180804) both have important shortcomings in providing a comprehensive approach to feeding problems. Persons with Alzheimer's disease show difficulty in initiating meals. Elimination of environmental factors that inhibit initiation of the meal and assistance in promoting eating are key factors in improving their caloric intake. When food is in their mouth, they may keep the food in the mouth without swallowing (swallowing apraxia). Soft music in the background at mealtimes can increase food intake. Occupational therapists should assess the need for assistive feeding devices such as heavy-handled spoons, built-up handles for forks or spoons, knife and fork combinations, stainless steel food bumpers, gravity-assisted drinking cups, double-handed mugs with lids, comfort grip roller knife–forks, and adaptive chopsticks (Figure 14–5). Table 14–4 provides examples of common feeding problems and some possible management strategies.

Providing food between meals is one way to increase total caloric intake. Snack trolleys taken around by aides who can identify those who eat poorly or are at risk of dehydration can reduce weight loss (Figure 14–6). In persons with weight loss, there is no such thing as bad calories, so ice cream parlors open in the afternoon between meals increase food intake (Figure 14–7). Baking bread in a special needs unit can increase food intake because of the aroma of fresh bread.

Liquid caloric and protein supplements are important components of maintaining adequate food intake in persons with anorexia. They need to be given at least 1 hour before a meal. They should not be given with the meal because they reduce the amount of calories ingested at the meal when this happens. Vegetable juices mixed with fruits such as grapes or tomatoes can be prepared in the nursing home. Ice cream shakes and chocolate milk represent other cheap supplemental drinks that can be given to residents.

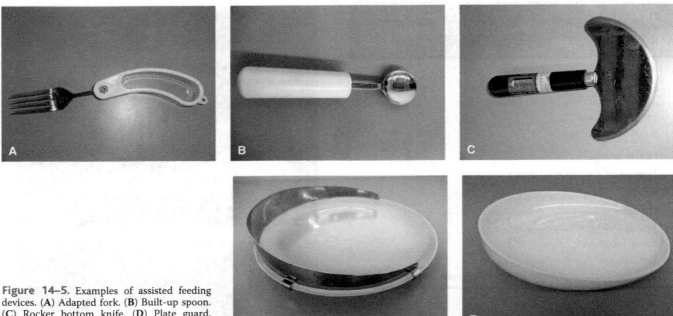

Figure 14–5. Examples of assisted feeding devices. (**A**) Adapted fork. (**B**) Built-up spoon. (**C**) Rocker bottom knife. (**D**) Plate guard. (**E**) Adapted plate.

The ideal supplement is a leucine-enriched essential amino acid mixture that if given between meals will slow the rate of protein loss from muscle (Figure 14–8). It is recommended that during rehabilitation residents receive 1.2 g/kg of protein daily, spread equally over meals. Using caloric supplements or chocolate milk as the fluid with which medications are taken is another way to enhance caloric intake.

At present, two orexigenic agents appear to have some utility in increasing food intake. Megestrol acetate is a mixed progestagen–corticosteroid–anabolic agent that leads to demonstrable weight gain. It causes an increase in fat, which is similar to what is seen in starving children when they eat. Fat is a more available calorie source than muscle. Megestrol acetate is poorly absorbed on an empty stomach, leading to the development of a nanoparticle formulation (Megace ES), which is much better absorbed. Effective doses of megestrol acetate are between 600 and 800 mg of the liquid formulation. Megestrol acetate used in the long term suppresses adrenal function; thus, if the person becomes ill, he or she will need stress doses of corticosteroids. Because megestrol acetate is a progestagen, it should not be given to bedfast individuals to reduce the danger of developing deep vein thrombosis. It is more effective at increasing weight gain in women. Dronabinol is a tetrahydrocannabinol (cannabis) drug that causes a small increase in food intake. It should be started in low doses in older persons because it can induce delirium. Because it also improves taste of the food, has an antinausea effect, decreases pain, and enhances general well-being, it can be useful for palliation at the end of life. Ghrelin agonists increase food intake but are experimental at this stage.

SARCOPENIA

Sarcopenia is excessive age-related loss of muscle. Muscle loss is associated with an increase in functional disability. However, muscle loss alone is a poor predictor of muscle function, and as such, it has been suggested that the definition of sarcopenia should include a measurement of muscle strength or function. A comparison of the different international definitions is given in Table 14–5. Measurement of muscle loss can be carried out by measuring midarm muscle circumference, dual energy x-ray absorptiometry (using only appendicular skeleton and correcting for height), computed tomography, magnetic resonance image, or ultrasonography. Bioelectrical impedance is not recommended for individuals because of variability induced by hydration status. There are multiple causes of sarcopenia (Table 14–6). Treatment of sarcopenia should focus on resistance exercise for at least 1 year. Testosterone at high doses improves muscle mass and strength. Increased protein intake of 1.2 to 1.5 g/kg per day and possibly the addition of creatine slow loss of protein. Experimental drugs to treat sarcopenia include selective androgen receptor molecules, myostatin antibodies, and decoy receptors to the activin II receptor. Obese persons who lose muscle mass (i.e., obese sarcopenic or "fat frail" individuals) have particularly poor outcomes.

CACHEXIA

Cachexia is the excessive loss of muscle and adipose tissue caused by inflammatory cytokines produced in large amounts by illness. Besides weight loss, it is characterized by low albumin levels, anemia, and an elevated C-reactive

Table 14–4.   COMMON FEEDING PROBLEMS AND SOME POSSIBLE MANAGEMENT STRATEGIES

Feeding Difficulty	Management
Aspiration	See Table 14–10
Food refusal	If paranoid, use buffet dining.
	Encourage eating.
	Determine if food is acceptable to resident.
	Try to open resident's mouth without forcing.
	Consider use of low-dose antipsychotic.
Refuses assistance	Provide finger foods.
	Increase time to allow self-feeding.
Visual problems	Use color contrasts between food, plate, and table.
Agitation or hits feeding assistant	Encourage while keeping distance.
	Try to orientate about inappropriateness of behavior.
	Seek help from another aide.
	Offer to feed at another time.
Failure to start eating	Provide verbal encouragement.
	Help start eating behavior.
Failure to continue eating	Remind to eat.
	Remind to swallow.
	Remove environmental distractions.
	Offer food variety.
	Give appetite stimulants.
Wanders	Provide finger foods.
Too sleepy to eat	Discontinue medication.
	Touch and voice to remind to eat.
	Change mealtimes.
Cannot chew	Cut food into small bits.
Cannot keep food in mouth	Give larger amounts per bite.
	Use hands to hold in mouth.
Lacking motor skills	Try specialized feeding utensils.
	Allow hand feeding.

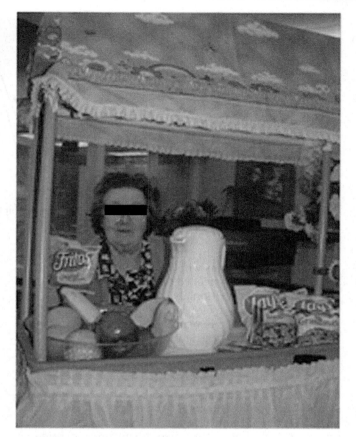

Figure 14–6. Snack and hydration cart.

The major exception is persons with gluten enteropathy. Lactose-deficient patients may also need some dietary restrictions. With aging, lactase deficiency becomes more common. Lactose can be added to dairy products or taken as a capsule, allowing digestion of milk products. Persons with specific food allergies need those foods to

protein. Treatment includes treatment of the underlying cause and attempting to maintain adequate caloric and protein intake. Table 14–7 provides a comparison of cachexia, sarcopenia, and anorexia as causes of weight loss.

THERAPEUTIC DIETS

In general, it is no longer believed that the majority of residents in nursing homes should be given therapeutic diets.

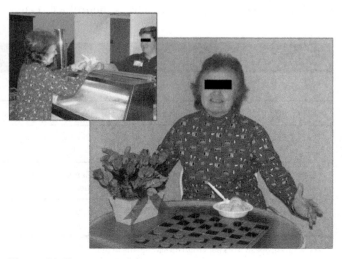

Figure 14–7. Ice cream parlors.

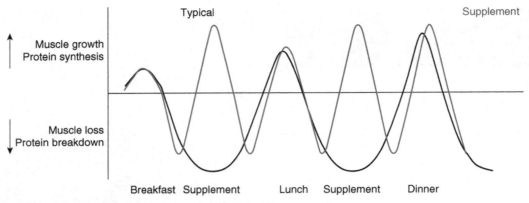

Figure 14–8. Maintaining muscle balance by giving a protein supplement between meals.

be restricted. Weight loss diets are considered inappropriate in nursing homes with minimal exceptions. "Heart healthy" diets are not needed because nursing home diets are on the whole nutritionally balanced.

Two studies have clearly shown no advantage of the American Diabetes Association diabetic diet. One of these suggested that restricting candy and cakes was also unnecessary.

The evidence for very low-salt diets for heart and renal failure is also relatively poor. Somewhere between 3 and 4 g of salt a day appears to be better for these persons. This allows them to eat the average nursing home diet. They should not have access to salt to add at mealtimes. Similarly, low-protein diets are no longer considered appropriate for persons with renal failure because they lead to protein energy undernutrition.

As a rule, therapeutic diets should not be allowed in a nursing home without specific permission of the medical director. This position is supported by the American Dietetic Society.

DYSPHAGIA AND FEEDING TUBES

Swallowing problems are present in about half of institutionalized persons. The majority of residents with oropharyngeal dysphagia have a neurologic cause (e.g., Parkinson's disease, stroke, dementia). This form of dysphagia presents with coughing while eating, a "wet voice," food regurgitation or food sticking in the throat, unexplained weight loss, refusal to eat, or recurrent chest infections. Drugs as a cause of swallowing difficulty should be considered (Table 14–8).

When a resident is noticed to have difficulty in swallowing, the nurse should assess:

- Alertness of resident (i.e., is this caused by delirium?)
- Speed and range of tongue movements
- Ability to cough and strength of cough
- Wet or gurgly voice
- Presence of a dry mouth (xerostomia)
- Severity of dysphagia (e.g., slow swallowing [>10 seconds to swallow a mouthful], pocketed food, drooling, or clear aspiration)

A full approach to the nursing assessment of dysphagia is given by the SWALLOWING . . . ON A PLATE protocol (www.cera.usyd.edu.au/manuals_plate.html). Following this approach should result in an individualized swallowing care plan.

A simple bedside test for swallowing consists of giving the patient 30 mL of water to swallow and (1) see that the pharyngeal swallow (elevation of hyoid) begins within 2 seconds, (2) exclude the presence of drooling,

Table 14–5. COMPARISON OF SARCOPENIA DEFINITIONS		
Group	**Screen**	**Definition**
EWG SOP	Gait speed <0.8 m/s	Low muscle mass (not defined)
IANA Sarcopenia Task Force	Gait speed <1.0 m/s	Low appendicular lean mass (<7.23 kg/m^2 in men; 5.67 kg/m^2 in women)
SIG: Cachexia-Anorexia in Chronic Wasting Diseases	Gait speed <0.8 m/s or other performance measure	Low muscle mass (2 SD)
Sarcopenia with Limited Mobility (SCWD)	6-min walk <400 m or gait speed <1.0 m/s	Low appendicular lean mass (2 SD) corrected for sex and ethnicity

EWG SOP, european working group on sarcopenia in older People; IANA, international association on nutrition and aging; SCWD, society on sarcopenia, cachexia and wasting diseases; SD, standard deviation; SIG, special interest group.

Table 14–6.   CAUSES OF SARCOPENIA

- Aging
- Decreased food or protein intake
- Decreased exercise or muscle use
- Decreased testosterone
- Decreased DHEA
- Decreased GH or IGF-1
- Increased cytokines (IL-6, IL-1, TNF-α)
- Decreased vitamin D
- Peripheral vascular disease
- Insulin resistance

DHEA, dehydroepiandrosterone; GH, growth hormone; IGF, insulinlike growth factor; IL, interleukin; TNF, tumor necrosis factor.

(3) observe for cough in first 60 seconds after swallowing, and (4) observe for dysphoria. Any of these observations suggest the presence of dysphagia requiring further evaluations. Some prefer to start with semisolid thickened fluids before water and then move to try dry toast.

A speech therapist or clinician can undertake videofluoroscopy (modified barium swallow) to determine whether the food is entering the respiratory tract and whether the swallowing muscles are working appropriately. This test can also be used to determine if different consistencies of food are swallowed more efficiently.

After either a formal or bedside swallow test, an appropriate diet such as pureed or thickened liquids (nectar, honey, or pudding consistency) can be recommended. Gel thickeners are also available. Thickened liquids have poor palatability, leading to poor compliance and often weight loss.

Table 14–7.   COMPARISON OF ANOREXIA, SARCOPENIA, AND CACHEXIA

	Anorexia	Sarcopenia	Cachexia
Weight loss	Moderate	Mild or even gain	Severe
Muscle loss	Moderate	Severe	Severe
Body fat	Severe	Gain	Severe
Food intake	Decreased	Unchanged	Decreased
Anemia	Mild	None	Moderate
Cytokines	Normal to mild increase	Mild increase	Marked increase
Albumin	Mild decrease	Normal	Marked decrease

Table 14–8.   DRUGS THAT AFFECT OROPHARYNGEAL SWALLOWING

Tricyclic antidepressants
Theophylline
Calcium channel blockers
Cholinesterase inhibitors
Carbachol
Cisapride
Metoclopramide
Oxybutynin

Numerous nursing techniques can decrease the risk of aspiration (Table 14–9).

A variety of swallowing exercises can be used to treat dysphagia. These are particularly effective in persons with Parkinson's disease. Electrical stimulation can be used to increase the strength of the gustatory muscles and retrain neurologic pathways. Angiotensin-converting enzyme inhibitors can enhance the cough reflex. Bromergocryptine improves swallowing in some older persons.

The major purpose of treating dysphagia is to avoid the risk of aspiration pneumonia. Aspiration can lead to pneumonitis (without bacterial infection) or pneumonia. In persons with dysphagia, aspiration pneumonia should be expected when a person develops tachypnea (>28 breaths/min), fever, cough when not eating, rales (crackles), chest pain, and increased confusion or falls (delirium).

Table 14–9.   NURSING TECHNIQUES TO REDUCE ASPIRATION

- Sit the resident upright.
- Use a chin tuck or head turn.
- Sit in front of the resident looking at him or her.
- Observe food and liquid consistencies that the resident handles best.
- Do not mix liquid and foods of different consistencies.
- Place food in the mouth on the unaffected side if the person has had a stroke.
- Feed small amounts slowly.
- Have the person swallow twice before the next mouthful.
- Check that the mouth is empty after each mouthful (e.g., look for pocketing).
- Keep teeth and mouth clean before and after meals.
- Reduce distractions.
- Stroke under chin downward to initiate swallowing.
- Check for food under dentures.
- Hold food in cheek on paralyzed side to assist swallowing.
- Enhance nondistracting social interaction during meals.
- Use artificial saliva in persons with xerostomia.

Feeding tubes can be the only way a person with a stroke or other neurologic condition can survive. In persons with dementia, there is no evidence that tube feeding improves survival or quality of life. Persons with tubes still aspirate secretions from their mouths, which often have more bacteria in them than persons who are feeding regularly. The use of tube feeding in many nursing home residents is an individual family decision that often involves cultural and religious beliefs. Tube feedings are greatly overused in nursing home residents in the United States, driven by the legal system. Ethically, removing a feeding tube is no different than inserting it, and removing an inappropriately inserted feeding tube should not be considered an act of "failing to feed" the resident. Residents who do not tolerate thickened liquids should have the quality of life choice of not having to have them even if this behavior increases aspiration risk.

DEHYDRATION

Dehydration is a key event in long-term care. When a resident becomes dehydrated, it is considered a mark of poor care. In reality, older persons are extremely vulnerable to becoming dehydrated, and an older person with a fever can become dehydrated very rapidly. Dehydration is defined as a reduction in total body water caused either by pure water loss (presenting with hypernatremia) or a loss of salt and water (which may be hyponatremic). When the osmolality is greater than 300 mmol/kg, it is considered to be dehydration. Values between 295 and 300 mmol/kg are defined as predehydration. Osmolality can be measured or calculated by using the following formula:

$$\text{Osmolality} = 2 \times (\text{Na} + \text{kmmol/L})$$
$$+ \frac{\text{Plasma glucose (ng/dL)}}{18} + \frac{\text{BUN (ng/dL)}}{28}$$

A ratio of blood urea nitrogen (BUN) to creatinine of greater than 20:1 is often used to detect dehydration. However, there are many other causes of an elevated BUN-to-creatinine ratio, requiring caution in the use of this ratio (Table 14–10).

Dehydration occurs in up to 30% of the older population. Recorded diagnosis of dehydration in nursing homes

is very rare (1.2% in Iceland; 1% in the United States; and 0.8% in Ontario, Canada). This suggests a major underdiagnosis of dehydration in nursing homes. A simple screen for residents to suggest a workup for dehydration is the DEHYDRATIONS mnemonic (Table 14–11).

The diagnosis of dehydration and appropriate therapy is driven by biochemical measurements (Table 14–12).

Pseudohypernatremia can be caused by hyperglycemia, hypertriglyceridemia, or mannitol infusion. Early diagnosis in the nursing home requires increasing staff awareness of the factors responsible for dehydration (fever, hot weather, diarrhea, vomiting, diuretics) and recognizing the relationship of dark urine, orthostasis, and incontinence to dehydration. A number of measures that reduce the incidence of dehydration in facilities are given in Table 14–13.

Fluid replacement requirement is calculated as fluid deficit (Table 14–14) + Urine loss + 500 ml/day (insensible loss, increase of fever, or hyperventilation). Because of the fear of cerebral-positive myelinolysis, fluid replacement should be at 1 MEqv/hr. The formula for calculating fluid deficit is as follows:

$$\text{Fluid deficit} = \left[\frac{\text{Serum sodium}}{140} \right]$$
$$\times \text{Baseline body weight (kg)} \times 0.5$$
$$- \text{Present body weight (kg)} \times 0.5$$

Table 14–11.	THE DEHYDRATIONS SCREEN FOR DEHYDRATION
Drugs (e.g., furosemide)	
End of life	
High fever	
Yellow urine turns dark	
Dizziness (orthostasis)	
Reduced oral intake (dementia, acute illness)	
Axilla dry	
Tachycardia	
Incontinence (fear of)	
Oral problems and thickened liquids	
Neurologic impairment (confusion)	
Sunken eyes	

Table 14–10.	CAUSES OF AN ELEVATED RATIO OF BLOOD UREA NITROGEN TO CREATININE

- Bleeding
- Muscle loss
- Increased protein intake
- Renal or heart failure
- Glucocorticoids
- Licorice (glycorrheic acid)[a]
- Dehydration

[a]In the United States, licorice is not true licorice.

Table 14–12.	BIOCHEMICAL MEASUREMENTS IN THE DIAGNOSIS OF DEHYDRATION

Biochemical Measurements			
Sodium	Osmolality	BUN/Creatinine	Treatment
↑	↑	↑	5% dextrose water
↓	↑	↑	Isotonic saline

Table 14–13.	TECHNIQUES TO REDUCE DEHYDRATION IN NURSING FACILITIES

- Education of CNAs
- Offer straws and sip cups
- Have fluid rounds
- Hydration cart
- Frozen juice bars
- Remind families to offer fluid when in facility
- Encourage fluid intake in incontinent residents
- Use swallowing techniques and cueing for residents receiving thickened fluids
- Check that adequate fluid is being administered with tube feedings

Fluid replacement can be oral when dehydration is mild (sodium <150 MEq/L). Most dehydrated residents require either subcutaneous infusion (hypodermoclysis) or intravenous infusion. There are a number of advantages of subcutaneous infusions in nursing homes (Table 14–14). Subcutaneous infusions can be initiated with or without hyaluronidase. The rate of subcutaneous infusion can vary from 50 mL to 125 mL/hr. Hyaluronidase reduces the occupancy of local edema.

VITAMIN D AND OTHER VITAMINS AND MINERALS

Vitamin D

Studies throughout the world have demonstrated that almost all nursing home residents are vitamin D deficient; these studies use a 25(OH) vitamin D level of 30 ng/mL(nmol/L). In addition, studies in Japan have shown that because of the poor creatinine clearance in nursing home residents, they tend to have even lower 1,25(OH) vitamin D levels, leading to an increased parathyroid hormone and increased loss of bone.

Low vitamin D levels are associated with poor quantity and quality of bone, resulting in hip fracture. Low vitamin D levels are also associated with decreased muscle strength, frailty, decreased cognition, increased disability, and increased mortality rates. In nursing homes, an increased mortality rate was associated with 25(OH) vitamin D levels below 14 nmol/L (35 ng/dL).

Replacement of 800 IU of vitamin D daily together with calcium supplementation decreased hip fracture in the nursing home. At present, the state of the art suggests replacement of 1000 to 2000 IU of vitamin D daily is appropriate for all nursing home residents who do not have hypercalcemia. Measurement of 25(OH) vitamin D does not appear to be cost effective. It is recognized that these replacement levels will not return all nursing home residents to normal levels.

Fortification of bread with vitamin D in nursing homes has been shown to be effective in maintaining vitamin D levels. A study in New Zealand determined that exposing nursing home residents to sunlight for 30 minutes a day increased 25(OH) vitamin levels. European studies have found exposure to 15 minutes a day of ultraviolet B levels equivalent to summer sunshine increases vitamin D levels and is cheaper than using oral vitamin D supplementation. Exposure to ultraviolet B weekly after showering also increased vitamin D levels.

Other Vitamins and Minerals

In developed nations, most persons who are eating the food in a nursing home have adequate vitamin status. Pyridoxine and riboflavin levels are low in some residents, but there is little evidence to support their replacement, with the exception of pyridoxine replacement in persons receiving isoniazid. Folate fortification of bread in the United States and Australia makes folate deficiency relatively rare, but in Europe, folate deficiency is more common and should be considered in persons with megaloblastic anemia and cognitive impairment. Folate deficiency can be caused by a number of medications (Table 14–15). Folate deficiency leads to an increase in homocysteine. In Europe (but not in the United States), elevated homocysteine levels are associated

Table 14–14.	ADVANTAGES OF SUBCUTANEOUS INFUSION (HYPODERMOCLYSIS) OVER INTRAVENOUS INFUSION

- Subcutaneous infusions easy to start, maintain and restart
- Less bruising
- Can deliver drugs such as morphine, insulin, hydrocortisone, penicillins
- Rarely causes infection
- Easier to use in confused patients
- Relatively cheap

Table 14–15.	DRUGS CAUSING FOLATE OR VITAMIN B_{12} DEFICIENCY	
Folate Deficiency	**Vitamin B_{12} Deficiency**
Anticonvulsants	Proton pump inhibitors
Metformin	Metformin
Methotrexate	Colchicine
Sulfasalazine	Mineral oil
Triamterene	
Trimethoprim	
Antacids	

with myocardial infarction, stroke, cognitive dysfunction, and osteoporosis. A recent meta-analysis showed that antioxidant vitamins are associated with increased mortality rates.

Vitamin B_{12} deficiency is common because of the high prevalence of pernicious anemia in older persons and malabsorption caused by use of drugs. Bacterial overgrowth in the gut and in some countries (tapeworm) results in vitamin B_{12} deficiency and weight loss. The presence of vitamin B_{12} deficiency is confirmed by demonstrating an elevated level of methylmalonic acid. All persons with cognitive dysfunction, megaloblastic anemia, and posterior column neuropathy (poor balance) should be screened for vitamin B_{12} deficiency. Vitamin B_{12} can be replaced by injection or orally with high doses.

Hypomagnesemia is relatively common in nursing home residents, especially those receiving diuretics and diabetics. In a German study, one third of nursing home residents had low magnesium levels. Low magnesium levels lead to alterations in parathyroid hormone release and abnormal calcium metabolism. It is also associated with calf cramps in the nursing home.

Zinc plays a central role in immune function, skin healing, and insulin secretion. Persons with diabetes mellitus, liver failure, or cancer and those taking diuretics are particularly prone to zinc deficiency. Zinc replacement should be considered in residents with vascular or pressure ulcers. Zinc deficiency can be measured by obtaining leukocyte zinc levels or a combination of low serum zinc and hyperzincuria. Low serum zinc level alone is an acute phase reactant and therefore cannot be used to diagnose zinc deficiency.

KEY POINTS

1. Weight loss is the most common nutritional problem in nursing homes.
2. Depression is responsible for one third of the weight loss in nursing home residents.
3. The MNA and SNAQ can be used to detect persons at risk of malnutrition.
4. Persons with swallowing problems should be carefully evaluated, and use of specific foodstuffs needs to take into account palatability and wishes of the resident.
5. Caloric supplements need to be given between meals.
6. Dining ambience, buffet meals, and a snack or hydration cart can all improve food intake.
7. Tube feedings have little efficacy in persons with dementia.
8. Dehydration is common in nursing homes and can be treated with subcutaneous fluid infusions.
9. Hypomagnesemia is associated with calf cramps.
10. Hypozincemia is associated with impaired wound healing.

SUGGESTED READINGS

Amella EJ, Stockdell R. How to try this: The Edinburgh Feeding Evaluation in Dementia Scale: Determining how much help people with dementia need at mealtime. *Am J Nurs.* 2008;108:46-54.

Argiles JM, Anker SD, Evans WJ, et al. Consensus on cachexia definitions. *J Am Med Dir Assoc.* 2010;11:229-230.

Aselage MB, Amella EJ, Watson R. State of the science: Alleviating mealtime difficulties in nursing home residents with dementia. *Nurs Outlook.* 2011;59:210-214.

Bauer JM, Kaiser MJ, Sieber CC. Sarcopenia in nursing home residents. *J Am Med Dir Assoc.* 2008;9:545-551.

British Association for Enteral and Parenteral Nutrition. *Nutrition Screening Survey in the UK in 2007: A Report by BAPEN.* http://www.bapen.org.uk/pdfs/nsw/nsw07_report.pdf. Published 2008. Accessed April 8, 2013.

Chang C-C, Roberts BL. Strategies for feeding patients with dementia: How to individualize assessment and intervention based on observed behavior. *Am J Nurs.* 2011;111:36-44.

Cote TR. How to perform subcutaneous hydration. *J Am Med Dir Assoc.* 2008;9:291.

Crecelius C. Dehydration: Myth and reality. *J Am Med Dir Assoc.* 2008;9:287-288.

Demontiero O, Herrmann M, Duque G. Supplementation with vitamin D and calcium in long-term care residents. *J Am Med Dir Assoc.* 2011;12:190-194.

Drinka PJ, Krause PF, Nest LJ, Goodman BM. Determinants of vitamin D levels in nursing home residents. *J Am Med Dir Assoc.* 2007;8:76-79.

Durnbaugh T, Haley B, Roberts S. Assessing problem feeding behaviors in mid-stage Alzheimer's disease: Clients with mid-stage Alzheimer's disease may be eating far less than their caregivers believe. *Geriatr Nurs.* 1996;17:63-67.

Evans WJ, Morley JE, Argiles J, et al. Cachexia: A new definition. *Clin Nutr.* 2008;27:793-799.

Gau JT. Prevalence of vitamin D deficiency/insufficiency practice patterns in nursing homes. *J Am Med Dir Assoc.* 2010;11:296.

Hamid Z, Riggs A, Spencer T, et al. Vitamin D deficiency in residents of academic long-term care facilities despite having been prescribed vitamin D. *J Am Med Dir Assoc.* 2007;8:71-75.

Kamel HK. Update on osteoporosis management in long-term care: Focus on bisphosphonates. *J Am Med Dir Assoc.* 2007;8:434-440.

Landi F, Laviano A, Cruz-Jentoft AJ. The anorexia of aging: Is it a geriatric syndrome? *J Am Med Dir Assoc.* 2010;11:153-156.

Landi F, Liperoti R, Fusco D, et al. Sarcopenia and mortality among older nursing home residents. *J Am Med Dir Assoc.* 2012;13:121-126.

Landi F, Russo A, Liperoti R, et al. Anorexia, physical function, and incident disability among the frail elderly population: Results from the ilSIRENTE study. *J Am Med Dir Assoc.* 2010;11:268-274.

Lippincott's Nursing Center.com. Better resources for better care. How to try this: Edinburgh Feeding Evaluation in Dementia Scale: Determining how much help people with dementia need at mealtime. http://www.nursingcenter.com/prodev/ce_article.asp?tid=807225. Accessed April 29, 2013.

Metheny NA, Davis-Jackson J, Stewart BJ. Effectiveness of an aspiration risk-reduction protocol. *Nurs Res.* 2010;59:18-25.

Metheny NA. Preventing aspiration in older adults with dysphagia. *ORL Head Neck Nurs.* 2011;29:20-21.

Morley JE. Weight loss in older persons: New therapeutic approaches. *Curr Pharm Des.* 2007;13:3637-3647.

Morley JE. Vitamin D redux. *J Am Med Dir Assoc.* 2009;10:591-592.

Morley JE. Anorexia, weight loss, and frailty. *J Am Med Dir Assoc.* 2010;11:225-228.

Morley JE. Hip fractures. *J Am Med Dir Assoc.* 2010;11:81-83.

Morley JE. Undernutrition in older adults. *Fam Pract.* 2012;29(suppl 1):i89-i93.

Morley JE. Undernutrition: A major problem in nursing homes. *J Am Med Dir Assoc.* 2011;12:243-246.

Morley JE, Argiles JM, Evans WJ, et al. Society for Sarcopenia, Cachexia, and Wasting Disease. *J Am Med Dir Assoc.* 2010;11:391-396.

Morley JE, Thomas DR, Wilson MM. Cachexia: Pathophysiology and clinical relevance. *Am J Clin Nutr.* 2006;83:735-743.

Munir J, Wright RJ, Carr DB. A quality improvement study on calcium and vitamin D supplementation in long-term care. *J Am Med Dir Assoc.* 2007;8(3 suppl 2):e19-e23.

Rolland Y, Perrin A, Gardette V, et al. Screening older people at risk of malnutrition or malnourished using the Simplified Nutritional Appetite Questionnaire (SNAQ): A comparison with the Mini-Nutritional Assessment (MNA) tool. *J Am Med Dir Assoc.* 2012;13:31-34.

Salva A, Coll-Planas L, Bruce S, et al. Nutritional assessment of residents in long-term care facilities (LTCFs): Recommendations of the Task Force on Nutrition and Ageing of the IAGG European region and the IANA. *J Nutr Health Aging.* 2009;13:475-483.

Sloane PD, Ivey J, Helton M, et al. Nutritional issues in long-term care. *J Am Med Dir Assoc.* 2008;8:476-485.

Tada A, Miura H. Prevention of aspiration pneumonia (AP) with oral care. *Arch Gerontol.* Geriatr 2012;55:16-21.

Thomas DR, Cote TR, Lawhorne L, et al. Understanding clinical dehydration and its treatment. *J Am Med Dir Assoc.* 2008;9:292-301.

Vellas B, Villars H, Abellan G, et al. Overview of the MNA—Its history and challenges. *J Nutr Health Aging.* 2006;10:456-463.

Virginia Henderson International Nursing Library. Midstage Alzheimer's feeding behavior inventory. http://hdl.handle.net/10755/180804. Accessed April 9, 2013.

Wilson MM, Philpot C, Morley JE. Anorexia of aging in long term care: Is dronabinol an effective appetite stimulant? A pilot study. *J Nutr Health Aging.* 2007;11:195-198.

Wilson MM, Thomas DR, Rubenstein LZ, et al. Appetite assessment: Simple appetite questionnaire predicts weight loss in community-dwelling adults and nursing home residents. *Am J Clin Nutr.* 2005; 82:1074-1081.

Wright RM. Use of osteoporosis medications in older nursing facility residents. *J Am Med Dir Assoc.* 2007;8:453-457.

Yeh SS, Lovitt S, Schuster MW. Pharmacological treatment of geriatric cachexia: Evidence and safety in perspective. *J Am Med Dir Assoc.* 2007;8:363-377.

MULTIPLE CHOICE QUESTIONS

14.1   The amount of time to adequately feed a resident with dementia is approximately:
a. 20 minutes
b. 30 minutes
c. 45 minutes
d. 60 minutes

14.2   The amount of protein required by a person undergoing rehabilitation or with sarcopenia is:

a. 0.4 g/kg/day
b. 0.8 g/kg/day
c. 12 g/kg/day
d. 18 g/kg/day

14.3   Which of the following is true regarding prevention or treatment of protein energy malnutrition?

a. Therapeutic diets (e.g., diabetic, heart healthy) have a role to play in nursing Homes.
b. Megestrol acetate increases food intake and produces weight gain.
c. Buffet dining is not recommended.
d. Families should not be allowed to feed residents.
e. Caloric supplements should be given at the initiation of the meal.

14.4   Which of the following is not an advantage of hypodermoclysis (subcutaneous fluid infusion) in nursing homes?

a. Easy to start and maintain
b. Commonly causes shin infections
c. Less bruising
d. Easier to use in confused patients compared with intravenous infusions
e. Easy to restart

14.5   Which of these drugs causes folate deficiency?

a. Protein pump inhibitors
b. Colchicine
c. Digoxin
d. Anticonvulsants
e. Mineral oil

14.6   Which of the following concerning vitamin D is *not* true?

a. Fortification of bread with vitamin D in nursing homes maintains vitamin D levels.
b. 30 minutes of sunlight exposure daily increases vitamin D levels.
c. 800 IU of vitamin D daily reduces hip fracture in nursing homes.
d. Exposure to ultraviolet B levels after shower increases vitamin D levels in nursing home residents.
e. 1,25(OH) vitamin D should be measured in all nursing home residents.

Chapter 15

SEXUALITY WITHIN THE NURSING HOME

Young love is about wanting to be happy. Old love is about wanting someone else to be happy.
—Mary Pipher, psychologist

Although, as explained in Chapter 5, sexual abuse is an unacceptable occurrence within all types of eldercare, it is important that practitioners recognize the place of sexuality and intimacy within the lives of older people. Our sexuality defines our identity, and age does not change this nor does admission to a nursing home. The World Health Organization (WHO) describes sexuality in terms of gender identity; social roles; sexual orientation; eroticism; pleasure; intimacy; and, of course, reproduction (http://www.who.int/reproductivehealth/topics/gender_rights/sexual_health/en). For older nursing home residents, sexuality means different things, including companionship, love, tenderness, affectionate talk, kissing, touch, and other rituals associated with a long-term intimate partnership. It can also be interpreted in terms of dignity, privacy, and respect in relation to a resident's state of dress and undress, touching, and exposure of what he or she considers to be private areas of the body to others, particularly to people of a different gender or faith. It is beyond the scope of this chapter to detail the array of cultural and faith differences and taboos in relation to dress, nakedness, and sanctions related to touch. However, we wish to stress that in resident-centered approaches, it is essential that staff appreciate the cultural codes and expectations of individuals and their communities to avoid offense and ensure that an appropriate respectful plan of care is developed. When a resident has a preference to be cared for by staff of a particular gender and this is difficult to accommodate on the duty schedule, it may be possible to work in partnership with the family, who may be able to directly contribute to selected acts of physical care. An example of this might be that a gentleman's son might be able to provide care that the resident believes is too intimate for a female nurse. Regardless of a person's unique and cultural expectations, it is always desirable to promote privacy and ensure minimal exposure of a person's genitalia and a woman's breasts during intimate care, toilet assistance, and physical examination and treatment. In these situations, doors or screens should be closed, window curtains drawn if the room is overlooked, and covers (sheets) used with discretion to minimize both the duration and extent of exposure.

However, sexuality and sexual expression by older people are not confined to issues of gender identity and cultural sensitivities; they are also about sexual desires and behaviors, although this is often overlooked by staff in long-term care settings. For some older nursing home residents, sexuality continues to be associated with physical desire and acts of sex, which may include masturbation. Sexual relationships are a manifestation of the human need to feel contact, affection, and intimacy in its broadest sense. A person-centered approach to sexual health and sexuality allows staff to understand the priorities and interests of individuals and agree on appropriate strategies. A balance is required to manage potential risks and the need to protect vulnerable individuals against the rights for self-determination, privacy, and the pursuit of intimate moments between consenting adults.

Young persons often find it difficult to believe that sexuality remains a core need of many older persons. Yet for many older persons, the loss of physical and emotional intimacy is a source of suffering. For many nursing home residents, social intimacy is more important than physical and sexual intimacy. Yet sexuality remains important as shown in one nursing home study in which 8% of persons had had sexual activity within a month, 17% expressed a desire for sexual activity, and nearly 90% had sexual thoughts and fantasies. Intimacy can be expressed in multiple forms (Table 15–1). There are three components of intimacy:

- Mutual choice and reciprocity
- Trust
- Delight

A study in Scotland found that in nursing homes where the staff supported the rights of the residents to intimacy, nonsexual flirtations were more common. This suggests that a nonsupportive environment causes suppression of sexuality.

Intimate relationships in nursing homes can be either heterosexual or homosexual. In some cases, this may be nonsexual and purely a way of obtaining comfort from closeness. In other cases, older persons who have repressed their true sexuality may "come out of the closet" for the first time in the nursing home. Others may have been practicing homosexuals without their families being aware of it. Homosexual relationships often cause more conflict with families and staff than do heterosexual relationships.

Table 15–1.   EXPRESSIONS OF INTIMACY IN NURSING HOMES

- Compliments (with or without a sexual undertone)
- Flirtations
- Smiling
- Touching
- Hugging
- Enjoyment of another's company
- Caressing
- Kissing
- Hand holding
- Petting
- Caressing of genitals (one's own or others)
- Masturbation
- Use of a vibrator
- Sexual intercourse

Some older residents deliberately abstain from forming intimate relationships because of the fear of the emotional pain potentially associated with the high possibility of their loved one's dying.

There are numerous barriers to developing intimate relationships in nursing homes (Table 15–2).

In all nursing homes, there should be an ability to allow persons who wish to have sexual experiences by themselves or with another to have privacy. Staff needs to respect this right by not entering a resident's room unannounced and to be sensitive to times when it should not be entered. Persons who have inappropriate sexual displays in public (e.g., masturbation) should be redirected to an appropriate area in their room and given privacy.

Deciding whether or not a person with cognitive decline can enter into a relationship with another is often

Table 15–2.   BARRIERS TO DEVELOPING INTIMATE AND SEXUAL RELATIONSHIPS IN NURSING HOMES

- Lack of privacy
- Staff attitudes
- Family attitudes
- Lack of an accepting partner
- Cognitive decline and the problem of consent
- Feelings of not being attractive
- Poor health
- Functional limitations
- Decreased libido (low testosterone)
- Erectile dysfunction
- Loss of vaginal lubrication and elasticity
- Dyspareunia

a difficult decision because of issues of the capacity to consent. Sometimes it can be very difficult to determine if one resident is taking advantage of another, particularly with mood fluctuations, emotional lability, and inconsistent behaviors. This can be a major problem when one or both of the residents are still married to another. Not all spouses can be as accepting of the situation as Sandra Day O'Connor, a United States Supreme Court Justice, who was happy for her husband when he developed a loving relationship with another individual with dementia in the nursing home. Figure 15–1 provides an outline to approaching acceptable relationships in nursing homes. The family or legal guardian should be involved in all decisions as should staff members. In many cases, this may require prolonged discussions to allow the family to perceive the appropriateness of the relationship. At all times, these decisions should be documented and remain within the acceptable legal framework of the area. The WHO has affirmed the right of all persons to decide whether or not to be sexually active and to enter into a desirable sexual relationship free from coercion.

More than half of men and three quarters of women in nursing homes believe that they are sexually undesirable. Staff members should help residents with grooming and self-esteem to diminish this feeling.

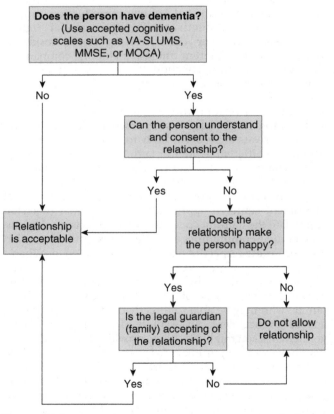

Figure 15–1. Approach to approving an intimate or sexual relationship of a cognitively impaired individual in a nursing home. MMSE, Mini Mental Status Examination; MoCA, Montreal Cognitive Assessment; VA-SLUMS, VA-St. Louis University Mental Status.

Decreased libido caused by a decline in testosterone can be treated with testosterone injections (testosterone cypionate or enanthate 200 mg intramuscularly every 2 weeks) when desired. This should be limited to persons with a documented low testosterone level. Moving testosterone levels into the normal range rarely causes problematic sexual behavior. The increased recognition that frailty and sarcopenia are caused in part by a deficit in anabolic hormones will lead to an increase in testosterone or selective androgen receptor molecules in the nursing home, with an increase in libido. When desired, phosphodiesterase inhibitors or vacuum tumescence devices can be supplied to reverse erectile dysfunction. For many men, the ability to have an erection is more important than the need to use it!

Another thorny issue is the use of pornographic material in the privacy of one's room. In general, this is acceptable. However, it may be disturbing to other residents and staff. The advent of the Internet has made this easier to access in a more private way.

In Holland, residents can invite prostitutes into the nursing home and have a variety of sexual acts with them. This is much less acceptable in the United States and would be illegal if officially condoned. However, a number of nursing homes have allowed family to employ prostitutes, especially for younger residents, without officially condoning the behavior.

All nursing homes should have a written policy regarding sexuality (Table 15–3). Staff need education in sexuality and should be receptive and open to discussing it with residents. The facility needs to determine whether or not a cognitively intact resident's sexual activity should be discussed with family or guardians.

In many cases, it will be apparent that the behavior is appropriate for the individual resident but not for others. In most cases, this should lead to the intervention's

Table 15–3.	NURSING HOME POLICY ON INTIMACY AND SEXUALITY

- All residents are entitled to express intimacy and sexuality in an appropriate manner.
- Sexuality may be with other residents or visitors.
- Two residents with an intimate relationship should be entitled to share a room.
- Materials of a sexual nature that are legal may be kept in the nursing home and used in the privacy of the resident's room.
- Staff needs to be aware of intimate relations and to determine with the social worker, physician, and administrator if it is coercive.
- Residents need to have access to private space to undertake sexual acts by themselves or with others.
- The facility shall or shall not inform family of a resident's sexual behavior when it is appropriate.
- The facility has a plan to deal with inappropriate sexual behavior.

Table 15–4.	BEHAVIOR MODIFICATION TO DEAL WITH INAPPROPRIATE SEXUAL BEHAVIOR

- Prevent staff from saying or doing inappropriate things.
- Ignore behavior when possible.
- Firmly say "no" and remove an offending hand or other body part from contact.
- Make clear that the behavior is unacceptable.
- Remove the resident to an area away from the person of interest (resident or staff) and provide a staff member of the other sex.
- Use clothing that makes genital touching and exposing in public difficult.
- Provide psychological therapy (cognitive behavioral therapy).
- Have open discussions with staff on how to prevent behavior.

being directed to alleviate the others and allow the resident expression of his or her sexuality.

Dealing with inappropriate sexual behavior begins by educating staff not to encourage flirtatious behavior from residents and to politely but firmly rebuff any advances. Much inappropriate behavior is caused by either frontal lobe strokes or Lewy body dementia. Some residents with dementia develop delusional jealousy. Another common problem is false sexual allegations against staff and other residents. The basics of behavioral therapy are outlined in Table 15–4. Drug therapy should rarely be used. Antipsychotics are ineffective. Medroxyprogesterone reduces behaviors but is associated with increased venous and arterial thrombosis (e.g., deep vein thrombosis, stroke, myocardial infarction).

With the advent of the baby boomers, who have more open sexual viewpoints, coming into nursing homes, staff needs to recognize that engagement in "kinky" behaviors will increase. As an example, in one nursing home, the partner of a male resident took him out of the nursing home. After returning, he was noted on a number of occasions to have linear lacerations on his buttocks. In discussion with the partner and resident, it became clear that they had a long history of mutually satisfying sadomasochistic behavior. After further discussion, the administrator and director of nursing thought that this behavior should not continue because of possible difficulties in explaining to inspectors why this was not abuse. This plan was mutually agreed to. Whether or not this was the correct quality of life decision had no satisfactory answer.

When sexual behavior is considered inappropriate, the first decision to be made is for whom is it inappropriate?

- For the resident
- For other residents
- For staff
- For family
- For the organization
- For others (e.g., visitors)
- For legal or religious systems

KEY POINTS

1. Many persons continue to have sexual feelings when they are in nursing homes.
2. Persons need privacy to act on their sexual feelings.
3. There are many forms of expression of intimacy.
4. Nursing homes need to have an approach to approving intimate and sexual relationships in a nursing home.
5. The recognition of the right for a person to have a relationship with one of the same sex is a human right.
6. Behavior modification should be used to treat inappropriate sexual behavior.
7. Decreased libido in men can be safely treated with testosterone.

SUGGESTED READINGS

Bardell A, Lau T, Fedoroff JP. Inappropriate sexual behavior in a geriatric population. *Int Psychogeriatr.* 2011;23:1182-1188.

Hajjar RR, Kamel HK. Sex and the nursing home. *Clin Geriatr Med.* 2003;19:575-586.

Hajjar RR, Kamel HK. Sexuality in the nursing home, part 1: attitudes and barriers to sexual expression. *J Am Med Dir Assoc.* 2004; 5(2 suppl):S42-S47.

Heath H. Older people in care homes: sexuality and intimate relationships. *Nursing Older People.* 2011;23(6):14-16.

Kamel HK, Hajjar RR. Sexuality in the nursing home, part 2: managing abnormal behavior—legal and ethical issues. *J Am Med Dir Assoc.* 2004;5(2 suppl):S48-S52.

Pioneering Change: Sexuality in Nursing Homes Education Module. http://www.agingkansas.org/longtermcare/PEAK/modules/sexuali tymodule.pdf. Accessed May 16, 2012.

Roach SM. Sexual behaviour of nursing home residents: staff perceptions and responses. *J Adv Nurs.* 2004;48:371-379.

Tsai SJ, Hwang JP, Yang Ch, Liu KM. Delusional jealousy in dementia. *J Clin Psychiatry.* 1997;58:492-494.

Ward R, Vass AA, Aggarwal N, et al. A kiss is still a kiss? The construction of sexuality in dementia care. *Dementia.* 2005;4:49-72.

WHO (World Health Organization). Defining Sexual Health: Report of a Technical Consultation on Sexual Health, 28-31 January 2002, Geneva. http://www.who.int/reproductivehealth/topics.gender_ rights/sexual_health/en. Accessed April 10, 2013.

MULTIPLE CHOICE QUESTIONS

15.1   Which of the following should *not* be a barrier in nursing homes to residents' developing intimate relationships?

a. Lack of an accepting partner
b. Feelings of not being attractive
c. Poor health
d. Homosexuality
e. Dyspareunia

15.2   Which of the following should *not* by itself make it unacceptable for two persons in a nursing home to have an intimate or sexual relationship?

a. Cognitive impairment
b. Relationship makes the person happy
c. Not approved by the administrator
d. Inability to clearly consent to the relationship
e. Not approved of by nurses

15.3   Which of the following is *not* an effect of testosterone?

a. Improves libido
b. Can improve erections
c. Lowers hematocrit
d. Increases muscle mass
e. Improves dysphoria

15.4   Which are appropriate treatments for inappropriate sexual behavior?

a. Medroxyprogesterone
b. Antipsychotics
c. Not discussing it with staff
d. Make clear that behavior is unacceptable
e. Staff saying inappropriate things

15.5   Many older persons in nursing homes feel unattractive, and this inhibits them from seeking comforting, intimate relationships.

a. True
b. False

Chapter 16

INCONTINENCE

Incontinence is often the factor that precipitates admission of an older person to long-term care. The stigma associated with loss of continence has an immense impact on self-esteem, quality of life, and mood. Incontinence of urine and or feces thus sets off a cascade of emotional responses associated with shame, embarrassment, and loss of dignity. It is important for nursing home practitioners to distinguish between transient and acute challenges to continence and established conditions. Managing continence problems in nursing homes is a multidisciplinary endeavor, but the majority of continence-related activities are undertaken by nurses and nurses' aids. There are a number of models of continence promotion spanning medical curative strategies that might include medications or surgical intervention to social models with a focus on containing leakage. The rehabilitation model aims to restore control and function, focusing on education and other supportive behavior change activities. Each of these models has a place within the nursing home, and the approach should be selected after a comprehensive assessment to understand the nature of the problem, the resident's condition, and his or her continence care preferences.

URINARY INCONTINENCE

Urinary incontinence is extremely common in nursing homes with a prevalence ranging from 37% to 77%. Women are more likely to be incontinent than men largely as a result of damage to the pelvic floor during childbirth. Other factors associated with incontinence are impaired cognition, being bedfast, constipation, and having limited ambulatory capacity. Depression and schizophrenia are also associated with incontinence. Persons with incontinence are more likely to fall and fracture a hip; have pressure ulcers, a variety of skin conditions (especially cutaneous fungal infections), and urinary tract infections (UTIs); and be socially isolated. Incontinence represents a major reason why older persons come to live in nursing homes. Management of incontinence in a nursing home requires an institutional focus on maintaining continence (organizational culture), stability in staff (i.e., low turnover), and group support of all the staff. For successful continence promotion, a continence specialist, usually an advanced nurse practitioner or continence advisor, is necessary.

Transient (Reversible) Incontinence

The causes of transient incontinence are given in Table 16–1. UTIs should always be excluded in persons with new onset of acute incontinence. Older persons often have white blood cells or bacteria in the urine; as such, unless there are both excess white blood cells (>5 per high-power field [hpf]) and bacteria (>100,000 per ml), the person should not be treated for a UTI. For similar reasons, a culture should be obtained after antibiotic use. In persons with transient incontinence, a toileting diary that records incontinent episodes, fluid intake, and toileting episodes should be maintained and regularly reviewed.

Persistent Incontinence

The basic causes of persistent incontinence are stress, urge, overflow, and functional. Many nursing home residents have mixed forms of incontinence. There are a number of principles of management of chronic incontinence that apply to all persons regardless of the cause of incontinence (Table 16–2). Drug therapy can be understood when one remembers that urination occurs when the parasympathetic nervous system stimulates detrusor muscle and the sympathetic nervous system (PIS) is inhibited, which opens the internal urethral sphincter.

Functional Incontinence

Functional incontinence is caused by a failure to recognize the need to use the toilet or failure to remember to use the toilet (dementia), lack of motivation to use the toilet (depression), or when physical and mobility limitation decreases the ability to use the toilet (stroke or frailty). Treatment of functional incontinence requires a bladder diary to determine when toileting and prompted voiding should occur (Table 16–3). Exercise together with every two hours incontinence care during the waking hours decreases urinary incontinence and skin wetness but has limited improvement in enhancing skin health, especially pressure ulcers. Although prompted voiding with exercise improves incontinence in nursing homes, exercise alone has little effect. When necessary, toileting regimens need to be supplemented by the use of absorbent pads. However, long-term trials on the best methods for managing functional incontinence do not currently exist.

Table 16–1.	CAUSES OF TRANSIENT INCONTINENCE	
Delirium		Drugs
Retention of urine with overflow		Restricted mobility
Infection		Impaction (fecal)
Polyuria		Prostatism

Table 16–2. BASIC MANAGEMENT OF INCONTINENCE

- Persons with incontinence should use the toilet frequently (every 3 to 4 hours).
- Constipation should be treated with sorbitol or lactulose.
- Smoking should be stopped to decrease coughing.
- Persons with incontinence should avoid the cold because it decreases arginine vasopressin levels.
- Alcohol should be limited because it decreases arginine vasopressin levels.

Table 16–3. PROMPTED VOIDING PROTOCOL

Goal: To reduce the frequency of wetness in selected residents from 7 AM to 7 PM

Assessment Period (3 Days)

1. Contact the resident every 2 hours from 7 AM to 7 PM.
2. Focus the resident's attention on voiding by asking whether he or she is wet or dry.
3. Check the resident for wetness, record in the bladder record, and give feedback on whether the resident is correct or incorrect.
4. Whether wet or dry, ask the resident if he or she would like to use the toilet, bedpan, or urinal.
   a. If the resident says yes:
      i. Assist the resident.
      ii. Record the results on the bladder record.
      iii. Give the resident positive reinforcement by spending an extra minute or two talking with him or her.
   b. If the resident says no, prompt and encourage him or her to toilet two more times.
   c. If the resident continues to say no, inform him or her that you will be back in an hour and request that the resident try to delay voiding until then.
5. Offer the resident a drink of fluid before leaving.
6. Every other hour, check the resident for wetness (without prompting the resident) and record the results in the bladder record.
   a. If the resident spontaneously requests toileting assistance, provide it and record the results in the bladder record.
   b. Offer the resident a drink of fluid before leaving.
7. During the 3-day assessment period:
   a. Collect a clean urine specimen for urinalysis and culture (if indicated).
   b. Perform a postvoid residual (PVR) determination.
   c. Perform bladder stress tests in women until either the test result is positive or the test result is negative and the resident's total bladder (voided volume plus PVR) exceeds 150 to 200 mL.

Targeting

1. Prompted voiding is more effective in some residents than others. Between 25% and 40% of residents respond well.
2. The best candidates for a long-term prompted voiding program are residents who show the following characteristics during the assessment period:
   a. Have an average of one or less episode of urinary incontinence per day.
   b. Have an hourly wet check percentage of 20% or less.
   c. Have an appropriate toileting rate of more than 66% (calculated by the number of voids into the toilet divided by the total number of voids).
3. Residents who do not meet these criteria but who attempt to toilet at least twice a day should be considered for further evaluation and other more specific treatments.
4. Residents who fail to respond and attempt to toilet infrequently should be considered for a supportive check and change program.

Prompted Voiding (Ongoing Protocol)

1. Contact the resident every 2 hours from 7 AM to 7 PM.
2. Use the same procedures as for the assessment period (see 1–4 above).
3. For nighttime management, use either a modified prompted voiding schedule or a containment device.
4. A quality assurance nurse should perform random wet checks to ensure that responsive residents are maintaining expected levels of dryness.
5. If a resident who has been responding well has an increase in incontinence frequency despite adequate staff implementation of the protocol, he or she should be evaluated for reversible factors.

Adapted with permission from Ouslander JG, Osterweil D, Morley J. *Medical Care in the Nursing Home.* New York: McGraw-Hill; 1991:241.

Overflow Incontinence (Incontinence Associated with Incomplete Bladder Emptying)

When the postvoid residual urine volume is greater than 200 mL, overflow incontinence is assumed to occur. Autonomic neuropathy, spinal cord injury, lower urinary tract symptomatology (LUTS), and bladder outlet obstruction can cause overflow incontinence, in which the bladder fills and leakage of urine is a result of an overspill.

Neuropathic incontinence is most commonly caused by diabetes mellitus. Parasympathomimetics, such as bethanechol, can be tried but work poorly. In most cases, intermittent urinary catheterization is the management of choice but is challenging to implement in older nursing home residents.

Spinal cord damage results in incontinence by preventing inhibitory signals from the central nervous system from preventing the normal urinary reflex arc. Intermittent catheterization is the appropriate therapy, although it can be challenging to achieve in a nursing home. In older persons in a nursing home, spinal cord metastases (from prostate and other cancers) and lumbar spinal stenosis are the major causes. There is often a concomitant increase in falls. These residents are at increased risk of bladder cancer, stones, infections, and upper urinary tract dysfunction. Persons who have dementia (wacky), have a gait disturbance (wobbly), and are incontinent (wet) should be worked up for normal-pressure hydrocephalus.

Lower urinary tract symptomatology (bladder dyssynergy) is very common in older men and occurs in 8% of older women. In men, this is often associated with an enlarging prostate. Symptoms in men consist of difficulty in initiating the stream, poor quality of the stream, splitting or spraying of urine, intermittency, and postvoid dribble. These symptoms can also be caused by UTI; thus, it is important to rule this out from the beginning. The American Urological Association Symptom Score (Table 16–4) should be used to highlight the nature and severity of specific LUTS experienced and can help in identifying successful treatment. A variety of medications are available for LUTS (Table 16–5). α_1-Adrenergic blockers are the most efficacious. These agents often cause hypotension, orthostatic hypotension, and fatigue. They can be used on an as required basis with fewer side effects.

Men with large prostates causing bladder outlet obstruction may also respond to treatment with 5α reductase inhibitors such as finasteride and dutasteride. Saw palmetto is a phytotherapy that works in some older persons. Prostate surgery can be efficacious in many men but may not be offered to those in nursing homes. The insertion of artificial urinary sphincters can improve continence after surgery.

In women, bladder outlet obstruction can occur after pelvic floor surgery. Urethral strictures can also lead to bladder outlet obstruction.

Urge Incontinence (Overactive Bladder)

Urge incontinence, leakage arising from the inability to suppress an urgent desire to urinate, is very common. It is associated with large volumes of urine loss. Treatment involves teaching the person to try to inhibit the urge to

Table 16–4.   AMERICAN UROLOGICAL ASSOCIATION SYMPTOM INDEX

Use the following point scale to answer each of the questions. Total the score from all the questions.

0 = Not at all

1 = Less than once in five times you have urinated

2 = Less than half the time

3 = About half the time

4 = More than half the time

5 = Almost always

Over the past month, how often have you:

Had the sensation of not completely emptying your bladder after you finished urinating?

Had to urinate again less than 2 hours after you finished urinating?

Found that you stopped and started again several times when you urinated?

Found it difficult to postpone urination?

Had a weak urinary stream?

Had to push or strain to begin urination?

Had to get up to urinate from the time you went to bed at night until you got up in the morning?

(For this question, use the following point scale: 0 = none, 1 = 1 time, 2 = 2 times, 3 = 3 times, 4 = 4 times, 5 = 5 times or more)

Total score from all questions _____

Score	Severity
0–7	Mild
8–19	Moderate
20–35	Severe

Table 16–5.   TREATMENTS AVAILABLE FOR LOWER URINARY TRACT SYMPTOMATOLOGY

α_1-Blockers

Terazosin

Doxazosin

Tamsulosin

Alfuzosin

5α Reductase Inhibitors

Dutasteride

Finasteride

Phosphodiesterase Inhibitors

Sildenafil

Phytotherapy

Saw palmetto (*Serenoa repens*)

Prostate Surgery

Minimally invasive (microwave or radiofrequency)

Transurethral resection of prostate

Table 16–6.   EXAMPLES OF BEHAVIORAL INTERVENTIONS FOR URINARY INCONTINENCE

Procedure	Definition	Types of Incontinence	Comments
Patient Dependent			
Pelvic muscle (Kegel) exercises	Repetitive contraction of pelvic muscles	Stress and urge	Requires adequate function and motivation Biofeedback may be useful in teaching the exercises
Biofeedback	Use of bladder, rectal, or vaginal pressure recordings to train resident to contract pelvic floor muscles and relax bladder	Stress and urge	Requires equipment and trained personnel Relatively invasive Requires adequate cognitive and physical function and motivation
Bladder training	Use of pelvic muscle exercises with or without biofeedback and other strategies to manage urgency	Urge	Requires a trained therapist, adequate cognitive and physical functioning, and motivation
Bladder retraining (see Table 16–12)	Progressive lengthening or shortening of intervoiding interval, with adjunctive techniques[a] such as intermittent catheterization Used in residents recovering from bladder overdistension with persistent retention	Acute (e.g., post-catheterization with urge or overflow, poststroke)	Goal is to restore normal pattern of voiding and continence Requires adequate cognitive and physical function and motivation
Caregiver Dependent			
Prompted voiding (see Table 16–3)	Regular (every 2 h during the day 7 AM–7 PM) Prompts to void with positive reinforcement	Urge, stress, and functional	Goal is to prevent wetting episodes Can be used in residents with impaired cognitive or physical functioning Requires staff or caregiver availability and motivation
Habit training	Variable toileting Schedule based on pattern of voiding with positive reinforcement	As above	As above

[a]Adapted with permission from Ouslander JG, Osterweil D, Morley J. *Medical Care in the Nursing Home*. New York: McGraw-Hill; 1991:239.

urinate or to distract him- or herself, thus reducing the urge. Examples of behavioral interventions for urinary incontinence are given in Table 16–6. Bladder retraining can be somewhat successful in community-dwelling older persons but has poor success in nursing home residents because of the need for the person to be motivated, with sufficient cognitive ability to understand what is asked of him or her and apply it. Biofeedback has more success, but nursing home residents require continuous training. A variety of anticholinergic drugs have been used with varying success (Table 16–7). Most of these drugs decrease cognition to a small degree. In addition, they cause a dry mouth, constipation, blurred vision, and often orthostatic hypotension. Although electrical stimulation can work, it is rarely used in nursing homes. Intravesical injection of botulinum toxin or the vanilloids capsaicin and resiniferatoxin can decrease detrusor hyperreflexia but are not commonly available to nursing home residents because those treated

need to be able to self-catheterize as botulinum toxin in particular may result in urinary retention. In some nursing homes in the United States, nurses regularly carry out intermittent catheterization. The benefits of augmentation cystoplasty are again far more likely to accrue in younger persons.

Stress Incontinence

Stress incontinence occurs when intraabdominal pressure is increased by sneezing or coughing, overcoming the ability of the urethral sphincter to remain closed. It is significantly more common in women than men because of weakened pelvic floor musculature from childbirth and factors such as obesity. It occurs in 10% of men who have had a radical prostatectomy. Pelvic floor muscle exercises (Kegel exercises) can be very effective when performed regularly. Unfortunately, it is difficult to get

Table 16–7.	MANAGEMENT OF URGE INCONTINENCE (DETRUSOR HYPERCONTRACTILITY)

- Behavioral intervention and physical therapy: bladder training and pelvic floor muscle training
- Biofeedback
- Anticholinergic medication
  - Oxybutynin (IR, ER, Patch)
  - Tolterodine (IR, ER)
  - Trospium
  - Solifenacin
  - Darifenacin
  - Fesoterodine
- B$_3$ adrenoreceptor agonist mirabegron (filed for approval)
- Sacral nerve stimulation or percutaneous posterior tibial nerve stimulation
- Intravesical therapy
- Botulinum A toxin
- Augmentation cystoplasty

ER, extended release; IR, immediate release.

cognitively impaired nursing home residents to perform these exercises on a regular basis. A study in a Turkish nursing home did show that behavior therapy with Kegel exercises can be successful with results lasting up to 6 months. α-Adrenergic agonists have a small effect but may increase blood pressure. Duloxetine has mild efficacy; however, it is not first-line treatment. Pessaries can be useful, but there is a lack of good-quality evidence of efficacy. Although surgery is successful in younger women, it is a poor option for most nursing home residents (Table 16–8).

Mixed Incontinence

Any combination of the different forms of incontinence can occur, often making drug treatment problematic. One example is detrusor hypercontractility and impaired contraction.

Table 16–8.	MANAGEMENT OF STRESS INCONTINENCE

- Pelvic floor muscle training (Kegel exercises)
- Weighted cone exercises
- α Agonists (e.g., pseudoephedrine)
- Serotonin–norepinephrine uptake inhibitor (duloxetine)
- Pessaries
- Injection of bulking agents (collagen)
- Surgery
  - Colposuspension
  - Slings: bladder neck or mid-urethral
  - Artificial urinary sphincter
- Estrogen

Absorbent Products for Incontinence

For light to moderate urinary incontinence, the following types of pads are available:

- Disposable pads
- Washable pads with an integral pad
- Washable diapers
- Disposable diapers
- Disposable pull-ups
- Disposable T-shaped diapers (have a waistband)

For light incontinence, disposable insert pads have the least leakage but are the most expensive. Skin health is affected equally by all types.

For moderate incontinence, pull-ups (most expensive) perform best. During the day, however, women prefer disposable inserts. In men, diapers perform better. Nursing home caregivers find pull-ups and inserts easier to apply and quicker to change. Women find washable products unacceptable, but the majority of men do not find them objectionable.

Incontinence-Associated Dermatitis

Chronic exposure of skin to urine leads to redness, which can be associated with erosion or blistering. This leads to the loss of skin barrier function. This then results in skin infections such as candidiasis. Incontinence associated dermatitis needs to be differentiated from pressure ulcers and treated appropriately. The approach to the treatment of dermatitis caused by incontinence and prevention is outlined in Tables 6–9 and 6–10.

Urinary Catheters

Both urinary catheters and condom catheters increase UTIs, and urinary catheters can produce trauma to the urinary tract. Intermittent urinary tract catheterization has a much lower rate of UTI than indwelling urinary catheters; unfortunately the use of intermittent catheters

Table 16–9.	COMPARISON OF INCONTINENCE-ASSOCIATED DERMATITIS AND PRESSURE ULCERS	
	Incontinence Associated Dermatitis	**Pressure Ulcers**
Site	Any area	Over prominence
Shape	Different superficial areas or spots	One area or ulcer
Edges	Irregular	Distinct
Depth	Superficial	Skin loss
Necrosis	None	Can be present
Blanchable	Yes, with white surrounding maceration	No

Table 16–10.	SKIN CARE TO PREVENT INCONTINENCE-ASSOCIATED DERMATITIS

- Use a no-rinse skin cleanser with pH of healthy skin (pH 5.4–5.9).
- Cleansing should be as close as possible to time of incontinence episode.
- Use a soft cloth.
- DO NOT use soap and water.
- If skin is macerated, use an emollient-based moisturizer.
- Protectants (petrolatum, dimethicone, zinc oxide, acrylates) have a small and variable ability to prevent dermatitis.
- Absorptive products decrease dermatitis.

Table 16–11.	INDICATIONS FOR A LONG-TERM INDWELLING URINARY CATHETER

- Urinary retention characterized by the following:
  - Causes persistent overflow incontinence, symptomatic infections, or renal dysfunction
  - Cannot be corrected surgically or medically
  - Cannot be managed practically with intermittent catheterization
- Skin wounds, pressure sores, or irritations that are being contaminated by incontinent urine
- Care of terminally ill or severely impaired persons for whom bed and clothing changes are uncomfortable or disruptive
- Preference of patient or caregiver when patient has not responded to more specific treatments

Adapted with permission from Ouslander JG, Osterweil D, Morley J. *Medical Care in the Nursing Home.* New York: McGraw-Hill; 1991:246.

Table 16–12.	KEY PRINCIPLES OF MANAGING LONG-TERM INDWELLING URINARY CATHETERS

- Maintain the sterile, closed, gravity drainage system and avoid breaking the closed system.
- Use clean techniques in emptying and changing the drainage system; wash hands between patients in institutional settings.
- Secure the catheter to the upper thigh or lower abdomen to avoid perineal contamination and urethral irritation caused by movement of the catheter.
- Avoid frequent and vigorous cleaning of the catheter entry site; washing with soapy water once per day is sufficient for personal hygiene.
- Do not routinely irrigate unless repeated obstructions occur.
- If bypassing occurs in the absence of obstruction, consider the possibility of bladder spasms, which can be treated with a bladder relaxant.
- Change the catheter according to the manufacturer's instructions.
- If catheter obstruction occurs frequently, increase the patient's fluid intake and acidify the urine if possible (diluting acetic acid irrigations maybe helpful).
- Do not routinely use prophylactic or suppressive urinary antiseptics or antimicrobials.
- Do not do routine surveillance cultures to guide management of individual patients because all chronically catheterized patients have bacteriuria (which is often polymicrobial, and the organisms change frequently).
- Do not treat infection unless symptoms develop; symptoms may be nonspecific, and other possible sources of infection should be carefully excluded before symptoms are attributed to the urinary tract.
- If a symptomatic infection occurs, the catheter should be changed before a specimen is collected for culture. (Specimens obtained from the old catheter may be misleading because of colonization of the catheter lumen.)
- If symptomatic urinary tract infections frequently develop, a genitourinary evaluation should be considered to rule out pathology conditions such as stones, periurethral or prostatic abscesses, and chronic pyelonephritis.

Adapted with permission from Ouslander JG, Osterweil D, Morley J. *Medical Care in the Nursing Home.* New York: McGraw-Hill; 1991:246.

is not common in some nursing homes. Silver alloy catheters (but not silver oxide) decrease infection in the short term. Antimicrobial impregnated catheters reduce asymptomatic bacteriuria in the short term but not necessarily infections. Purple urine bag syndrome occurs in long-term catheterized persons with asymptomatic bacteriuria and a high tryptophan diet. Other complications of long-term indwelling urinary catheters besides UTI and asymptomatic bacteriuria are bladder stones, periurethral abscesses, and bladder cancer.

Suprapubic catheters can be used when a chronic indwelling catheter is needed and if:

- Urinary catheterization is difficult or potentially dangerous
- The person has neurologic disease such as multiple sclerosis or spinal cord injury
- The person has intractable urinary incontinence and other methods have failed
- The person needs it for palliative use
- It is the choice of the patient or caregiver when the advantages and disadvantages have been explained

Contraindications include bladder cancer, use of anticoagulants or antiplatelet therapy, abdominal wall sepsis, and a subcutaneous vascular graft in the suprapubic region.

In all persons with a suprapubic catheter, a catheter valve as an alternative to free drainage needs to be considered. When persons with a suprapubic catheter have severe abdominal pain spreading from the catheter insertion site, they should be immediately sent to a urologist. Staff members in nursing homes need to be trained to change suprapubic catheters because these catheters can dislodge or fall out, and if not reinserted quickly, the insertion site may close. Antibiotics should be given for cellulitis in the catheter site or symptomatic UTI. Antibiotics are not used for pericatheter discharge or asymptomatic bacteriuria. Residents with urine bypassing the catheter or a blockage need a urology referral.

The indications for a chronic indwelling bladder catheters are outlined in Table 16–11. Table 16–12 provides the principles of managing chronic indwelling urinary catheters. After removal of an indwelling catheter, a bladder retraining protocol should be initiated (Table 16–13).

Table 16–13.   BLADDER RETRAINING PROTOCOL FOR USE AFTER THE REMOVAL OF AN INDWELLING CATHETER

Goal: To restore a normal pattern of voiding and continence after the removal of an indwelling catheter

1. Monitor the resident's urine output every 4 hours for 1 or 2 days.
2. Remove the indwelling catheter (clamping the catheter before removal is not necessary).[a,b]
3. Initiate a toileting schedule
   a. Begin by taking the resident to the toilet:
      i. Every 2 hours during the day and evening
      ii. Before getting into bed
      iii. Every 4 hours at night
   b. Instruct the resident on techniques to trigger voiding (e.g., running water, stroking the inner thigh, suprapubic tapping) and to help completely empty the bladder (e.g., bending forward, suprapubic pressure, double voiding).
4. If the resident is unable to void by the time the expected bladder volume is 500 mL (or at his or her functional bladder capacity, on the basis of monitoring in step 1, or if the postvoid residual is greater than 400 mL, reinsert the catheter and consider a urodynamic evaluation or the use of a permanent catheter.
5. If the postvoid residuals are 100 to 400 mL, continue to monitor until they are consistently less than 200 mL.[c]
6. Monitor the resident's voiding and continence pattern with a systemic record that allows the recording of:
   a. Frequency, timing, and amount of incontinence episodes
   b. Fluid intake pattern
   c. Postvoid or intermittent catheter volume
7. If the resident is voiding frequently (i.e., more often than every 2 hours), encourage him or her to delay voiding as long as possible and instruct him or her (if possible) to use pelvic muscle exercises and techniques to help empty the bladder completely; consider the use of biofeedback if available.
8. If the resident continues to have incontinence:
   a. Rule out reversible causes.
   b. Consider urodynamic evaluation to determine care and appropriate treatment.

[a]Indwelling catheters should be removed from all residents who do not have an indication for their short- or long-term use. For those who have had significant retention (>400 mL), the catheter should be kept in for several days to decompress the bladder.

[b]Clamping routines have never been shown to be helpful and are not appropriate for residents who have had overdistended bladders.

[c]A precise value cannot be recommended on the basis of available data. Residual volumes less than 200 mL generally do not cause upper urinary tract complications.

Adapted with permission from Ouslander JG, Osterweil D, Morley J. *Medical Care in the Nursing Home.* New York: McGraw-Hill; 1991:240.

FECAL INCONTINENCE

More than half of residents in nursing homes have some degree of fecal incontinence. In the majority of cases, these residents also have urinary incontinence. Fecal incontinence is a major reason for institutionalization. Fecal

Table 16–14.   CAUSES OF FECAL INCONTINENCE

- Fecal impaction
- Cognitive impairment
- Depression
- Stroke
- Arthritis with limited mobility
- Paraplegia
- Local disease
  - Pudendal nerve damage
  - Anorectal trauma
- Excess use of laxatives
- Radiation
- Neoplasm

incontinence increases the cost of care in the United States by approximately $9000 a year per resident.

There are a number of causes of fecal incontinence (Table 16–14). After a physical examination, a number of diagnostic tests may be considered. These include a flexible sigmoidoscopy, colonoscopy, anorectal manometry, electromyography, anal ultrasonography, magnetic resonance imaging, and defecating portography. Other than the first two, these are rarely used in nursing homes.

Conservative management of fecal incontinence includes a high-fiber diet, antidiarrheals for diarrhea, and a postmeal toileting regimen. Prompted voiding increases the number of continent bowel movements. Biofeedback can play a role in improving fecal incontinence in residents with the cognitive ability to be able to be involved in the procedures. Anal irrigation systems are popular and provide effective management for a large number of people, especially those with spinal injuries; however, good-quality evidence of effect is lacking. If these measures fail, disposable absorbent pads can be used but must be fitted for the purpose of containing fecal incontinence because urinary pads are not designed for this purpose and are not as effective. Rarely, surgical procedures such as sphincter repair or injection of glutaraldehyde cross-linked collagen may be useful. Sacral nerve stimulation has been used successfully in younger persons. If fecal incontinence is severe, a diverting colostomy is the surgical procedure of choice.

FUTURE CONTINENCE TECHNOLOGIES

Current continence management in many nursing homes relies heavily on the use of absorbent pads to contain urine and feces, which some older residents find undignified. Pads and other absorbent products can also be expensive and do not treat the underlying cause of the bladder or bowel dysfunction. There is clearly a need to develop new conservative treatment technologies for older people, particularly for nursing home residents. One such technology that shows promise is transcutaneous posterior tibial nerve stimulation (TPTNS). TPTNS is a technique of noninvasive peripheral electrical neuromodulation for the treatment of LUTS, urinary incontinence, and fecal incontinence. The

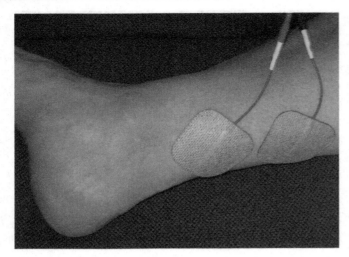

Figure 16–1. Positioning transcutaneous posterior tibial nerve stimulation electrodes.

technique modulates the sacral plexus indirectly via the sensory, motor, and autonomic fibers of the posterior tibial nerve, although the exact mechanism of action has yet to be fully understood. Although the potential for TPTNS as a first-line treatment option for bladder and bowel dysfunction in the nursing home population has yet to be established, a recent feasibility study of nursing home residents shows encouraging results. The TPTNS treatment involves 30 minutes of therapy twice a week for 6 weeks. Therapy involves positioning two self-adhesive surface electrodes on the lower leg; thus, this is a dignified treatment with high user acceptability. The negative electrode is positioned behind the medial malleolus and the positive electrode 10 cm proximal to it. Correct positioning is determined by noting a hallux reaction (plantar flexion of the great toe or fanning of all toes) or the person's description of tingling, pulsing, or movement in the great toe (Figure 16–1). Stimulation is delivered at fixed frequency of 10 Hz and pulse width of 200 ms in continuous mode. The intensity level of the stimulation current (range, 0–50 mA) is determined when correct positioning has been established, according to the comfort level of the person. Further research is needed to establish the criteria for determining which nursing home residents are most likely to benefit from TPTNS, and definitive trials are warranted to strengthen the evidence base before implementation. Development of such conservative interventions could transform the future of continence care within nursing homes.

KEY POINTS

1. Optimal management of incontinence requires the availability of a continence specialist nurse or continence advisor.
2. New-onset incontinence is often caused by UTI.
3. Management of all forms of incontinence should include an individually assessed toileting program.

4. Neuropathic (overflow) incontinence is best treated with intermittent catheterization.
5. LUTS occurs most commonly in men and is treated with α_1-blockers, 5-α reductase inhibitors, or prostate surgery.
6. Behavioral therapy with Kegel exercises can improve stress and urge incontinence in nursing home residents.
7. Anticholinergic drugs are used to treat urge incontinence.
8. Stress incontinence may be treated with serotonin–norepinephrine uptake inhibitors and pessaries.
9. A variety of absorbent products are available for incontinence and perform reasonably well.
10. Appropriate skin care is necessary to prevent incontinence-associated dermatitis.
11. Indwelling urinary catheters should be avoided whenever possible.
12. Urinary catheters can be used for persons in hospice care for comfort and quality of life.
13. Fecal incontinence is common in nursing home residents and needs to have its cause identified.
14. Conservative measures can often improve fecal incontinence.

SUGGESTED READINGS

Amarenco G, Sheikh Ismael S, Even-Schneider A, et al. Urodynamic effect of acute transcutaneous posterior tibial nerve stimulation in overactive bladder. *J Urol.* 2003;169:2210-2215.

Aslan E, Komurcu N, Beji NK, Yalcin O. Bladder training and Kegel exercises for women with urinary complaints living in a rest home. *Gerontology.* 2008;54(4):224-231.

Bates-Jensen BM, Alessi CA, Al-Samarrai NR, Schnelle JF. The effects of an exercise and incontinence intervention on skin health outcomes in nursing home residents. *J Am Geriatr Soc.* 2003;51:348-355.

Beeckman D, Woodward S, Rajpaul K, Vanderwee K. Clinical challenges of preventing incontinence-associated dermatitis. *Br J Nurs.* 2011;20:784-786.

Booth J, Hagen S, McClurg et al. A feasibility study of transcutaneous posterior tibial nerve stimulation for bladder and bowel dysfunction in older adults in residential care homes. *J Am Med Dir Assoc.* 2013;14:270-274. Video of TPTNS procedure available at www.jamda.com.

Booth J, Kumlien S, Zang Y. Promoting urinary continence. In Tolson D, Booth J, Schofield I (eds). *Evidence Informed Nursing with Older People.* Oxford, UK: Wiley-Blackwell; 2011.

Chen YT, Lin MH, Lai HY, et al. Potentially inappropriate urinary catheter indwelling among long-term care facilities residents. *J Eval Clin Pract.* 2009;15:592-594.

Fader M, Cottenden AM, Getliffe K. Absorbent products for moderate-heavy urinary and/or faecal incontinence in women and men. *Cochrane Database Syst Rev.* 2008;(4):CD007408.

Fader M, Cottenden A, Getliffe K, et al. Absorbent products for urinary/faecal incontinence: a comparative evaluation of key product designs. *Health Technol Assess.* 2008;12:iii-iv, ix-185.

Fader M, Cottenden AM, Getliffe K. Absorbent products for light urinary incontinence in women. *Cochrane Database Syst Rev.* 2007;(2):CD001406.

Findlay JM, Maxwell-Armstrong C. Posterior tibial nerve stimulation and faecal incontinence: a review. *Int J Colorectal Dis.* 2011;26:265-273.

Fink HA, Taylor BD, Tacklind JW, et al. Treatment interventions in nursing home residents with urinary incontinence: a systematic review of randomized trials. *Mayo Clin Proc.* 2008;83:1332-1343.

Jonsson K, Emanuelsson-Loft AL, Nasic S, Hedelin H. Urine bladder catheters in nursing home patients: a one-day point prevalence study in a Swedish county. *Scand J Urol Nephrol.* 2010;44:320-323.

Lin SY, Wang RH, Lin CC, Chiang HY. Competence to provide urinary incontinence care in Taiwan's nursing homes: perceptions of nurses and nurse assistants. *J Wound Ostomy Continence Nurs.* 2012;39:187-193.

Lyons SS. How do people make continence care happen? An analysis of organizational culture in two nursing homes. *Gerontologist.* 2010;50:327-339.

Morley JE. Urinary incontinence and the community-dwelling elder: a practical approach to diagnosis and management for the primary care geriatrician. *Clin Geriatr Med.* 2004;20:427-435.

Offermans MP, Du Moulin MF, Hamers JP, et al. Prevalence of urinary incontinence and associated risk factors in nursing home residents: a systematic review. *Neurourol Urodyn.* 2009;28:288-294.

Ouslander JG. *Medical Care in the Nursing Home*, 2nd ed. New York: McGraw-Hill; 1991.

Roe B, Flanagan L, Jack B, et al. Systematic review of descriptive studies that investigated associated factors with the management of incontinence in older people in care homes. *Int J Older People Nurs.* 2013;8(1):29-49.

Shamliyan T, Wyman J, Bliss DZ, et al. Prevention of urinary and fecal incontinence in adults. *Evid Rep Technol Assess.* 2007;(161):1-379.

Schnelle JF, Leung FW, Rao SS, et al. A controlled trial of an intervention to improve urinary and fecal incontinence and constipation. *J Am Geriatr Soc.* 2010;58:1504-1511.

Schreiner L, Santos T, Knorst M. Randomised trial of transcutaneous tibial nerve stimulation to treat urge urinary incontinence in older women. *Int Urogynecol J.* 2010;21:1065-1070.

Tariq SH, Morley JE, Prather CM. Fecal incontinence in the elderly patient. *Am J Med.* 2003;115:217-227.

Walid MS. Prevalence of urinary incontinence in female residents of American nursing homes and association with neuropsychiatric disorders. *J Clin Med Res.* 2009;1:37-39.

MULTIPLE CHOICE QUESTIONS

16.1   For urination to occur, which of the following is correct?

    a. Both the parasympathetic and sympathetic nervous system stimulate the detrusor muscle.

    b. The sympathetic nervous system stimulates the detrusor muscle.

    c. The parasympathetic nervous system inhibits the internal urethral sphincter.

    d. The sympathetic nervous system inhibits the internal urethral sphincter.

16.2   An 80-year-old woman with mild dementia has incontinence every time she coughs. What type of incontinence does she have?

    a. Urge incontinence

    b. Stress incontinence

    c. Lower urinary tract symptomatology

    d. Neuropathic incontinence

    e. Functional incontinence

16.3   A 75-year-old man has incontinence. His postvoid residual is 300 cc. What kind of incontinence does he have?

    a. Functional

    b. Urge

    c. Stress

    d. Reflex

    e. Lower urinary tract symptomatology

16.4   Which of the following should not be used to prevent incontinence-associated dermatitis?

    a. Soft cloth

    b. Acrylates

    c. Soap and water

    d. Emollient-based moisturizer

16.5   Which of the following is an indication for a chronic indwelling catheter?

    a. Urge incontinence

    b. Stress incontinence

    c. Functional incontinence

    d. Care of a terminally ill patient for his or her comfort

Chapter 17

BOWEL CHANGES

For most adults, bowel function is a personal and private matter. Although bowel problems are not an inevitable concomitant of aging, many older nursing home residents have bowel care needs. Bowel changes are a source of discomfort, pain, and morbidity for residents; they can be embarrassing; and if they are not appropriately managed, relatively minor problems such as mild constipation can quickly worsen and have profound impacts on a person's health and well-being. It is not uncommon for staff to describe a resident as bowel obsessed, but for anyone who has experienced severe constipation, this behavior is understandable. In addition to impact on the resident's health, poorly managed bowel care is likely to cause an unpleasant work environment and may contribute to staff absentee and turnover rates. Bowel changes and fecal incontinence are often complex and multifaceted. Thus, nursing home staff needs to be knowledgeable and skilled in effective evaluation of bowel symptoms and bowel care interventions.

MANAGING CONSTIPATION

Constipation is an extremely common problem affecting 33 million persons in the United States and resulting in 92,000 hospitalizations a year. In older persons, nearly one in four complains of constipation. When the Rome Criteria for Constipation (Table 17–1) are used, 17% of older persons have constipation. Constipation is slightly more common in women, and one third of the community-dwelling population older than the age of 80 years uses a laxative at least once a month. In nursing homes, approximately 50% of residents complain of constipation. About half of these meet the Rome Criteria for constipation. The extra cost of caring for a resident with constipation in a nursing home is about $2000 per year.

Constipation causes a decreased quality of life, decreases functional status, increases pain, and causes urinary incontinence. It also is associated with fecal incontinence, stercoral ulcers, fecaloma, increased pain from hemorrhoids, and fecal impaction. Fecal impaction can lead to intestinal obstruction, necessitating surgery. Constipation can also lead to delirium and physical and verbal aggression. A number of conditions are known to increase the risk of constipation (Table 17–2).

The basic treatment for constipation is to increase fluid intake, use bulking agents (i.e., fiber) if mobile, exercise, and use the toilet within a half hour after eating to make maximum use of the gastro-colic reflex. Stool softeners (e.g., dioctyl sodium or calcium sulfosuccinate) have no evidence of efficacy. Stimulant laxatives such as senna and bisacodyl castor oil have a low rate of efficacy in truly constipated persons. Osmotic laxatives, such as sorbitol (not used in the United Kingdom), lactulose or polyethylene glycol (Miralax and Movicol), work in the majority of constipated patients. For persons with constipation, the starting dose is 50 mL before sleep, and the dosage can be increased to 100 mL twice daily. Miralax comes as a 17-g powder and Movicol as a 13-g powder that is dissolved in water. Most truly constipated persons need at least double the dose and, as such, sorbitol and lactulose are cheaper.

When a person still has severe constipation on high doses of osmotic laxatives, the choice is between enemas (tap water, saline, or oil) or more expensive but efficacious drugs. Colchicine is a cheap alternative to some of the more expensive drugs and often treats constipation. Lubiprostone (approved by the Food and Drug Administration) is an orally administered bicyclic fatty acid that activates the chloride-2 channel, producing a chloride rich intestinal fluid secretion. A number of controlled studies have found that it approximately doubles the weekly spontaneous bowel movements compared with placebo. It also decreases abdominal discomfort and improves stool consistency. Prucalopride is a high-affinity selective serotonin (5-HT_4) agonist that is approved in Europe and Canada for constipation. Linaclotide is a drug that works similarly to cholera toxin, increasing fluid into the bowel. It has a similar effectiveness to lubiprostone. Although some persons in nursing homes need these expensive drugs long term, most can have them discontinued after 1 to 4 weeks. Constipation caused by opiate use can usually be treated with osmotic laxatives but, when severe, methylnaltrexone or alvimopan can be used. Methylnaltrexone does not cross the blood–brain barrier, so it reverses the peripheral effect of opiates on the gut while allowing the opiate to still exert its central analgesic effect. Figure 17–1 provides an approach to treating constipation in nursing homes.

Table 17–1.   ROME CRITERIA FOR CONSTIPATION
• Straining at defecation for at least a quarter of the time
• Lumpy or hard stools for at least a quarter of the time
• A sensation of incomplete evacuation for at least a quarter of the time
• Two or fewer bowel movements per week

UNDERSTANDING AND MANAGING FECAL INCONTINENCE

Fecal incontinence is not a disease; rather, it is a sign or symptom, and management should commence with the identification of the cause or causes. Initial assessment involves relevant medical history, a general examination, anorectal examination, and cognitive assessment.

Approximately 20% of community-dwelling older adults have fecal incontinence. Within the nursing home population, the prevalence is increased to 50%. Fecal incontinence occurs in nearly 80% of persons with end-stage dementia. Half of older persons with fecal incontinence also have urinary incontinence.

The most common reason for fecal incontinence is overflow associated with fecal impaction. Cognitive and mobility impairment may also contribute to overflow incontinence. A variety of surgical procedures, radiation, rectal ischemia, and inflammatory bowel disease are associated with fecal incontinence. Rectal prolapse can also cause fecal soiling. Multiple sclerosis and spinal cord injury (e.g., spinal stenosis) are neurologic causes of fecal incontinence. Autonomic neuropathy associated with diabetes mellitus also results in fecal soiling.

Simple management techniques include habit training in which a routine for bowel evacuation is established. This should occur immediately after breakfast. Ensuring that

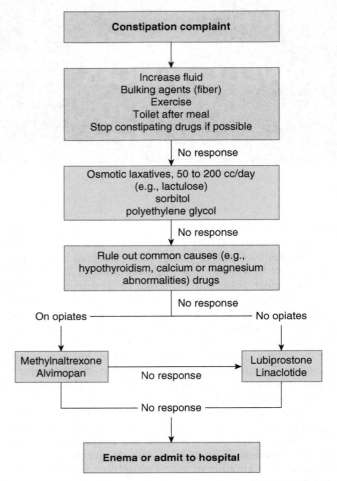

Figure 17–1. An approach to treating constipation in nursing homes.

Table 17–2.   FACTORS ASSOCIATED WITH CONSTIPATION IN NURSING HOMES
• Immobility
• Decreased fluid and nutrient intake (particularly fiber)
• Colonic and rectal cancers
• Parkinson's disease
• Diabetes mellitus
• Hypercalcemia or hypomagnesia
• Pneumonia
• Hypothyroidism
• Drugs: Iron and calcium supplements
▪ Antidepressants
▪ Antipsychotics
▪ Antihistamines
▪ Calcium channel antagonists
▪ Drugs for urge incontinence
▪ Diuretics
▪ Opiates
▪ Nonsteroidal antiinflammatory drugs

older people feel comfortable and safe and that they are confident that their privacy will not be disturbed are key elements in establishing a bowel routine. Learning forward with the forearms on thighs and a foot stool to raise the feet and relax the anorectal angle often works. Increasing evacuation requires diaphragmatic breathing coupled with bracing of abdominal muscles. Pelvic floor muscle training and biofeedback may also decrease fecal soiling. Anal plugs, when tolerated, can be highly effective in the short term but are not recommended for long-term use. Pads and incontinence underwear can also be used. For frequent and large-volume fecal incontinence, collection devices that attach to the skin around the rectum may be effective. Use of loperamide or codeine can be useful when diarrhea is a contributing factor.

Frequent fecal incontinence is damaging to the skin. Use of wet wipes, cleaning agents with a barrier cream, or a bidet shower with gentle drying of skin with a towel can all protect skin integrity. When local ulcers develop, a colloid dressing can protect them from fecal soiling.

Surgical therapies have been successful in younger persons. Gracioplasty with electrical stimulation has been successful in younger persons but has not been studied in older persons. Artificial sphincters have shown some success. Injections of bulking agents (glutaraldehyde, cross-linked collagen, and Durasphere F1) into the submucosa have been used in small numbers of individuals. Sacral nerve stimulation is successful in selected cases but is not routinely available.

DIARRHEA

Diarrhea is a common problem in nursing home residents. Diarrhea can have disastrous effects on the quality of life of older persons. Older persons in nursing homes are four times as likely to die when they have diarrhea compared with community-dwelling elders. However, the majority of diarrhea episodes are self-limiting, lasting less than 48 hours.

Acute diarrhea in older persons is most commonly caused by infections, drugs, or fecal impaction. Other causes to be considered are food poisoning, ischemic colitis, and large bowel obstruction. Any cause of chronic diarrhea can present for the first time in an older person as acute diarrhea. Viruses are the most common causes of acute diarrhea. These include rotavirus, Norwalk virus, calicivirus, and enteric adenoviruses. Besides *Clostridium*, bacterial causes of diarrhea include *Escherichia coli*, *Campylobacter*, *Salmonella*, *Shigella*, *Vibrio*, and staphylococcus. In some parts of the world, parasites such as amoeba need to be considered.

Antibiotic-associated diarrhea is a common problem in nursing homes. Roughly one in four nursing home residents have *Clostridium difficile* in their stool after 2 weeks of antibiotic therapy. The majority of these residents do not have diarrhea. Those with diarrhea can progress to pseudomembranous colitis and toxic megacolon. The diagnosis can be made by detecting either cytotoxin A or B in the stool, but it can take up to 48 hours after diarrhea starts for these to be detectable. Culture of *C. difficile* in the stool is highly sensitive in making the diagnosis, but because of commensal occurrence, is less specific. If *C. difficile* is identified, it should be tested for in vitro toxin production. Primary treatment of *C. difficile* is metronidazole, or in difficult-to-treat cases, vancomycin. Other treatments to resistant infection are fidaxomicin and rifaximin. Donor fecal transplantation and antibodies against *C. difficile* toxin can also be used. Prevention of spread requires careful hand washing with detergent (because alcohol gels and rubs are ineffective against spores) and environmental cleaning with detergent and hypochlorite solutions. *Saccharomyces boulardii* is a probiotic that can prevent *C. difficile* infection.

Specific regional guidance for control of *C. difficile* infection should be followed, and the English Department of Health recommends that a protocol represented by the acronym SIGHT is applied in all cases of diarrhea including nursing homes:

- **S**uspect that a case may be infective where there is no clear alternative cause for diarrhea.
- **I**solate the patient while determining the cause of the diarrhea
- **G**loves and aprons must be used for all contacts with the patient and their environment.
- **H**and washing with soap and water should be carried out before and after each contact with the patient and his or her environment.
- **T**est the stool for toxin by sending a specimen immediately.

Table 17–3. CAUSES OF CHRONIC DIARRHEA IN OLDER PERSONS

Drugs	Osmotic laxatives
	Magnesium-containing antacids
	Colchicine
	Proton pump inhibitors
	Theophylline
Tube feedings	
Lactose deficiency (Lactose malabsorption)	
Microscopic colitis (collagenous or lymphocytic)	
Endocrine	Hyperthyroidism
	Adrenal insufficiency
	Systemic mastocytosis
Neoplasms	Colon cancer
	Villous adenoma
Diverticulitis	
Bacterial invasion	Small intestine bacterial overgrowth
	Tuberculosis
	Yersiniosis
Ischemic colitis	
Inflammatory bowel disease	Crohn's disease
Ulcerative colitis	
Radiation colitis	
Celiac disease	
Pancreatic exocrine insufficiency	

Nursing home managers should ensure that standards for infection control are upheld in line with current national guidance. These standards should include ensuring staff have had adequate infection control training and updates, policies for infection control (including management of diarrhea and outbreaks), adequate waste management facilities, and adequate monitoring of unwell residents. Outbreaks should be reported to the local public health authority.

The causes of chronic diarrhea are listed in Table 17–3. Lactose deficiency becomes more common as we age. Celiac disease is common in older persons and is underdiagnosed. Persons with celiac disease may present with iron-deficiency anemia, cognitive problems, ataxia, polyneuropathy, or osteoporosis. Persons with diabetes mellitus or hypothyroidism are at high risk for developing celiac disease. The diagnosis is made by measuring antiendomysial or transglutaminase antibodies.

HEMORRHOIDS

More than half of persons older than 50 years of age have hemorrhoidal symptoms at some time. Hemorrhoids are swollen veins in the submucosal space of the anus or rectum.

Table 17–4.	SURGICAL APPROACHES TO TREATMENT OF HEMORRHOIDS

Office-based procedures
- Rubber band ligation
- Injection of micronized purified flavonoid fraction (phlebotonics)
- Sclerotherapy

Surgical procedures
- Harmonic scalpel
- LigaSure Vessel Sealing System
- Doppler-guided transanal ligation
- Milligan-Morgan open hemorrhoidectomy
- Circular stapled hemorrhoidopexy

They are often itchy or painful, and they may bleed, leaving blood spots on the toilet paper. Besides bleeding, they can also produce mucous discharge or the feeling of failure to completely empty the rectum. Thrombosed external hemorrhoids present as a very painful lump around the anus.

Most hemorrhoids can be managed by simple measures. Altering the diet and increasing fluids will produce a soft bulky stool and decrease straining during defecation. A warm water (40°C) bath (Sitz bath) may relieve symptoms. Classically, Preparation H (a combination of phenylephrine and mineral oil, shark liver oil, and petrolatum), Anusol, and Germaloids decrease itching and protect the inflamed anal mucosa and, by producing vasoconstriction, may decrease bleeding. Either suppositories or creams containing a topical anesthetic, nifedipine, or corticosteroids will relieve acute pain.

A number of surgical procedures are available when the hemorrhoid symptoms become unacceptable or bleeding leads to anemia (Table 17–4).

KEY POINTS

1. Constipation is common in nursing homes and is prevented by increasing fluids, exercise, bulking agents (fiber) if the resident is mobile, and toileting after meals.
2. Osmotic laxatives (sorbitol, lactulose, and polyethylene glycol) are the treatment of choice for constipation. Unresponsive constipation can be treated with lubiprostone. Methylnaltrexone is the treatment of choice for severe opiate constipation. Stool softeners should not be used.
3. Fecal incontinence is very common in nursing home residents. A number of conservative treatment approaches can be successful. Appropriate skin care is important to prevent ulceration.
4. Most hemorrhoids can be treated by producing a soft, bulky stool and by creams with local anesthetics, hydrocortisone, or phenylephrine.

SUGGESTED READINGS

Akhtar AJ. Acute diarrhea in frail elderly nursing home patients. *J Am Med Dir Assoc.* 2003;4:34-39.

Akhtar AJ, Padda M. Fecal incontinence in older patients. *J Am Med Dir Assoc.* 2005;6:54-60.

Akpan A, Gosney MA, Barret J. Factors contributing to fecal incontinence in older people and outcome of routine management in home, hospital and nursing home settings. *Clin Interv Aging.* 2007;2:139-145.

Crogan NL, Evans BC. *Clostridium difficile*: an emerging epidemic in nursing homes. *Geriatr Nurs.* 2007;28:161-164.

Deneve C, Janoir C, Poilane I, et al. New trends in clostridium difficile virulence and pathogenesis. *Int J Antimicrob Agents.* 2009; 33(suppl 1):S24-S28.

Department of Health. *Clostridium difficile* infection: how to deal with the problem. London: Department of Health, December 2008.

Durrant J, Snape J. Urinary incontinence in nursing homes for older people. *Age Ageing.* 2003;32:12-18.

Hyman NH. Anorectal disease: how to relieve pain and improve other symptoms. *Geriatrics.* 1997;52:75-76.

Johanson JF, Irizarry F, Doughty A. Risk factors for fecal incontinence in a nursing home population. *J Clin Gastroenterol.* 1997;24:156-160.

Leung FW, Rao SS. Fecal incontinence in the elderly. *Gastroenterol Clin North Am.* 2009;38:503-511.

NICE. Faecal incontinence: the management of faecal incontinence in adults. NICE Clinical Guideline 49. http://www.nice.org.uk. Accessed April 8, 2013.

Pekmezaris R, Aversa L, WolfKlein G, et al. The cost of chronic constipation. *J Am Med Dir Assoc.* 2002;3:224-228.

Phillips C, Polakoff D, Maue SK, Mauch R. Assessment of constipation management in long-term care patients. *J Am Med Dir Assoc.* 2001; 2:149-154.

Simor AE, Bradley SF, Strausbaugh LJ, et al. SHEA Long-Term-Care Committee. *Clostridium difficile* in long-term-care facilities for the elderly. *Infect Control Hosp Epidemiol.* 2002;23:696-703.

Slotwiner-Nie PK, Brandt LJ. Infectious diarrhea in the elderly. *Gastroenterol Clin North Am.* 2001;30:625-635.

Stahl TJ. Office management of common anorectal problems. *Postgrad Med.* 1992;92:141-146.

Tariq SH. Constipation in long-term care. *J Am Med Dir Assoc.* 2007;8: 209-218.

Tariq SH. Fecal incontinence in older adults. *Clin Geriatr Med.* 2007; 23:857-869.

Volicer L, Lane P, Panke J, Lyman P. Management of constipation in residents with dementia: sorbitol effectiveness and cost. *J Am Med Dir Assoc.* 2005;6(3 suppl):S32-S34.

MULTIPLE CHOICE QUESTIONS

17.1   Which of the following is an osmotic laxative?

    a. Dioctyl sodium
    b. Lactulose
    c. Senna
    d. Bisacodyl
    e. Lubiprostone

17.2   Specific drugs used to treat opioid-induced constipation include:

    a. Lubiprostone and colchicine
    b. Senna and bisacodyl
    c. Lactulose and polyethylene glycol
    d. Alvimopan and methylnaltrexone

17.3   What is the most common cause of fecal incontinence?

a. Constipation
b. Rectal prolapse
c. Spinal stenosis
d. Autonomic neuropathy
e. Surgical procedures of the rectum

17.4   Which of the following is *not* true concerning celiac disease?

a. Can produce iron-deficiency anemia
b. Transglutaminase antibodies is a diagnostic test
c. Is associated with osteoporosis
d. Is more common in persons with diabetes mellitus
e. Is caused by antibiotic therapy

17.5   Which of the following is *not* true concerning *C. difficile* diarrhea?

a. Diagnosis is made by detecting cytotoxin A or D in stool
b. Is associated with antibiotic therapy
c. Can be treated with fidaxomicin
d. Culture of *C. difficile* in stool is less specific than cytotoxin identification
e. Hand washing and environmental cleaning with hypochlorite solutions are key to prevent spread

Chapter 18

MOBILITY AND FALLS PREVENTION

Walking speed and balance in older persons are highly predictive of death. Men 85 years and older with a gait speed of 1.4 m/sec have a 93% 5-year survival rate compared with 49% for those with a speed less than 0.8 m/sec. In women 85 years and older, a gait speed of 0.6 m/sec or greater, the 5-year survival rate is 74% compared with 47% for those less than 0.4 m/sec. Gait speed also predicts cognitive impairment, disability, falls, and institutionalization. Besides age, weight, lower lean body mass, muscle strength, self-reported physical activity, body mass index, chronic diseases (especially cardiovascular disease), stride length, and inflammatory markers are predictors of gait speed. As shown in Figure 18–1, new robotic walking aides are being developed to help keep people mobile.

GAIT DISTURBANCES

Gait disturbances are common in nursing home residents (Table 18–1). In residents, there is often more than one cause of the gait disturbance. Features of a normal gait are the outside of the heel strikes ground first, during gait a space is present between both legs from a side view, knees are flexed, arms swing, and feet are 2 to 4 inches apart.

When there is a decline in executive function, persons find it difficult to walk and talk at the same time. This is called "dual tasking." An inability to "dual task" leads to increased falls and is common in persons with dementia. It can be detected by asking the person a simple question while walking such as "What is the capital of the United States?" Besides persons with dementia, dual tasking is a particular problem in those with Parkinson's disease. A physical therapist can enhance a person's ability to dual task by having him or her count backwards while walking.

FALLS

One in six nursing home residents fall each year, and those who fall tend to fall frequently. Thus, there are roughly 1.7 falls per nursing home bed per year. Falls lead to hip fractures, head trauma, lacerations, fractures, and soft tissue injuries. In the United States, falls account for two thirds of nursing home liability cases. It is important to recognize that falls are inevitable, so the goals in a nursing home are to decrease the number of falls and prevent injuries when possible. Fear of falling leads to social isolation, depression, and increased disability because the resident decreases his or her walking. Falls can be either extrinsic or intrinsic (Table 18–2).

When a resident has a new-onset fall, it should be considered to be caused by delirium until proven otherwise. Persons with dementia are twice as likely to fall compared with similar aged persons who are cognitively intact. This is caused by disturbances of gait and balance, greater step to step variability, and an inability to "dual task." Numerous medications lead to increased falls (Table 18–3). Selective serotonin reuptake inhibitors are more likely to cause falls than are tricyclic antidepressants. Dopamine agonists used for restless legs syndrome are an important cause of falls.

Persons with diabetes mellitus are at an increased risk of falls because of peripheral neuropathy, the possibility of hypoglycemia, and executive function problems. Fall risk is increased regardless of frailty status if HbA_1C is below 7%. Residents on kidney dialysis are at high risk of falls, and a fall markedly increases their risk of death.

The relative risk for falls in persons with lower extremity weakness is between 2.4 and 8.4. Resistance exercise and balance training represent a major approach to preventing falls. Tai chi decreases falls because it increases balance. Poor vision is an important cause of falls. Persons with bifocal glasses are at particular risk of falling.

There are a number of causes of syncope or presyncope in older persons. Older persons have amnesia for syncopal events. The major causes of syncope are given in Table 18–4. Approximately 30% of the time, syncope is caused by carotid sinus hypersensitivity. There are two types of carotid sinus hypersensitivity, namely cardioinhibitory (asystole >3 sec) and vasodepressor (>50 mm Hg fall in blood pressure) during carotid sinus massage. The cardioinhibitory form is treated with pacemaker insertion. Orthostasis is present in up to 25% of all nursing

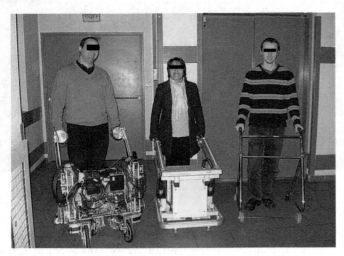

Figure 18–1. Three generations of walkers.

home residents; thus, standing blood pressure needs to be obtained in all residents. In persons who fall, the possibility of postprandial hypotension should be considered. Seizures, especially petit mal and partial complex seizures, should be always considered as a cause of falling.

A number of scales to identify fallers have been developed. Although these scales identify those at risk of falling, they do not appear to reduce falls. The Mini Falls Assessment has been developed to pinpoint areas in the individual that increase their risk of falling and are treatable (Table 18–5).

Falls onto wooden or carpeted surfaces have been shown to result in the least fractures per 100 falls in residential facilities. This has led to a search to find the ideal compliant (low stiffness) flooring that is cost effective and does not alter balance. A variety of foam floors that attenuate force by 15% to 50% are commercially available. Clinical

Table 18–1.	GAIT DISTURBANCES IN OLDER PERSONS	
Type	**Description**	**Cause**
Retropulsion	Leans backward as walks	Aging
Dementia gait		
Mild	Cautious gait	Loss of executive function
Severe	Short steps, dysequilibrium, shuffling, and apraxia of starting and turning	Frontal lobe damage
Ataxic	Wide based; cannot do tandem walk	Cerebellar
Spastic		
Hemiparetic	Stiff leg that swings in hemicircle while walking with toe hitting floor before heel	Stroke
Paraparetic	Stiff legs, waddling with scissors gait	Spinal cord lesion
Steppage	Marked hip flexion on side of gait	Foot drop
Antalgic	Limping	Pain
Hypokinetic	Difficulty in initiation with shuffling and limited arm swing	Parkinson's disease
Dyskinetic	Involuntary movements during walking	Chorea
Circumduction	Lumbar lordosis, waddling, and cannot climb stairs	Proximal muscle weakness
Sensory deficit	Broad based with short steps	Peripheral neuropathy
Anxiety or psychogenic	Hesitant, which improves with distraction or unusual patterns	Psychological states
Stenotic gait	Pain with walking; walks with flexed position; easier to walk uphill; pain improves with sitting	Lumbar spinal stenosis
Claudication	Increasing pain with walking; slow gait	Peripheral vascular disease
Arthritic	Decreased gait speed, less knee movement, increased hip movement, loss of knee locking	Osteoarthritis
Vestibular	Unsteady gait worse on unsteady surface or in the dark with movement of visual image while walking	Vestibulopathy
Hydrocephalic	Small-stepped, shuffling gait with normal arm swing	Normal-pressure hydrocephalus

Table 18–2.	OVERVIEW OF THE MAJOR CAUSES OF FALLS IN NURSING HOMES
Extrinsic	Uneven surfaces
	Poor lighting
	Clutter
	No grab bars in the toilet
	Poor contrast with steps
Intrinsic	Delirium
	Dementia
	Medications
	Lower extremity weakness (sarcopenia or dynapenia)
	Poor balance
	Poor vision
	Gait problems
	Depression
	Orthostasis
	Postprandial hypotension
	Loss of consciousness

	• Syncope
	  ▪ Carotid sinus hypersensitivity
	  ▪ Arrhythmias
	• Stroke (transient ischemia attack)
	• Seizures
	  ▪ Grand mal
	  ▪ Petit mal
	  ▪ Partial complex seizures

trials are needed to confirm that these floors reduce fractures and are cost effective.

An approach to fall prevention is given in Chapter 5. Table 18–6 provides a list of the treatments that have been proven to be effective for reducing falls.

Table 18–3.	MEDICATIONS ASSOCIATED WITH INCREASED FALLS

Psychotropic medications
- Neuroleptics
- Sedative hypnotics
- Benzodiazepines
- Any antidepressant

Anticonvulsants

Nonsteroidal antiinflammatory drugs

Propoxyphene

Dopamine agonists

Diuretics

Antihypertensives

Hypoglycemia agents

Nitrates

Antiarrhythmias

Table 18–4.	CAUSES OF SYNCOPE

Vasovagal

Carotid sinus hypersensitivity

Cardiac arrhythmia

Dehydration

Anemia

Vasodilation

Autonomic dysfunction

Drug induced

Orthostasis

Postprandial hypotension

HIP FRACTURES

In Japan, the incidence of hip fractures in nursing home residents is 1.5% per year for women and 1.0% for men. In Germany, the rates are higher at 5.1% for women and 3.3% for men. In Washington State, the overall incidence of hip fracture is 2.3%. Residents with a previous fracture have twice the risk of a subsequent fracture over the next 2 years. The 1-year mortality rate after a hip fracture is about 30% with men being more likely to die than women. Vertebral fractures are present in more than one third of nursing home residents. Pressure ulcers occur in up to one third of hip fracture patients. Most of these pressure ulcers develop while the person is in the hospital, not during the nursing home stay.

A study in 256 Bavarian nursing homes involving 13,653 residents as the intervention group and 893 nursing homes with 31,668 residents as the control groups showed that a fall prevention program could reduce femoral fractures. The intervention program is outlined in Table 18–7. This program produced an adjusted relative risk of 0.82 in the intervention group.

A study in Australia on older persons with hip fracture showed that twice-a-week resistance training, a geriatric assessment, and vitamin D resulted in a decrease in mortality rate, hospitalization, and nursing home stay. A somewhat less aggressive program in the United States had minimal benefits.

Hip protectors, when good compliance with their use is obtained, can decrease hip fractures. It is now recognized that not all hip protectors are constructed adequately to provide protection. When an individual has fallen on the hip protector, the seal is broken, and it is no longer effective. After being washed, hip protectors need three cycles through the dryer to remove all water or they are no longer protective.

Calcium and vitamin D have been shown to reduce hip fracture in nursing homes. The average resident needs 1000 mg of calcium a day and ingests in meals about 600 mg of calcium (slightly less in Southeast Asian countries). Calcium can be increased by adding yogurt or milk to the diet. Calcium interferes with the absorption of most medications and as such cannot be given

Table 18–5.   MINI FALLS ASSESSMENT

Name	Sex	Age	Place of Residence	
			No	Yes
1. Fewer than seven medicines			0	1
2. **Not receiving:**				
Antipsychotics *or*			0	1
Antidepressives *or*			0	1
Benzodiazepines			0	1
3. Receiving vitamin D or 25(OH) vitamin D level > 25 ng/mL			0	1
4. Systolic blood pressure >130 mm Hg			0	1
5. **No standing blood pressure drop:**				
On standing <10 mm Hg			0	1
At 3 min <20 mm Hg			0	1
6. Sitting with buttocks behind trunk			0	1
7. **Able to rise from chair:**				
With assistance			0	1
Without assistance			0	1
8. **Balance:**				
Center of balance not backward			0	1
Stand with eyes shut			0	1
Stand on one leg			0	1
Obvious body sway standing still			0	1
9. **Gait:**				
Lifts foot off ground			0	1
Space between feet			0	1
No knee flexion			0	1
Heel strike			0	1
Step over keys			0	1
Turns without loss of balance			0	1
Does not stop when asked capital of country			0	1
10. No fear of falling			0	1
11. No foot deformity			0	1
12. No cataracts or bifocals			0	1
13. Not fatigued			0	1
14. Can walk one block			0	1
15. Can climb one flight of stairs			0	1
16. Not lost >5% of weight in 6 months			0	1
17. No fall in last 6 months			0	1

Table 18–6.   EFFECTIVE TREATMENT APPROACHES FOR FALLS

- Multidisciplinary, multifactorial programs
- Muscle strengthening and balancing exercises
- Environmental hazard modification
- Withdrawal of psychotropic medications
- Tai chi exercise intervention
- Cardiac pacing for falls with cardioinhibitory carotid sinus hypersensitivity

Table 18–7.   COMPONENTS OF THE BAVARIAN NURSING HOME INTERVENTION PROGRAM TO REDUCE HIP FRACTURES

- Education of fall and fracture prevention strategies
- Progressive strength and balance training
- Advice on environmental adaptations with a focus on fitting the environment to the resident
- Education on hip protectors

Table 18–8. DRUGS USED TO TREAT OSTEOPOROSIS

Class	Drug	Comments
Bisphosphonates (Inhibits osteoclasts)	Alendronate	Take weekly; generic and cheap
	Ibandronate	Take monthly; relatively cheap
	Risedronate	Take weekly; expensive
	Zoledronic acid	Yearly intravenous infusion; expensive
RANK ligand antagonists (inhibits osteoclast)	Denosumab	Take as injection every 6 months; very expensive; can cause severe infections and possibly cancer
PTH (enhances osteoblast activity)	Teriparatide	Daily injections; extremely expensive
Anabolic (enhances osteoblast activity)	Testosterone	Injections every 2 weeks, gel, or oral

Cheap to expensive |
| Inhibits sclerostin (enhances osteoblast activity) | Sclerostin antibody | Under development |
| Calcitonin | Calcitonin | Less effective than bisphosphonates; useful for vertebral fracture pain |

PTH, parathyroid hormone; RANK, receptor activator of nuclear factor kappa-B.

with other drugs. We suggest that calcium is given at bedtime because the nighttime is when most calcium comes out of bones, and calcium at bedtime will reduce this. Vitamin D should be given at approximately 1000 IU/day. There is no clear indication to measure 25(OH) vitamin D levels, and if this is done, it is most probably not cost effective.

Approximately 80% of women and 60% of men in nursing homes in the United States have osteoporosis. The use of oral bisphosphonates in institutionalized individuals with osteoporosis was shown to reduce hip fracture and all-cause mortality rate. Table 18–8 provides the different drugs available for the treatment of osteoporosis. Oral bisphosphonates or intravenous zoledronic acid appear to be the drugs of choice. Zoledronic acid can be given in hospital before discharge in persons with hip fracture and can then be given yearly. Oral bisphosphonates need to be given with the resident fasting and standing or sitting up for half an hour after administration. Long-term use of bisphosphonates may lead to atypical fractures, so some do not use them after 5 years.

KEY POINTS

1. Slow walking is associated with an increased mortality rate.
2. Gait disorders need to be recognized and treated.
3. "Dual tasking" deficits and retropulsion need to be treated to reduce falls.
4. All fallers should have a pharmacy consult to reduce fall associated medications and a physical therapy consult for resistance and balance exercises.
5. Carotid sinus hypersensitivity, orthostasis, and postprandial hypotension cause syncope.
6. An interdisciplinary falls prevention program reduces falls.
7. Hip fractures can be reduced with an educational intervention.
8. After a hip fracture, a geriatric assessment coupled with vitamin D and resistance exercise improves outcomes.
9. All persons with osteoporosis should receive calcium, vitamin D, and bisphosphonates.
10. Calcium cannot be given with other medications.

SUGGESTED READINGS

Allali G, Assal F, Kressig RW, et al. Impact of impaired executive function on gait stability. *Dement Geriatr Cogn Disord.* 2008;26:364-369.

Axer H, Axer M, Sauer H, et al. Falls and gait disorders in geriatric neurology. *Clin Neurol Neurosurg.* 2010;112:265-274.

Becker C, Rapp K. Fall prevention in nursing homes. *Clin Geriatr Med.* 2010;26:693-704.

Cameron ID, Murray GR, Gillespie LD, et al. Interventions for preventing falls in older people in nursing care facilities and hospitals. *Cochrane Database Syst Rev.* 2010;(1):CD005465.

Choi M, Hector M. Effectiveness of intervention programs in preventing falls: a systematic review of recent 10 years and meta-analysis. *J Am Med Dir Assoc.* 2012;13:188.e13-21.

Cronin H, Kenny RA. Cardiac causes for falls and their treatment. *Clin Geriatr Med.* 2010;26:539-567.

Edwards BJ, Perry HM III, Kaiser FE, et al. Relationship of age and calcitonin gene-related peptide to postprandial hypotension. *Mech Ageing Dev.* 1996;87:61-73.

Gunby MC, Morley JE. Epidemiology of bone loss with aging. *Clin Geriatr Med.* 1994;10:557-574.

Hampton JL, Brayne C, Bradley M, Kenny RA. Mortality in carotid sinus hypersensitivity: a cohort study. *BMJ Open.* 2011;1(1):e000020.

Hommel E, Ghazi A, White H. Minimal trauma fractures: lifting the specter of misconduct by identifying risk factors and planning for prevention. *J Am Med Dir Assoc.* 2012;13:180-186.

Ijmker T, Lamoth CJ. Gait and cognition: the relationship between gait stability and variability with executive function in persons with and without dementia. *Gait Posture.* 2012;35:126-130.

Kamel HK, Hussain MS, Tariq S, et al. Failure to diagnose and treat osteoporosis in elderly patients hospitalized with hip fracture. *Am J Med.* 2000;109:326-328.

Kerr SR, Pearce MS, Brayne C, et al. Carotid sinus hypersensitivity in asymptomatic older persons: implications for diagnosis of syncope and falls. *Arch Intern Med.* 2006;166:515-520.

Lam R. Office management of gait disorders in the elderly. *Can Fam Physician.* 2011;57:765-770.

Messinger-Rapport BJ, Morley JE, Thomas DR, Gammack JK. Intensive session: new approaches to medical issues in long-term care. *J Am Med Dir Assoc.* 2007;8:421-433.

Messinger-Rapport BJ, Thomas DR, Gammack JK, Morley JE. Clinical update on nursing home medicine: 2009. *J Am Med Dir Assoc*. 2009;10:530-553.

Miller DK, Lui LY, Perry HM III, et al. Reported and measured physical functioning in older inner-city diabetic African Americans. *J Gerontol A Biol Sci Med Sci*. 1999;54:M230-M236.

Miller DK, Morrison MJ, Blair SD, et al. Predilection for frailty remedial strategies among black and white seniors. *South Med J*. 1998;91:375-380.

Morley JE. A fall is a major event in the life of an older person. *J Gerontol A Biol Sci Med Sci*. 2002;57:M492-M495.

Morley JE. An overview of diabetes mellitus in older persons. *Clin Geriatr Med*. 1999;15:211-224.

Morley JE. Clinical practice in nursing homes as a key for progress. *J Nutr Health Aging*. 2010;14:586-593.

Morley JE. Falls and fractures. *J Am Med Dir Assoc*. 2007;8:276-278.

Morley JE. Falls—where do we stand? *Mo Med*. 2007;104:63-67.

Morley JE. Hip fractures. *J Am Med Dir Assoc*. 2010;11:81-83.

Morley JE. Hot topics in geriatrics. *J Am Med Dir Assoc*. 2008;9:613-616.

Morley JE. Osteoporosis and fragility fractures. *J Am Med Dir Assoc*. 2011;12:389-392.

Morley JE. Should all long-term care residents receive vitamin D? *J Am Med Dir Assoc*. 2007;8:69-70.

Morley JE. The elderly type 2 diabetic patients: special considerations. *Diabet Med*. 1998;15(suppl 4):S41-S46.

Morley JE, Rolland Y, Tolson D, Vellas B. Increasing awareness of the factors producing falls: the mini falls assessment. *J Am Med Dir Assoc*. 2012;13:87-90.

Morley JE, Silver AJ. Nutritional issues in nursing home care. *Ann Intern Med*. 1995;123:850-859.

O'Dwyer C, Bennett K, Langan Y, et al. Amnesia for loss of consciousness is common in vasovagal syncope. *Europace*. 2011;13:1040-1045.

Quigley P, Bulat T, Kurtzman E, et al. Fall prevention and injury protection for nursing home residents. *J Am Med Dir Assoc*. 2010;11:284-293.

Roush K. Prevention and treatment of osteoporosis in postmenopausal women: a review. *Am J Nurs*. 2011;111:26-35.

Sanders AB, Morley JE. The older person and the emergency department. *J Am Geriatr Soc*. 1993;41:880-882.

Scherder E, Eggermont L, Swaab D, et al. Gait in ageing and associated dementias: its relationship with cognition. *Neurosci Biobehav Rev*. 2007;31:485-497.

Studenski S, Perera S, Patel K, et al. Gait speed and survival in older adults. *JAMA*. 2011;305:50-58.

Task Force for the Diagnosis and Management of Syncope; European Society of Cardiology (ESC); European Heart Rhythm Association (EHRA); Heart Failure Association (HFA); Heart Rhythm Society (HRS), et al. Guidelines for the diagnosis and management of syncope (version 2009). *Eur Heart J*. 2009;30:2631-2671.

Thynne K. Normal pressure hydrocephalus. *J Neurosci Nurs*. 2007;39:27-32.

Villars H, Oustric S, Andrieu S, et al. The primary care physician and Alzheimer's disease: an international position paper. *J Nutr Health Aging*. 2010;14:110-120.

Von Haehling S, Morley JE, Anker SD. An overview of sarcopenia: facts and numbers on prevalence and clinical impact. *J Cachexia Sarcopenia Muscle*. 2010;1:129-133.

MULTIPLE CHOICE QUESTIONS

18.1   Which of the following is true of normal gait?

a. Inside of the heel strikes the ground first
b. Outside of the heel strikes the ground first
c. Forefoot strikes the ground first
d. Knees do not flex

18.2   An 83-year-old man walks with a flexed position and finds it easier to walk up hill, and his pain improves with sitting. What kind of gait does he have?

a. Retropulsive
b. Antalgic
c. Claudication
d. Sensory deficit
e. Stenotic gait

18.3   The average number of falls per nursing home bed each year is:

a. 0.6 to 1
b. 1.1 to 1.5
c. 1.6 to 2
d. 2 to 2.5
e. 2.6 to 3.0

18.4   Which of the following statements regarding falls is true?

a. Delirium is an unusual cause of new onset falls.
b. Persons with dementia are twice as likely to fall.
c. SSRIs rarely cause falls.
d. Falls in nursing home are virtually never from extrinsic causes.
e. Dopamine agonists used to treat restless legs do not cause falls.

18.5   Which of the following do/does *not* protect against hip fracture?

a. Calcium and vitamin D
b. Hip protectors
c. Calcitonin
d. Bisphosphonates
e. Resistance exercises

Chapter 19

SLEEP DISTURBANCE

Individuals vary greatly in their apparent need for sleep, and the length of time people believe they need to sleep alters over their life course. Feelings of being able to function efficiently and a person's sense of vitality and well-being are influenced by their perceptions of taking adequate sleep and rest. Over time a number of theories have emerged to explain the function of sleep in humans; in simple terms, sleep can be understood in terms of an activity implicated in brain health. Sleep is a surprisingly complex phenomenon involving four stages and different states that make up the sleep cycle. Studies of adults have shown that on average, people experience between four and six sleep cycles in which they move between different stages and states of sleep each night. The sleep–wake activity pattern of an individual is a circadian rhythm (around a day), and there is much to learn about how it is affected by the aging process and changes in later life in response to fluctuations in core body temperature. Such changes may explain daytime napping and disordered sleep patterns. Inadequate levels of sleep—and in the extreme, sleep deprivation—affect functional performance, mood, and well-being. There are many health, emotional, age-related, and environmental factors that increase the likelihood of sleep disturbance in older nursing home residents. For example, auditory threshold awakening changes so that older people are more easily awoken by noise. This often surprises staff who assume that because so many residents have age-related hearing loss that they are less likely to be disturbed by nighttime noise.

Sleeplessness and behavioral disturbances at night are a common reason for older persons to be institutionalized. On average, nursing home residents spend 6.2 hours asleep when in bed at night and 2.1 hours awake. Most nursing home residents sleep for short periods of time (about 22 minutes) and then awaken and go back to sleep. Persons with mild to moderate dementia are awake more often than other residents, but persons with severe dementia tend to sleep for longer periods. These awakenings lead to more stage 1 and 2 sleep and less rapid eye movement (REM) and slow-wave sleep.

INSOMNIA

A nursing home study in Canada found that 6.2% met the *Diagnostic and Statistical Manual of Mental Disorders,* edition IV, criteria for insomnia disorder and 17% had one or more symptoms of insomnia. Both disruptive behavior and psychological distress were strongly associated with insomnia disorder. In Norwegian nursing homes, residents spend more than 13 hours in bed with lying awake 1 hour before falling asleep and being awake for at least 2 hours during the night. In German nursing homes, 37.3% of residents had insomnia and 30% nonrestful sleep. In Egyptian geriatric homes, 65% of residents had trouble falling asleep and more than 50% could not maintain their sleep or had nonrestful sleep. In Japanese residents institutionalized in a geriatric hospital, insomnia and delay of onset of sleep were associated with an increased death rate. In the United States, one large study based on the Minimum Data Set reported that insomnia occurred relatively rarely with severe insomnia (6 or more nights a week) at 0.8% and moderate insomnia (1 to 5 times a week) at 5.5%. In this study, insomnia was associated with increased hip fracture. Another study in the United States showed that 29% of residents had a least one awakening in the previous week.

There are numerous reasons for sleep disturbances in nursing homes (Table 19–1). Noise and switching on of lights account for about half of the sleep disturbances. Care, such as regularly turning of patients confined to their beds, or toileting incontinent patients, is also disruptive. This occurs regardless of whether the resident is asleep, and caregivers tend to switch on the lights and talk to one another during care. A study in Germany showed that nighttime surveillance by nurses and nurse assistants decreases the sleep quality in nursing home residents. Care plans need to be developed to recognize the need for reduced nighttime interventions, and nursing assistants should be educated about the reasons. Lack of bright light during the day in nursing homes disrupts sleep rhythms. Daytime napping is common and may further lead to disruption of nighttime sleep.

A number of diseases (Table 19–2) and medications (Table 19–3) can cause or aggravate insomnia.

Management of insomnia requires a sleep hygiene program (Table 19–4). Decreasing nighttime noise and sleep disruptive nursing care associated with increased physical activity has been shown to be effective. High-lux light (2000 lux) for at least 4 hours in the morning improves circadian rhythm and sleep. Keeping residents out of bed as much as possible during the day and allowing

Table 19–1.	NIGHTTIME BEHAVIORAL DISTURBANCES IN NURSING HOMES

- Getting up at night
- Waking early in morning
- Talking or yelling at night
- Wandering or pacing

them to go to bed later are key issues. A glass of warm milk before going to bed represents a proven method for decreasing sleep latency. Cognitive behavioral programs can improve sleep in the nursing home but are difficult to implement.

In nursing homes, benzodiazepines and sedative–hypnotics are commonly used, often in place of attempts at improving sleep hygiene (Figure 19–1). A meta-analysis has questioned the efficacy of the long-term sleep-promoting effects of sedative–hypnotics. A recent study has found that both benzodiazepine and sedative–hypnotic use are associated with increased mortality rates. These drugs are also commonly associated with falls. Table 19–5 provides a comparison of different drugs used to improve sleep. When used, these drugs should be given only after the resident has demonstrated an inability to fall asleep. Rarely should they be used chronically.

NOCTURIA

Nocturia is the need to wake up to void on at least one occasion at night. In octogenarians, 90% of men and 70% of women have nocturia. In nursing home residents, half of urine volume is passed at night compared with less than 15% in 20-year-old adults. Nocturia is one of the most common reasons for poor sleep, leading to daytime fatigue, poor concentrating ability, cognitive impairment,

Table 19–2.	CONDITIONS ASSOCIATED WITH INSOMNIA

Dyspnea
- Asthma
- Orthopnea and paroxysmal nocturnal dyspnea (heart failure)
- Emphysema

Pain

Sleep apnea

Restless legs syndrome

Periodic limb disorder

Depression

Itching

Hyperthyroidism

Urinary incontinence

Gastric acid reflux during sleep

Parkinson's disease

Table 19–3.	MEDICATIONS ASSOCIATED WITH INSOMNIA

Donepezil

Diuretics

Selective serotonin reuptake inhibitors

Steroids (given after noon)

Theophylline

β-Agonists

Pseudoephedrine

Histamine (H_2) receptor antagonists

Caffeine

dysphoria, and falls. Persons with nocturia have poor health and have greater risk of death.

Numerous physiologic changes with aging increase the propensity for older persons to have nocturia. Loss of the increase in plasma arginine vasopressin (AVP) at night leads to nocturia. Atrial natriuretic hormone (ANH) levels are five times higher in nursing home residents than in young persons. Elevated ANH levels antagonize AVP action and decrease aldosterone secretion, leading to an increase in salt and fluid. Whether these changes in ANH increase nocturia is controversial. Bladder capacity declines with aging, and increased detrusor overactivity and lower urinary tract symptomatology increase the need to void at night.

The major causes of nocturia are increased urine flow at night, polyuria, bladder storage problems, and primary sleep disorders (Table 19–6).

Table 19–4.	SLEEP HYGIENE TECHNIQUES IN NURSING HOMES

- Increase daytime social activity.
- Increase exposure to sunlight or high lux (2000-lux) light.
- Limit daytime napping in the afternoon and evening.
- Limit time in bed.
- Limit nighttime noise.
- Keep bedrooms as dark as possible.
- Limit nursing interventions at night.
- Have residents participate in physical activity during the day.
- Avoid caffeine at night.
- Put residents with similar sleeping patterns together (e.g., do not put a resident who watches television all night in the same room as one who does not).
- Establish a sleep routine.
- Minimize nocturia.
- Try a small glass of hot milk at sleep time.
- Create regular routines for going to sleep and waking up, observing residents' preferences.
- Keep a record of bed and awakening times.

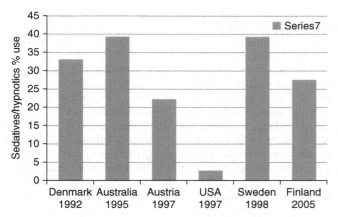

Figure 19–1. Variability of sedative–hypnotic use in different parts of the world.

Assessment of nocturia requires the utilization of a fluid intake and urinary output chart. This time chart should provide volumes whenever possible. Postvoid bladder volume needs to be assessed ideally by a bladder scan but in most places realistically by catheterization after voiding. A full history and examination may point to one of the causes identified in Table 19–6.

Simple lifestyle factors such as no longer taking fluid, alcohol, or caffeine for at least 2 hours before going to bed can improve sleep. Persons with edema should be encouraged to wear compression stockings, elevate their legs for 1 to 2 hours before going to bed, and take an afternoon nap. A diuretic taken 6 to 8 hours before sleep may reduce edema, leading to reduced nocturnal fluid volume. Serum sodium, creatinine, and blood urea nitrogen and

orthostasis need to be assessed regularly to avoid dehydration. The treatment may be limited to a few days a week if necessary. In persons with insomnia, a hypnotic agent not only may improve sleep but also reduces nighttime urine volume. In persons with urge incontinence, taking a short-acting anticholinergic drug will increase nighttime functional bladder capacity. Treatment of lower urinary tract symptomatology will decrease nocturia in some individuals. Intermittent catheterization before bed will help some individuals with increased postvoid residuals.

Low-dose desmopressin (0.1 mg) before sleep has been shown to decrease nocturia in a variety of patients, including those with prostatic hypertrophy. Desmopressin leads to a reduction in serum sodium, and long-term treatment can lead to hyponatremia. Residents taking desmopressin should have their serum sodium measure at 1 week and monthly while taking desmopressin.

SLEEP APNEA

In nursing homes, 43% of residents have at least five apneas per hour of sleep. Central sleep apnea was nearly twice as common as obstructive sleep apnea (OSA), which is the opposite of older persons in the community, in whom 80% have OSA. Sleep apnea in women, but not men, in nursing homes results in a higher mortality rate. In contrast to this formal study, sleep apnea in nursing home residents is diagnosed in fewer than 1%, suggesting marked underreporting of sleep apnea. Sleep apnea is most often diagnosed by the sleep partner complaining of excessive snoring or noticing apneic episodes. Because there is no bed partner in nursing homes, nurses and nurse aides need to be educated to recognize these signs and report them to the physician (Table 19–7).

Table 19–5. COMPARISON OF DRUGS USED TO TREAT INSOMNIA					
Class	Drug Name	Dose (mg)	Sleep Onset (min)	Increased Duration (min)	Recommendations
Benzodiazepams	Temazepam	15	15–30	60	Occasional use
	Triazolam	0.125–0.25	15–30	60	
Nonbenzodiazepine hypnotics (Z-drugs)	Zaleplon	16–20	20	60	Possibly safer and more efficacious long term
	Zolpidem	5–10	30–120	60	
	Zopiclone	7.5	60	60	
	Eszopiclone	1–2	25	60	
Antidepressants	Trazodone	50–150	?	?	Use only in depressed
Melatonin	Melatonin	1–3	120	5	Safe; limited effectiveness
	Ramelteon	4–8	30–60	11–14	
Antihistamines	Diphenhydramine	25–50	15–80	60–120	Do not use
Other	Chloral hydrate	500–2000	20–60	120	Do not use

Table 19–6. CAUSES OF NOCTURIA
Primary nocturia (increased urine flow at night)
• Loss of arginine vasopressin circadian rhythm
• Multisystem atrophy ($\downarrow$AVP)
• Alzheimer's disease ($\downarrow$AVP)
• Sleep apnea ($\uparrow$ANH at night)
• Edema ($\uparrow$fluid reabsorbed in recumbent position)
• Diuretics in evening
Polyuria
• Diabetes mellitus
• Hypercalcemia
• Diabetes insipidus
• Psychogenic polyuria
• Renal failure
• Lithium
Bladder storage problems
• Urge incontinence (detrusor overactivity)
• Lower urinary tract symptomatology
• Increased post void residual (e.g., prostate hypertrophy)
• Irradiation
• Pelvic surgery
• Constipation
• Cholinesterase inhibitors taken at night
• Anticholinergic drugs decreasing bladder capacity
Primary sleep problems
• Voiding of small volumes because awake

ANH, atrial natriuretic hormone; AVP, arginine vasopressin.

Sleep apnea is a condition in which the person stops breathing (apnea) or markedly decreases the breathing rate (hypopnea). Sleep apnea leads to excessive daytime sleepiness. It also causes nighttime sweating, morning headaches, and water retention. Sleep apnea is more common in persons with the ApoE4 Alzheimer's disease genotype. Persons with sleep apnea have an increased likelihood of having hypertension, heart disease, arrhythmias, stroke, diabetes mellitus, and executive function decline. Some improvement in these is seen with treatment of sleep apnea.

Table 19–7. SCREEN FOR NURSES AND NURSING ASSISTANTS TO REFER RESIDENT FOR TESTING FOR SLEEP APNEA
Check five times at night 1 hour apart:
• Resident snores: 1 point
• Abnormal breathing pattern: 1 point
• Resident has apneic episode: 2 point
• 2 or more points: Refer for testing

The diagnosis is made in a sleep laboratory using polysomnography, but nocturnal pulse oximetry, actigraphy, or transcutaneous capnography may be sufficient for most nursing home residents.

Continuous positive airway pressure (CPAP) is the treatment of choice. However, many persons struggle to use the face mask and refuse to use it. Older persons in nursing homes often have better outcomes if low-level CPAP settings are used. If a CPAP machine(s) is to be used in the nursing home, a respiratory or physical therapist needs to educate a small group of nurses in the appropriate use of the machine and how to encourage compliance. Nurses in the nursing home need special training in how to improve the acceptability of CPAP. Other treatments for OSA include dental appliances and surgery.

RESTLESS LEGS SYNDROME

Restless legs syndrome (RLS) is an urge to move one's legs in response to an uncomfortable sensation occurring mainly at night and resulting in poor sleep and increased daytime sleepiness. RLS is common in Lewy-Body dementia and persons with Parkinson's dementia. Periodic limb movement disorder is abnormal jerking or kicking of legs during sleep. These conditions are present in nearly one in five persons older than 80 years of age. The treatment of choice is the dopamine agonist ropinirole (0.25–4 mg). Its major side effects are orthostatic hypotension, headache, and fatigue. Benzodiazepines may also be helpful but have more side effects. In residents with low ferritin levels, intravenous iron may improve RLS.

PARASOMNIAS

Rapid eye movement sleep behavior disorder occurs in about 0.5% of persons older than 70 years of age. It is much more common in men. An increased prevalence is seen in persons with Parkinson's disease, Lewy body dementia, multiple system atrophy, and focal strokes. The symptoms of this disorder include shouting, singing, attempting to hit or strangle others, and jumping from bed. It appears that these patients are acting out their dreams during REM sleep. Clonazepam and melatonin have been the primary drugs used in these residents.

Tooth grinding (bruxism) is a common behavior that may lead to damage of teeth. A dental guard may be helpful.

Other parasomnias include hypnogogic hallucinations, nocturnal seizures, disorders of arousal (sleep walking), rhythmic movement disorder, and sleep onset paralysis.

NIGHTMARES

Nightmares occur in older persons at a rate of one in five compared with younger persons. Nightmares are particularly common in persons with post traumatic disorders such as Holocaust survivors. Cholinesterase inhibitors given to patients with Alzheimer's disease increase REM sleep and nightmares. Memantine also is associated with nightmares. Nightmares are not rare in persons with Parkinson's disease.

KEY POINTS

1. Nursing home residents spend at least a quarter of their time in bed awake.
2. Awakenings result in decreased slow-wave and REM sleep.
3. Insomnia is a major problem in nursing homes.
4. Nighttime surveillance by nursing staff decreases sleep quality of nursing home residents.
5. Donepezil and numerous other drugs cause insomnia.
6. Nurses need to be educated to implement sleep hygiene techniques in nursing homes.
7. The efficacy of sedative–hypnotic drugs for long-term use in nursing homes is questionable.
8. Nocturia is a major disrupter of sleep in nursing homes.
9. Sleep apnea is underdiagnosed in nursing homes.
10. A simple nursing screening test can be used to detect sleep apnea.
11. CPAP is underused in nursing homes.
12. RLS results in poor sleep and daytime sleepiness.

SUGGESTED READINGS

Aidabal L, BaHammam AS. Cheyne-Stokes respiration in patients with heart failure. *Lung.* 2010;188:5-14.

Altena E, Ramautar JR, Van Der Werg YD, Van Someren EJ. Do sleep complaints contribute to age-related cognitive decline? *Prog Brain Res.* 2010;185:181-205.

Bliwise DL, Carroll JS, Lee KA, et al. Sleep and "sundowning" in nursing home patients with dementia. *Psychiatry Res.* 1993;48:277-292.

Crowley K. Sleep and sleep disorders in older adults. *Neuropsychol Rev.* 2011;21:41-53.

Eyers I, Young E, Luff R, Arber S. Stroking the balance: night care versus facilitation of good sleep. *Br J Nurs.* 2012;21:303-307.

Gehrman PR, Martin JL, Shochat T, et al. Sleep-disordered breathing and agitation in institutionalized adults with Alzheimer disease. *Am J Geriatr Psychiatry.* 2003;11:426-433.

Koch S, Haesler E, Tiziani A, Wilson J. Effectiveness of sleep management strategies for residents of aged care facilities: findings of a systematic review. *J Clin Nurs.* 2006;15:1267-1275.

Martin JL, Ancoli-Israel S. Sleep disturbances in long-term care. *Clin Geriatr Med.* 2008;24:39-50.

Martin JL, Mory AK, Alessi CA. Nighttime oxygen desaturation and symptoms of sleep-disordered breathing in long-stay nursing home residents. *J Gerontol A Biol Sci Med Sci.* 2005;60:104-108.

McCurry SM, La Faza DM, Pike KD, et al. Managing sleep disturbances in adults family homes: recruitment and implementation of a behavioral treatment program. *Geriatr Nurs.* 2009;20:36-44.

Neikrug AB, Ancoli-Israel S. Sleep disturbances in nursing homes. *J Nutr Health Aging.* 2010;14:207-211.

Neikrug AB, Ancoli-Israel S. Sleep disorders in the older adults—a mini-review. *Gerontology.* 2010;56:181-189.

Norman D, Loredo JS. Obstructive sleep apnea in older adults. *Clin Geriatr Med.* 2008;24:151-165.

Raggi A, Ferri R. Sleep disorders in neurodegenerative diseases. *Eur J Neurol.* 2010;17:1326-1338.

Resnick HE, Phillips B. Documentation of sleep apnea in nursing homes: United States 2004. *J Am Med Dir Assoc.* 2008;9:260-264.

Van Cauter E, Leproult R, Plat L. Age-related changes in slow wave sleep and REM sleep and relationship with growth hormone and cortisol levels in healthy men. *JAMA.* 2000;284:861-868.

Vance DE, Heaton K, Eaves Y, Fazell PL. Sleep and cognition on everyday functioning in older adults: implications for nursing practice and research. *J Neurosci Nurs.* 2011;43:261-271.

Wolkove N, Elkholy O, Baltzan M, Palayew M. Sleep and aging: 2. Management of sleep disorders in older people. *CMAJ.* 2007;176:1449-1454.

MULTIPLE CHOICE QUESTIONS

19.1   Which of the following is the most common reason for poor sleep quality in nursing homes?

a. Severe Alzheimer's disease
b. Nighttime surveillance by staff
c. Lack of bright light during day
d. Daytime napping
e. Medications

19.2   Which of these drugs is *not* associated with insomnia?

a. β-Blockers
b. β-Agonists
c. Donepezil
d. Theophylline
e. Caffeine

19.3   Which of the following is *not* a part of a sleep hygiene program in nursing homes?

a. Increased daytime activity
b. A small glass of hot milk before sleep
c. Limit time in bed
d. Limit nursing interventions at night
e. A small cup of coffee before bed

19.4   Which of the following is a cause of nocturia?

a. Increased nighttime arginine vasopressin (AVP)
b. Decreased atrial natriuretic hormone
c. Diuretics in the morning
d. Diabetes mellitus

19.5   Which of these is *not* a symptom of sleep apnea?

a. Daytime sleepiness
b. Excessive snoring
c. Nighttime sweating
d. Morning headaches
e. Nightmares

19.6   Which of the following is true about use of continuous positive airway pressure for sleep apnea in nursing homes?

a. It does not improve function in patients with Alzheimer's disease.
b. There is minimal noise associated with use of the machine.
c. Using CPAP at low levels is more likely to be successful in nursing homes.
d. Humidifiers do not need cleaning.
e. Nurses do not need special training to use CPAP.

Chapter 20

SKIN DISORDERS AND PRESSURE ULCERS

With aging, there is a decrease in epidermal and dermal cell turnover, leading to a thinner skin with less production of oils and a decrease in subcutaneous adipose tissue. This makes the skin more vulnerable to a variety of pathogens and irritants. The skin is also more vulnerable to damage from shear forces. For these reasons, topical skin care assumes a major role in the care of nursing home residents.

A variety of skin care lotions have been developed for use in nursing home residents. Unfortunately, minimal studies have demonstrated their effectiveness. The use of disposable absorbent underpants to protect against incontinence has the best evidence of efficacy. However, they need to be changed on a regular basis to be effective. A combination of urine and stool can be especially damaging to skin. Thus, it is especially important to frequently check and change residents with double (both urine and stool) incontinence. Decreasing skin dryness and pressure sores is best done by using no-rinse cleansers. A mixture of zinc oxide, hydrous wool fat, benzyl benzoate, and benzyl alcohol appears to be capable to reducing skin redness.

SKIN DISORDERS

Skin conditions represent one of the most common sets of disorders facing health professionals in the nursing home setting. Many skin lesions are complex, and their diagnosis and skin care in general are major challenges. The lack of expertise on skin conditions in older persons among average physicians has led to rapid growth of teledermatology programs. These programs have been well accepted by nurses, physicians, and specialists. Most of these programs use a screening for skin lesions by nurses who then request a consult from the dermatologist for diagnosis and management. With the consult, the dermatologist receives a copy of the screening form (Table 20–1), a photograph of the skin lesion, and a medication list. The dermatologist can then either make a diagnosis or request a "live" consult by Skype or other telemedicine technique.

The new section M of the Minimum Data Set (MDS) 3.0 on skin conditions is double the size of MDS 2.0. An individualized assessment is required. Pressure ulcers must be differentiated from arterial, venous, other ulcers, wounds, and skin problems. Particular precaution is needed to not code spider or other insect bites as pressure ulcers. All new wounds should have a clinician's note describing them as avoidable or unavoidable. Documentation of all wounds or skin conditions should be completed when the resident first arrives in the nursing home.

The normal features of aged skin include fine and coarse wrinkles, purpura, dry skin, lentigines, telangiectasia, sebaceous hyperplasia, elastic skin, pigment changes, giant comedones, and blotchiness. Photoaging leads to actinic keratosis. The major causes of pruritus are given in Table 20–2. By far the most common cause of pruritus is dry skin or xerosis. This can lead to neurotic excoriations, especially among residents with dementia, which can in turn result in open lesions and superimposed infection. Thus, keeping residents' skin is a critical preventive measure. Staff also need to be educated on how scabies presents and to report if they develop pruritic lesions because scabies outbreaks in nursing homes can occur rapidly and be extremely disruptive to staff and their families in addition to the affected residents.

Flushing is not rare in older persons and has many causes (Table 20–3). About 15% of older persons have dermatographia. Fewer than 1% of them have systemic mastocytosis. Systemic mastocytosis can present with flushing, gastrointestinal reflux disease or peptic ulcers, syncope, and urticaria pigmentosa.

At least 18% to 38% of nursing staff members develop hand eczema. This is about double the prevalence in the general population. Not all of these cases are associated with occupational exposure. Excessive hand washing and use of gloves appear to be major occupational causes of hand eczema.

Common skin conditions and their diagnostic and management considerations are summarized in Table 20–4. The diagnostic approach to skin tumors is outlined in Figure 20–1. Examples of common skin conditions are given in Figure 20–2. Because of their prevalence and treatability, it is recommended that at least once a year a dermatologist or the medical director provide an inservice on skin diseases for the nursing staff. Skin infections such as scabies and cellulites are covered in Chapter 26.

SKIN TEARS

An international consensus panel defined skin tears as: "A wound caused by shear, friction and/or blunt force resulting in separation of skin layers. A skin tear can be

Table 20-1.	SKIN SCREENING FORM FOR NURSES

Name: _____ Date of Birth: _____

Location: _____

Skin tears:	Y/N	Location: _____
Rashes:	Y/N	Location: _____
Bruises:	Y/N	Location: _____
Pressure ulcer:	Y/N	Location: _____
Tumor (growths):	Y/N	Location: _____
Bullae:	Y/N	Location: _____
Dry skin:	Y/N	Location: _____
Reddened areas:	Y/N	Location: _____
Abscess:	Y/N	Location: _____
Red area:	Y/N	Location: _____
Skin flaking:	Y/N	Location: _____

NOTE: A picture of the lesion should be submitted with this report to the dermatologist

Table 20-2.	CAUSES OF PRURITUS

Local
- Xerosis
- Herpes zoster
- Dermatitis
- Scabies
- Pediculosis corpora
- Dermatitis herpetiformis
- Bullous pemphigoid
- Mycosis fungoides
- Urticaria

Systemic
- Diabetes mellitus
- Uremia
- Neurodermatitis (psychogenic)
- Carcinoid
- Systemic mastocytosis
- Cholestasis
- Lymphoma
- Polycythemia
- Infections (e.g., HIV, ascariasis, filariasis)

Medications
- Aspirin
- Opiates
- Vancomycin
- Antibiotic hypersensitivity

Table 20-3.	CAUSES OF FLUSHING

- Medication side effects (e.g., niacin)
- Spicy foods
- Carcinoid
- Systemic mastocytosis
- Medullary carcinoma of thyroid
- Renal cell carcinoma
- Bee sting
- Anaphylaxis

partial-thickness (separation of epidermis from dermis) or full thickness (separation of both the epidermis and the dermis from the underlying structures)."

The incidence of skin tears is about 0.9 per resident per year. However, a few residents can have multiple skin tears over the year. Both intrinsic and extrinsic factors lead to skin tears (Table 20–5). Skin tear prevention programs have been demonstrated to markedly decrease skin tears in nursing homes. The elements of a skin tear prevention program are outlined in Table 20–6.

The management of skin tears is outlined in Table 20–7. Cleansing of the wound requires irrigation with a syringe and 19-gauge needles using normal saline. This removes the biofilm and necrotic tissue. Bleeding needs to be controlled before the wound is dressed. Adhesive strips can be used for category I, adhesive strips and soft silicone foam dressings for category II, and silicone or low-tack foam dressing for category III skin tears. Hydrocolloids and traditional transparent film dressings are *not* to be used. Category I skin tears heal within 7 days, category II within 10 days, and category III within 14 days (Table 20–8).

SKIN CANCER

Skin cancer is the most common type of cancer. The three common types of skin cancer are basal cell cancer, squamous cell cancer, and melanoma (Figure 20–3). Nonmelanoma skin cancer rarely leads to death. Melanomas account for three quarters of skin cancer deaths. Factors suggestive of melanoma are outlined in Table 20–9.

Basal cell cancer has a pearly translucency and rounded edges and can ulcerate. Squamous cell cancer can present in many ways. Its characteristics are that it grows rapidly and is painful. The characteristics of malignant melanoma are given in Table 20–9.

Treatment for basal cell carcinoma is Mohs' surgery or complete circumferential peripheral and deep margin assessment. External radiation may be an alternative. In frail persons, watchful waiting may be the best approach.

For small squamous cell cancer, topical chemotherapy with imiquimod or 5-fluoruracil can control disease. Cryotherapy and radiation are alternatives. In most cases, curative therapy requires surgery.

Treatment of melanoma depends on the stage. Stage O (melanoma in situ) requires surgery with a wide margin excision. Stage I is surgery of tumor, possibly with lymph

Table 20–4.   COMMON SKIN DISORDERS SEEN IN NURSING HOMES

Actinic keratosis	Reddish brown scaly or crusty growth	• 5-Flurouracil ointment (0.5%–5%) • Imiquimod 5% cream • Ingenol mebutate • Cryosurgery or laser surgery
Bullous pemphigoid	Tense blisters with crusting after busting	• Systemic corticosteroids • Addition of immunosuppressants
Cherry angiomas	Round, red, nonblanching papules	• Laser treatment • Electrodissection • Surgical excision
Contact dermatitis	Inflamed skin with known contact with irritant	• Nonirritant soaps • Emollients • Topical steroid cream
Diabetic dermopathy	Pink or brown papular to macular eruption	• Treat diabetes
Drug eruption	Can be localized (fixed drug eruptions) or widespread occurring 1–10 days after a new drugs is started; rash type varies	• Stop drug • Local treatment of eruption • Systemic corticosteroids when required
Eczema	Erythema, scaling, or vesicles on hands or feet	• Emollients • Topical steroids • Occlusive dressings at night
Keratoacanthomas	Papular enlarging lesion that evolves to a hypopigmented scar	• Topical isotretinoin • Excision
Pemphigus	Blisters on skin, mouth, or genitals	• Corticosteroids • Azathioprine • Methotrexate
Postinflammatory hyperpigmentation	Brown hyperpigmentation	• Cosmetic dermatology
Psoriasis	Erythematous plaques with silver scaling	• Coal tar cream or paste topically • Topical steroids • Phototherapy • Calcipotriene • Anthralin • Methotrexate or cyclosporine • Biologicals
Sebaceous hyperplasia	Yellow, dome-shaped papules ± central umbilication	• Oral isotretinoin • Electrodessication • Laser therapy • Topical bichloracetic acid
Seborrheic dermatitis	Scaly red lesion of face and body flexures; can be associated with blepharitis or conjunctivitis	• Topical steroids • Tar-containing shampoos for scalp involvement
Stasis dermatitis	Pigmentation with associated varicosities and edema	• Support stockings
Tinea versicolor	Dark or light scaly lesions	• Topical selenium sulfide shampoo • Antifungals
Toxic epidermal necrolysis	Generalized eruption with tender skin and erythema leading to blisters	• Stop drug causes • Systemic steroids • Severe cases transfer to hospital
Xerosis	Dry skin; scales; cracks; flaking; fissures complicated by excoriations and pruritus	• Increased fluid intake • Moisturizing creams or lotions • Crisco oil to lower extremities at night • Soft, nonirritant clothing • Avoid steroid creams and antihistamines when possible • Do not dry skin vigorously after washing

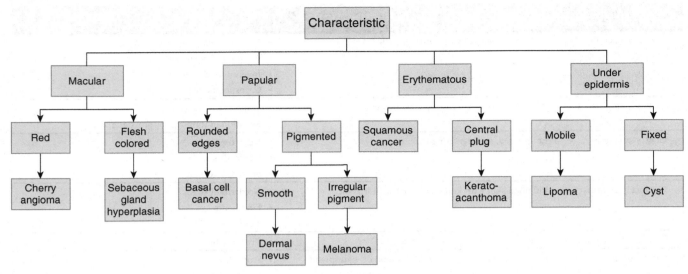

Figure 20–1. Diagnostic approach to skin tumors.

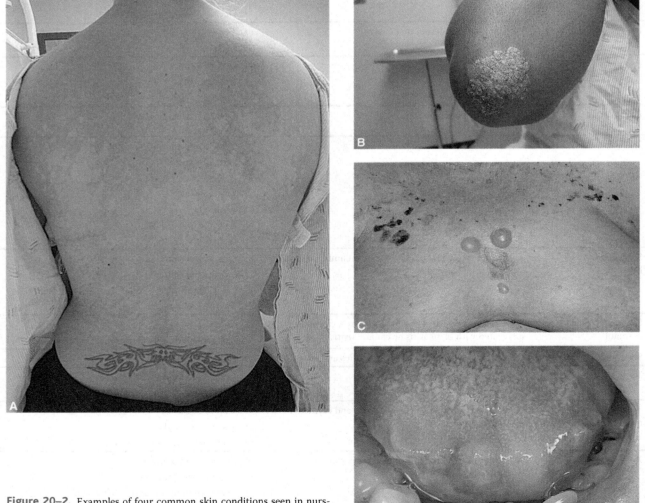

Figure 20–2. Examples of four common skin conditions seen in nursing homes. (**A**) Tinea versicolor. (**B**) Psoriasis. (**C**) Bullous pemphigoid. (**D**) Pemphigus. (Permission received from Dr. Nicole Burkemper, MD, Department of Dermatology, Saint Louis University.)

Table 20–5.	RISK FACTORS FOR DEVELOPMENT OF SKIN TEARS

Intrinsic
- Senile purpura
- Ecchymosis
- Edema
- Poor nutritional state
- Neuropathy
- Vascular disease
- Advanced age (>90 years)
- Hematoma
- Previously healed skin tears

Extrinsic
- Trauma
- Corticosteroid use
- Skin cleansers
- Tape removal
- Transfers
- Excess bathing

node removal. Stage II is surgery and lymph node mapping with removal if cancer is present. Stage III is surgery followed by interferon. Stage IV treatment is ipilimumab or vemurafenib with biologic therapy with interleukin-2. Outcomes are poor, and all persons should be offered the opportunity to enter a clinical trial. See Table 20–9 for the list of characteristics that suggest melanoma.

PRESSURE ULCERS

International advisory groups (European Pressure Ulcer Advisory Panel and National Pressure Ulcer Advisory Panel 2009) define pressure ulcers as localized injury to the skin or underlying tissue (or both) usually over a bony prominence as a result of pressure or pressure in combination with shear.

Table 20–6.	ELEMENTS OF A SKIN TEAR PREVENTION PROGRAM

- Assess all residents on admission for skin tear risk factors.
- At risk individuals should protect skin: wear sleeves, long pants, and long socks.
- Shin guards should be worn by persons who have skin tears.
- Apply moisturizers (emollients) twice a day.
- Educate staff on appropriate transfer strategies to avoid skin tears.
- Identify environmental causes and cover with protective devices.
- Avoid daily bathing and non-emollient soaps.
- Lotions containing humectants and barrier ingredients can be used judiciously.

Table 20–7.	MANAGEMENT OF SKIN TEARS

- Assess the wound using the STAR or Payne-Martin classification (see Table 20–8).
- Clean wound with saline applied from a syringe.
- Remove blood clots, slough, and foreign bodies.
- Use adhesive strips to obtain juxtaposition of epidermis in category I and II tears.
- Apply a moist wound dressing.
- Do not remove dressing for 2 to 3 days to allow healing.
- Consider tetanus prophylaxis.

Pressure ulcers cause pain and distress. Wound healing may be prolonged, which if poorly managed can have serious complications that can lead to life-threatening infections. It is important that nurses and nursing aides are aware of the risk factors for pressure ulceration and know how to minimize risk for individual residents. Nurses are also educators and as such need to make sure that residents and visitors are aware of pressure ulcers and of the importance of prevention. For example, if a family is taking a resident for an outing that involves prolonged sitting in a wheelchair, the nursing team should advise them on the use of an appropriate gel pad or other device.

About one in 10 residents in a nursing home has a pressure ulcer, although incidence rates as high as 39% have been reported from Brazil. Nearly two thirds of these pressure ulcers have their origin in acute care facilities. Pressure ulcers have a large cost burden. In the United States, this is $11 billion and in the United Kingdom £2.4 billion. The predisposing factors to the development of pressure ulcers in nursing homes are outlined in Table 20–10.

Table 20–8.	COMPARISON OF SKIN TEAR CLASSIFICATION SYSTEMS	
	Payne-Martin Classification	**STAR Classification**
Category 1A	Linear tear with skin pulled apart No tissue loss	Edges can be realigned to a normal anatomical position
Category 1B	Epidermal flap covers the dermis within 1 mm of margin	Edges can be realigned, but skin is pale, dusky, or darkened
Category IIA	Loss of <25% of epidermal flap	Edges cannot be realigned
Category IIB	>25% loss of epidermal flap	Non-realignment with pale, dusky, or darkened skin
Category III	Lack of epidermal flap	Skin flap is completely absent

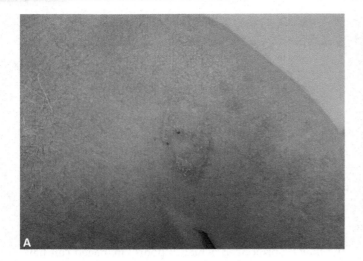

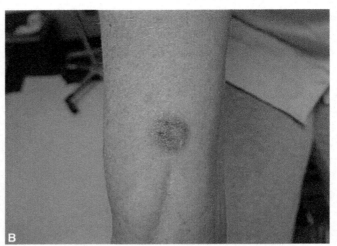

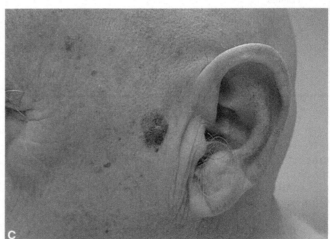

Figure 20–3. Three common types of skin cancer. (**A**) Basal cell carcinoma. (**B**) Squamous cell carcinoma. (**C**) Melanoma. (Permission received from Dr. Scott Fosko, MD, Department of Dermatology, Saint Louis University.)

Three pressure ulcer scales are commonly used. These are the Norton, Braden, and Waterlow scales. All of the scales include mobility and moisture exposure. The Norton and Braden scales include a measure of physical activity, and the Waterlow and Norton scales have a measure of general activity. The Braden and Waterlow scales examine nutrition and appetite, respectively. The Braden estimates function or shear forces and sensory perception. There is little evidence that using these scales results in fewer pressure ulcers than good nursing practices and increase preventive measures when a stage I pressure ulcer develops.

Both the National Pressure Ulcer Advisory Panel (United States) and the European Pressure Ulcer Advisory Panel have produced very similar pressure ulcer

Table 20–9.	CHARACTERISTICS SUGGESTIVE OF MELANOMA
Multiple colors: tan, blue, black, red, brown	
Evolving in size, shape, or color	
Local growth	
Asymmetry	
New spot (metastases)	
Outline irregular	
Mole is itchy or bleeding	
Area: >6 mm in diameter	

Table 20–10.	FACTORS THAT PREDISPOSE TO PRESSURE ULCERS	
Intrinsic Factors		**Extrinsic Factors**
Limited mobility		Pressure
Chronic diseases		Shear forces
Poor nutrition		Friction forces
Thinning of skin		Urine incontinence
Bony prominences		Fecal incontinence
		Corticosteroid use

Table 20–11.   PRESSURE ULCER STAGING/CATEGORY

Stage or Category	Clinical Features
Suspected deep tissue injury	Purple discoloration or a blood-filled blister due to underlying tissue damage
I	Intact skin with nonblanchable redness
II	Partial-thickness loss of dermis with red or pink wound bed and no slough
III	Full-thickness tissue loss without exposure of bone, muscles, or tendon; slough can be present; tunneling can be present
IV	Full-thickness tissue loss with exposed bone, tendon, or muscle; do not remove eschar on heels
Unstageable	Full-thickness tissue loss with base covered with slough or eschar in the wound bed

Table 20–13.   DIFFERENTIAL DIAGNOSIS OF ULCERS

Ulcer Type	Distinguishing Feature
Pressure ulcer	Occurs over a bony prominence
Venous ulcer	Located medially above or below the malleolus; presence of varicosities
Arterial ulcer	Punched-out, dry ulcer on a cool, shiny leg with little hair; pain relieved when leg is dependent
Diabetic foot wound	Occur in areas of pressure associated with peripheral neuropathy
Malignant ulcers	A single nodular ulcer that heals poorly

classification systems. The main features of these two staging categories are summarized in Table 20–11. The MDS 3.0 uses this categorization, but MDS 2.0 does not meet best practices staging.

The Pressure Ulcer Scale for Healing (PUSH) is a validated method to measure healing of pressure ulcers. It is now included in the MDS 3.0. The physician or advanced practice nurse may prefer to give his or her own description of the wound using the MEASURE mnemonic (Table 20–12).

It is important to make a proper diagnosis of a pressure ulcer and distinguish it from other causes of ulcers. Pressure ulcers are often considered a marker of poor care, although there is little evidence to support this concept. In the United States, they also often lead to lawsuits. The differential diagnosis of pressure ulcers is given in Table 20–13.

Table 20–12.   THE MEASURE MNEMONIC TO DESCRIBE PRESSURE ULCERS

Measure size accurately using ruler or computer assisted techniques

Exudate volume

Anatomic location

Suffering, including pain, odor, and effect of drainage on clothes

Undermining along wound edges

Reevaluation on a regular basis

Edge is or is not macerated

The basic strategies to prevent pressure ulcers are to turn the resident regularly and prevent excessive wetness of the skin. Most programs turn residents every 2 hours, but this is an empirical approach with no data to support it. Healthy older persons develop skin redness after 90 minutes of lying in one position. All persons in nursing homes should be encouraged to move every 15 minutes.

Pressure-reducing devices need to reduce pressure to less than 32 mm Hg, which is capillary closing pressure. Australian Medical Sheepskin has been shown to successfully prevent sacral pressure ulcers. Other pressure reducing devices include static (e.g., foam mattresses or devices filled with water) and dynamic (e.g., alternative pressure devices or air fluidized beds). All of these devices reduce pressure ulcers by half compared with standard hospital beds. There appears to be little advantage of the static over the dynamic pressure-relieving devices, making the choice of the device to be driven by cost and ease of use. None of these devices can adequately reduce pressure over heels and the trochanter. When pressure-relieving devices are used in conjunction with turning, it appears the optimum turning time is 4 hours.

Protein energy undernourished persons have a higher risk of developing pressure ulcers. A leucine-enriched balanced essential amino acid protein mix of 1.2 to 1.5 g/kg/day is recommended to decrease pressure ulcers. Low albumin in most nursing home residents reflects cytokine excess with third spacing of albumin rather than protein energy undernutrition. In persons who are zinc deficient, zinc replacement may accelerate wound healing. Residents at risk for zinc deficiency are those with diabetes mellitus, lung cancer, or cirrhosis or receiving furosemide.

The approach to healing of pressure ulcers is outlined in Table 20–14. The different types of occlusive dressing available are described in Table 20–15. In general, hydrocolloids appear to produce the best healing rate and, as such, are the dressing of choice. When there is excessive exudate, alginates may be preferred. Biomembranes are very expensive and not easy to obtain. A number of topical growth factors (e.g., nerve growth factor, platelet-derived

Table 20–14.   MANAGEMENT OF PRESSURE ULCERS

- Pressure reduction
  - Low air-loss bed
  - Frequent turning (90 min–4 hr)
  - Other static pressure-relieving devices
- Occlusive dressings (see Table 20–5)
- Debridement
  - Surgical sharp
  - Wet-to-dry gauze dressings removed when dry (not recommended)
  - Enzyme debridement: Papain (no longer on U.S. market) better than collagenase
- Topical growth factors (minimal effect)
- Nutritional support
  - 1.2–1.5g/kg/day of protein
  - Zinc in zinc deficient
- Bacterial management
  - Topical silver compounds
  - Topical cadexomer iodide
  - Antibiotics for signs of systemic infection

growth factor, and fibroblast-derived growth factor) are available. They are expensive and at best produce small advantages in wound healing. Similarly, vacuum-assisted closure devices have not been found to accelerate healing of pressure ulcers.

Superficial bacterial cultures from pressure ulcers are valueless, can be misleading, and result in unnecessary healthcare costs. Clinical leadership should not allow them to be done in their facilities. The Levine technique, in which a swab is pressed against the ulcer floor, expressing fluid and then rotated 360 degrees, may have more value, but this remains questionable. In general, an antibiotic should only be used when there are clear signs of systemic infection. The possible effect of bacteria on pressure ulcers is outlined in Figure 20–4.

Factors that are supportive of wound healing are hydrocolloid or alginate dressing use, less wound debridement (unless necessary to remove necrotic tissue) and staying with one dressing type. Topical antiseptics and antibiotic use are associated with poorer wound healing. An interdisciplinary pressure ulcer program led by a wound care specialist can reduce the occurrence of pressure ulcers and accelerate healing. However, it should be recognized that it is the focus on pressure ulcers, rather than any specific technique or intervention, that produces this positive outcome.

FOOT ULCERS IN DIABETES

One in four people with diabetes is likely to have a foot ulcer in his or her lifetime (Figure 20–5). The cost of managing a diabetic foot ulcer is approximately $6000 (£19,000). They occur because of the combined effects of neuropathy and peripheral vascular disease (ischemia). Total contact casting, but not other forms, enhances healing. Hydrogel treatment is more effective than surgical debridement. Maggots can reduce Methicillin-resistant *Staphylococcus aureus* (MRSA) in diabetic foot ulcers. Vacuum-assisted closure (125 mm Hg negative pressure) has not been shown to be more effective at wound healing. Topical recombinant human platelet-derived growth factor β (β homodimer) increased the time to wound healing and the probability of complete wound healing. Some evidence suggests that hyperbaric oxygen may reduce the requirement for amputation in diabetic foot ulcers. Ampicillin–sulbactam intravenously or oral amoxicillin–clavulanate produced equivalent wound healing to linezolid. No controlled trials have demonstrated the usefulness of antibiotics in most diabetic foot ulcers. Diabetic shoes with customized insoles have a role in preventing diabetic foot ulcers. All residents with severe diabetic foot ulcers should have vascular studies to determine the degree of peripheral vascular disease. In the United Kingdom, it is recommended that all persons with a diabetic foot ulcer have a referral to a diabetic foot clinic within 24 hours of the development of the ulcer. Table 20–16 provides available approaches to the management of diabetic ulcers.

Table 20–15.   COMPARISON OF WOUND DRESSINGS AVAILABLE TO TREAT PRESSURE ULCERS (+YES, –NO)

	Wet Saline Gauze Alginates	Hydrocolloids	Polymer	Films	Hydrogels
Water permeable	+	–	+	+	+
Easy to apply	+	+	–	+	+
Bacterial resistant	–	+	–	–	+
Damage epithelial cells	+/–	–	+	–	–
Pain relief	+	+	+	+	+
Maceration of skin	+/–		+/–	–	–

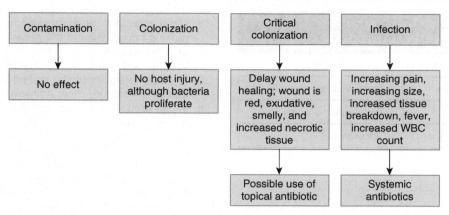

Figure 20–4. Effect of bacteria in pressure ulcers. WBC, white blood cell.

VASCULAR ULCERS

Vascular ulcers can be either arterial or venous. These ulcers need to be differentiated from pressure ulcers and their cause documented. Ischemic (arterial insufficiency) ulcers are caused by poor blood flow through the capillary beds of the legs. They classically occur on the lateral surface of the ankle or the distal digits. These ulcers have a "punched-out" appearance with small, round borders. They are associated with a cold, hairless limb and a lack of peripheral pulses. The limbs tend to be red when dangling and paler when elevated. The ulcers are painful, especially when the limb is exercised. The differential diagnosis of arterial leg ulcers is shown in Table 20–17. Treatment of arterial ulcers includes keeping the wound dry. Cadexomer iodine can absorb fluid draining from the ulcer. Occlusive dressings should be used. Topical antibiotics need to be avoided. The resident should not smoke. Treatment of pain is critical. Improving circulation can be done medically or by surgical revascularization. Pumps that increase perfusion to the limb can be considered.

Varicose leg ulcers occur on the lower leg. They are associated with skin varicosities and red-brown skin discoloration. About three quarters of venous ulcers are healed at 16 weeks. Wound dressings and wound compression (>25 mm Hg) are the cornerstones of treatment. No dressing has been shown to be superior.

OSTOMY CARE

There are three types of ostomies:

1. **Colostomy:** Formed from the large bowel or colon. They are closed and can be one or two piece.
2. **Ileostomy:** Formed from the small bowel or ileum. They pass about 800 mL of feces a day and require a drainable appliance that can be emptied three to six times a day.
3. **Urostomy (Ileal conduit):** Formed from ileum, which acts as a bladder into which the ureters can be implanted. Appliances need to be drainable and can be connected to a drainage bag at night.

Appliances used for ostomies can be clear or opaque and either a single piece or two pieces. The choice of an appliance depends on the size and type of ostomy, the resident's ability to manually change it, and the resident's preferences. Biodegradable stomas have been developed that can

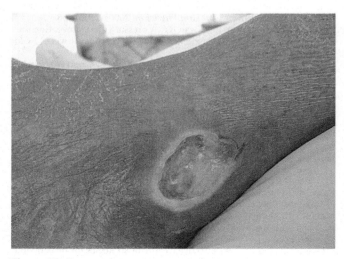

Figure 20–5. Foot ulcer.

Table 20–16.	APPROACHES TO MANAGING DIABETIC FOOT ULCERS

- Use an appropriate dressing
- Relieve pressure off the wound area
- Debridement where appropriate (evidence is poor, and debridement should be avoided if tissue hypoxia is present)
- Negative-pressure wound therapy (limited positive data)
- Hyperbaric oxygen can be used in those with low transcutaneous (partial) oxygen pressure
- Oral or intravenous antibiotics if wound is infected
- Epidermal growth factor (expensive; small effect)
- Stem cell application most probably helps
- Bioengineered fibroblast–keratinocyte co-culture
- Revascularization surgery

Table 20–17.	DIFFERENTIAL DIAGNOSIS OF ARTERIAL LEG DISEASE
Calciphylaxis	Spider Bite
Pyoderma gangrenosum	Pressure ulcers
Venous ulcers	Eosinophilic vasculitis
Traumatic	Scleroderma

3. Hand eczema is much more common in nurses in nursing homes than in the general population.
4. Skin tear classifications are available and should be used to determine the management.
5. Pressure ulcers should be staged by the National or European Pressure Ulcer Advisory Panel.
6. When used with a pressure-relieving device, the optimum turning time to prevent pressure ulcers is every 4 hours.
7. Do not get bacterial cultures of wounds.
8. Arterial, venous, and diabetic ulcers need to be differentiated from pressure ulcers.
9. Nurses and physicians need to have knowledge of how to care for stomas and to help decrease flatus and odor.

be flushed down the toilet. The adhesive (flange) is formed of hydrocolloid dressing–like material. There should be no creases in the flange. The hole in the flange should be 2 to 3 mm larger than the stoma. Two-piece appliances are joined either by adhesive or rings that click in place. The two-piece should never be used without the flange.

The problems associated with stomas consist of leakage, prolapse, parastomal herniation, bleeding, necrosis, and stenosis. If there is leakage, a flexible or convex barrier should replace the basic flat wafer. Peristomal problems include mucocutaneous separation, caput medusae formation, alteration in the abdominal plain, allergy to the appliances and dermatitis, fungal infections, and folliculitis. Persons with stomas need nurses to take a positive attitude to the stoma and need to receive psychological support to allow adaptation to the stoma. The resident–nurse relationship represents an important component in the success of ostomy care.

Two problems can be particularly vexing for persons with ostomies. These are flatus and odor. Reducing flatus requires eating small amounts slowly and chewing well. Yogurt, buttermilk, applesauce, white rice, and ripe bananas reduce flatus. Overeating, gum chewing, and smoking increase flatus. Foods such as beans, cabbage, broccoli, eggs, Brussels sprouts, and carbonated beverages increase flatus. In addition, many older nursing home residents are lactose intolerant, and avoidance of milk products should be attempted to determine if flatus is reduced. Flatus can cause a conspicuous bulge, and residents and nurses need to be able to remove flatus from the bag without causing spillage.

Deodorants can be used to reduce stool odor. A number of foods increase stool odor; these foods include asparagus, garlic, spices, onions, and most of the foods associated with increased flatus. Buttermilk, cranberry juice, yogurt, and parsley may reduce odor. Determining which foods have the major effect on flatus and odor is very individualized and thus requires trial and error.

KEY POINTS

1. Skin lesions are common and often difficult to diagnose.
2. Skin cancers need to be recognized and treated.

SUGGESTED READINGS

Anonymous. Topical skin care in aged care facilities. *Aust Nur J.* 2007;15(5):27-30.

Armstrong DG, Lavery LA, Wunderlich RP. Risk factors for diabetic foot ulceration: a logical approach to treatment. *J Wound Ostomy and Continence Nurse.* 1998;25:123-128.

Bianchi J. Preventing, assessing and managing skin tears [review]. *Nurs Times.* 2012;108(13):12, 14, 16.

Burch J. Essential care for patients with stomas. *Nurs Times.* 2011;107:45:12-14.

De Souza DM, de Gouveia Santos VL. Incidence of pressure ulcers in the institutionalized elderly. *J Wound Ostomy Continence Nurs.* 2010;37:272-276.

Dorman C. Ostomy basics. *RN.* 2009;July:22-24.

Dorner B, Posthauer ME, Thomas DR. The role of nutrition in pressure ulcer prevention and treatment: National Pressure Ulcer Advisory Panel White Paper. *Adv Skin Wound Care.* 2009;22:212-221.

European Pressure Ulcer Advisory Panel and National Pressure Ulcer Advisory Panel. *Prevention and Treatment of Pressure Ulcers: A Quick Reference Guide.* Washington, DC: National Pressure Ulcer Advisory Panel; 2009.

Game FL, Hinchliffe RJ, Apelqvist J, et al. A systematic review of interventions to enhance the healing of chronic ulcers of the foot in diabetes. *Diabetes Metab Res Rev.* 2012;2(suppl 1):119-141.

Janardhanan L, Leow YH, Chio MTW, et al. Experience with the implementation of a web-based teledermatology system in a nursing home in Singapore. *J Telemed Telecare.* 2008;14:404-409.

Jerant AF, Johnson JT, Sheridan CD, Caffrey TJ. Early detection and treatment of skin cancer. *Am Fam Physician.* 2000;62:357-368.

Kwong EW, Lau AT, Lee RL, Kwan RY. A pressure ulcer prevention programme specially designed for nursing homes: does it work? *J Clin Nurs.* 2011;20:2777-2786.

LeBlanc KA, Christensen D. Demystifying skin tears, part 2. *Nursing.* 2011;41:16-7.

LeBlanc K, Baranoski S; Skin Tear Consensus Panel Members. Skin tears: state of the science: consensus statements for the prevention, prediction, assessment, and treatment of skin tears. *Adv Skin Wound Care.* 2011;(9 suppl):2-15.

Levine JM, Ayello EA. MDS 3.0 Section M: skin conditions: what the medical director needs to know. *J Am Med Dir Assoc.* 2011;12:179-183.

Londahl M, Fagher K, Katzman P. What is the role of hyperbaric oxygen in the management of diabetic foot disease? *Curr Diab Rep.* 2011;11:285-293.

Luba MC, Bangs SA, Mohler AM, Stulberg DL. Common benign skin tumors. *Am Fam Physician.* 2003;67:729-738.

McInnes E, Dumville JC, Jammali-Blasi A, Bell-Syer SE. Support surfaces for treating pressure ulcers. *Cochrane Database Syst Rev.* 2011;(12):CD009490.

Millington T, Norris TW. Effective treatment strategies for diabetic foot wounds. *J Fam Pract.* 2000;49(suppl):S40-S48.

Mistiaen P, Achterberg W, Ament A, et al. Cost-effectiveness of the Australian Medical Sheepskin for the prevention of pressure ulcers in somatic nursing home patients: study protocol for a prospective multi-centre randomised controlled trial (ISRCTN17553857). *BMC Health Serv Res.* 2008;8:4.

Markova A, Mostow EN. US skin disease assessment: ulcer and wound care. *Dermatol Clin.* 2012;30:107-111.

Ndip A, Ebah L, Mbako A. Neuropathic diabetic foot ulcers—evidence-to-practice. *Int J Genl* Med 2012;5:129-134.

Norman RA. Long-term care dermatology. *Dermatol Ther.* 2003;16:186-194.

O'Meara SM, Bland JM, Dumville JC, Cullum NA. A systematic review of the performance of instruments designed to measure the dimensions of pressure ulcers. *Wound Repair Regen.* 2012;20:263-276.

Skudlik C, Dulon M, Wendeler D, et al. Hand eczema in geriatric nurses in Germany: prevalence and risk factors. *Contact Dermatitis.* 2009;60:136-143.

Stephen-Haynes J, Callaghan R, Bethell E, Greeenwood M. The assessment and management of skin tears in care homes. *Br J Nurs.* 2011;20(11):S12, S14, S16 passim.

Stulberg DL, Clark N, Tovey D. Common hyperpigmentation disorders in adults: part II. Melanoma, seborrheic keratoses, acanthosis nigricans, melasma, diabetic dermopathy, tinea versicolor, and postinflammatory hyperpigmentation. *Am Fam Physician.* 2003;68:1963-1968.

Tilley C. Caring for the patient with a fecal or urinary diversion in palliative and hospice settings: a literature review. *Ostomy Wound Manage.* 2012;58:24-34.

Tippett AW. Reducing the incidence of pressure ulcers in nursing home residents: a prospective 8-year evaluation. *Ostomy Wound Manage.* 2009;55:52-58.

Vig S, Dowsett C, Berg L, et al. International Expert Panel on Negative Pressure Wound Therapy (NPWT-EP). Evidence-based recommendations for the use of negative pressure wound therapy in chronic wounds: steps towards an international consensus. *J Tissue Viability.* 2011;20(suppl 1):S1-S18.

Williams J. Flatus, odour and the ostomist: coping strategies and interventions. *Br J Nurs.* 2008;17(suppl 2):S10-S12.

MULTIPLE CHOICE QUESTIONS

20.1 Which skin lesion has a papular enlarging lesion that evolves to a hypopigmented scar?

a. Cherry angioma
b. Pemphigus
c. Pemphigoid
d. Keratoacanthomas
e. Tinea versicolor

20.2 Which of the following is used to treat actinic keratosis?

a. 5-Flurouracil ointment
b. Corticosteroids
c. Isotretinoin
d. Coal-tar
e. Selenium sulfide shampoo

20.3 Which of the following foods can reduce ostomy odor?

a. Beans
b. Garlic
c. Asparagus
d. Onions
e. Yogurt

20.4 Which of the following is true concerning skin tears?

a. If the skin flap is completely absent, it is a category III in the Payne-Martin and STAR classifications.
b. Lack of more than 25% epidermal flap is a category IIA.
c. No tissue loss with a linear tear is category IB.
d. When the skin is pale, dusky, and darkened and the edges cannot be realigned, it is a category IIB.

20.5 In pressure ulcer staging, which is the earliest stage in which tunneling can be present?

a. Stage I
b. Stage II
c. Stage III
d. Stage IV

20.6 Which wound dressing is not water permeable, does not macerate skin or damage epithelial cells, and is bacterial resistant?

a. Polymer films
b. Hydrogels
c. Hydrocolloids
d. Alginates
e. Wet saline gauze

20.7 Which of the following is not suggestive of a melanoma?

a. Multiple colors
b. Asymmetry
c. New spots
d. Pearly translucency
e. Itchy or bleeding

Chapter 21

ORAL HEALTH

Oral health contributes substantially to health and well-being in older people. It is important to appreciate the role it plays in personal and social comforts that influence self-esteem and body image and communication, including talking and smiling, of nursing home residents. A neglected mouth at any age can lead to disease and distress, and the complexity of the aging mouth means that nursing home practitioners need to be familiar with common conditions and be effective in the management of the soft and hard tissues of the mouth. Good oral health implies comfort, hygiene, and the absence of disease.

Throughout life, we are conditioned to believe that a "perfect smile" requires a full set of perfectly straight white teeth and fresh breath. A quick glance at the Internet will support the pervasiveness of this idea, yet the dental health of older people in care homes is known to be poor, and standards of oral hygiene variable. In Scotland, it is recommended that residents who are admitted into nursing homes who have not seen a dental practitioner in the preceding year should be referred within the first week of admission to a dentist. Although it should be recognized that a proportion of people admitted to nursing homes will have poor oral health, a failure to prioritize oral health and hygiene by the nursing and medical team contributes to the further deterioration and avoidable problems. Standards of oral hygiene care are said by some authorities to be indicative of the overall quality of nursing care. In the United States and many other parts of the world, finding a dentist to work with older persons, especially those with dementia, is often very difficult.

Concerns about body image appear to remain relatively stable across the lifespan, and there is no reason to assume that the condition of the mouth and cleanliness of the postmealtime face is less of a concern for a resident than for others. It is easy to understand the impact on psychological health of facial disfigurement, yet we can easily overlook in a nursing home the impact on residents of tooth loss, ill-fitting dentures, and halitosis on a person's self-confidence and social interaction. In addition to the impact of well-being and sense of identity, clinicians have become increasingly interested in the links between physical health, disease, and risks associated with problems in the aging mouth. It is estimated that more than 100 systemic diseases have oral manifestations. For example, studies have demonstrated links between severe periodontal disease, diabetes mellitus, ischemic heart disease, and chronic respiratory disease to name but a few.

Common age-related changes of the mouth are shown in Table 21–1; in combination, these changes, which may be insidious in onset, compromise the ability for recovery from trauma, caries, and infections. These changes predispose frail older people to mucosal, gingival, and periodontal inflammation and other problems that can be compounded through poor oral hygiene and low intake of oral fluids. With increasing age, teeth may become brittle and stained. Surface enamel may be lost, and teeth may become loose as a result of breakdown of supporting tissues and bone loss. Teeth may be stained by food and drink (particularly tea and coffee), by nicotine from smoking, or by oral iron supplements. Teeth grinding (bruxism) wears down the surface of teeth and can be a problem in agitated residents.

Dental caries, mucosal pathology, and denture problems are extremely common among older people. Among older residents in care homes, untreated dental caries and soft tissue disease have been found to be almost universal in Glasgow and elsewhere. Oral pathology increases risk of aspiration of infectious material and saliva, leading to respiratory infection, which can be life threatening in vulnerable patients. Oral infections may have detrimental effects on systemic health. A recent study completed within 11 nursing homes in Japan found that brushing teeth after meals significantly reduces the risk of pneumonia. A recent systematic review on this topic concluded that one in 10 deaths from pneumonia in institutionalized older subjects could be prevented by frequent and efficient oral hygiene measures.

Dehydration is a significant risk factor for poor oral health through its effect on saliva flow. Diabetes mellitus, Sjogren's syndrome, and radiotherapy are also major causes of xerostomia. Clinical studies suggest up to 50% of the older population experience oral dryness and related complaints. Long-term medication and polypharmacy compound problems, because salivary gland hypofunction is exacerbated by many of the medications associated with frailty.

The oral side effects of drugs are the most common cause of xerostomia (dry mouth) in older patients and are a particular risk of polypharmacy. There are known to be more than 500 drugs that cause salivary gland dysfunction

Table 21–1.	AGE-RELATED CHANGES IN THE MOUTH

- Loss of mucosal elasticity
- Submucosal tissue and tactile sensitivity around the mouth
- Loss of mass and strength of orofacial muscles (jaw muscles)
- Decrease in pulp of vital teeth
- Increase in secondary dentine deposits
- Loss of bone support around the teeth
- Slight relocation of periodontal attachment
- Attrition of occlusal surfaces and erosion of other tooth surfaces
- Diminished taste sensation

Table 21–3.	TREATMENTS FOR XEROSTOMIA

- Avoid drugs that cause xerostomia
- Fluid intake of >2 L/day
- Frequent sips of water
- Artificial saliva: mucin-based products are better than methyl cellulose
- Sugar-free chewing gum (xylitol)
- Vitamin C or malic acid
- Parasympathomimetic drugs (e.g., pilocarpine, cevimeline, bethanechol, carbachol, pyridostigmine)
- Amifostine given with radiotherapy

(Table 21–2). Table 21–3 provides available approaches to treating xerostomia.

Some drugs also have other oral side effects, such as gingival overgrowth and glossitis. Although these are hard to counteract, the side effects need to be managed, and there is an increased need to carry out effective oral hygiene.

Figure 21–1 shows some of the most common threats to oral health in older nursing home residents, drawing attention to role of oral hygiene, which for dependent older people should be provided daily by the nursing team working in collaboration with physicians and dental services.

DENTAL CARIES AND TOOTH LOSS

Dental decay occurs because a combination of factors that make a tooth susceptible to acid attacks that occurs when the bacteria in plaque metabolize dietary sugars. The acid

attacks and demineralizes the tooth surface, causing caries. Other erosive conditions that contribute to tooth wear include:

- Alcohol abuse
- Hiatus hernia
- Duodenal ulceration
- Certain medications

Figure 21–2 shows typical wear and erosion that can present in older nursing home residents.

Recession of the gums also increases the risk of root caries, which is a particularly painful condition. Tooth loss is common in later life. Although not inevitable, tooth loss remains a clinical reality in the oldest old. However, in industrialized countries, more and more older people are retaining their natural teeth until late in life, and more are choosing tooth replacement with partial dentures than in previous generations. Table 21–4 shows the key considerations for dental care for edentulous, partially dentate, and dentate nursing home resident.

Providing oral hygiene to partially dentate residents is more complex and time consuming than cleaning an edentulous mouth with complete dentures, and this increases the time required per resident for effective oral hygiene to be achieved.

Dentures can become ill fitting, and areas around clasps on partial dentures can catch and rub, mucosa causing ulceration (Figure 21–3); these areas should be checked at regular intervals.

Caries in older people can advance considerably before the person recognizes or reports a painful tooth. This is caused by secondary dentine increasing the distance from the outer surface of the tooth to the pulp; large holes can develop within teeth before they are felt. It is therefore important that regular checkups (ideally every 6–12 months) are undertaken by a skilled practitioner such as a dental hygienist or dentist. It is important for the nursing and medical team to remember that although a resident may not display obvious signs of oral pain, such as refusal to eat, that this is no guarantee of the absence of dental problems. For dentate and partially dentate residents, the nursing home team should look out for discolored teeth, particularly around old fillings, because they are a potential sign that caries has started under the filling.

Table 21–2.	SOME OF THE MORE COMMON DRUGS THAT COMPROMISE SALIVARY SECRETIONS

Antibiotics

Anticholinergics

Anticonvulsants

Antidepressants (both SSRIs and tricyclics)

Antiemetics

Antihistamines

Antihypertensives

Antipsychotics

Some analgesics

Diuretics

Drugs for urinary incontinence

Parkinson's disease medications

Chemotherapeutic agents

Bronchodilators

SSRI, selective serotonin reuptake inhibitor.

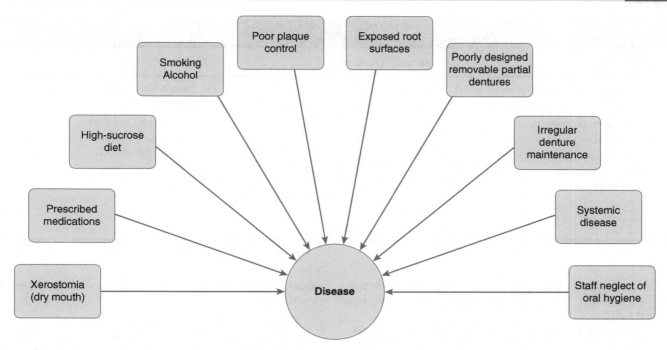

Figure 21–1. Threats to nursing home residents' oral health.

GUM DISEASE

Most adults experience mild gum disease from time to time; this is often mild and resolved with appropriate attention to oral hygiene. Signs of periodontal disease include:

- Gum recession is when the gums recede exposing the roots of teeth
- Gums bleeding when the teeth are brushed
- Red, swollen, or tender gums
- Detachment of the gums from the teeth
- Chronic bad breath or bad taste
- Mobile teeth

As the condition progresses, teeth may become loose or change their positions (Figure 21–4).

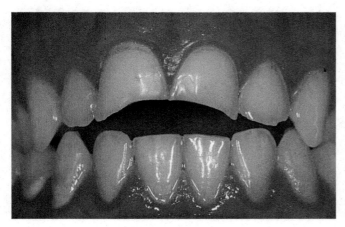

Figure 21–2. Tooth wear and erosion.

CHEWING AND SWALLOWING

There is a clear association between natural teeth and chewing ability, with dentures reducing chewing ability because of lower bite forces. Other conditions that may be associated with chewing difficulty include loose (mobile), broken, or chipped teeth; pain in the mouth; tooth sensitivity; sore "gums"; and pain in the face, jaw, temple, or front of the ear or earache. Unless these problems are acute in presentation, some of them maybe trivialized by older people, who are unaware of the potential impact on their health, including enjoyment of eating and drinking. The association between a change in dental status and low intake of essential nutrients is well established. Pain in the mouth, dry mouth (xerostomia), and inadequate dentition contribute most to chewing difficulties (dysphasia) in older people.

In the event of a person collecting food in the mouth and drooling, a practitioner with specific competencies can undertake a simple swallowing ability screening test and when appropriate refer the person to speech and language therapy. A further discussion of swallowing difficulties after stroke is found in Chapter 24.

XEROSTOMIA-DRY MOUTH

Saliva plays a central role in oral health throughout life. It has bacteriostatic and bactericidal properties that are protective. Saliva contributes to the comfort of the mouth. It is an essential lubricant, flushing the oral cavity to facilitate ingestion of food, and it acts to neutralize acids and strengthen tooth surfaces. Salivary flow and composition can be greatly altered by drugs and by disease processes. Lack of saliva can cause opportunistic

Table 21–4.   DENTAL CARE CONSIDERATIONS

Endentulous	Partially Dentate	Dentate
• Complete replacement dentures	• Removable partial denture	• Tooth maintenance
• Implant-retained prostheses	• Fixed prostheses Implant retained Tooth retained	• Minimal treatment intervention
• Removable over denture	• Stabilize existing dentition	• Effective daily oral hygiene
• Effective oral hygiene	• Over dentures or controlled progression to complete denture	• Regular inspection of mouth by registered nurse or physician
• Regular inspection of mouth by registered nurse or physician	• Effective daily oral hygiene	• Dental consultations
• Dental consulations	• Regular inspection of mouth by registered nurse or physician	
	• Dental consultations	

infections, particularly candidiasis and increased risk of periodontitis and caries, particularly at the cervical (gum) margin.

Preventing dry mouth is an important part of nursing care because the condition is uncomfortable and gives rise to swallowing difficulty and changes in taste sensation that reduce appetite. For further information about the nutritional impacts, see Chapter 14. Oral mucosa friability (susceptibility to damage) increases dramatically with dry mouth, whether it is caused by dehydration, neglect of oral hygiene, disease, medication, or other treatment side effects. Figure 21–5 shows dry mouth–associated radiotherapy and drug-induced dry mouth.

The risk of ulceration or laceration increases, and care is required from skilled practitioners to limit damage. Ulceration, no matter how small, is a painful condition, which if not treated can lead to serious problems and disease. Persistent dry mouth also makes talking difficult and makes the wearing of dentures problematic. Importantly, dry mouth makes the nursing home resident susceptible to oral infections, gum disease, caries, and halitosis (bad breath). Nursing interventions should aim to prevent dry mouth and protect lips and the corners of the external mouth from cracking:

- Regular rinses with water are important
- Regular application of Vaseline to lips is recommended

Treatments for dry mouth will vary depending on the underlying cause and overall health status of the person. For some residents, medication review can be the answer, and pharmacy advice should be sought. Hydration status should be considered, and when appropriate, staff might need to monitor fluid intake and take steps to encourage regular drinks. A minority of residents with severe problems that cannot be resolved by other interventions might benefit from artificial saliva. Salivary stimulants such as chewing gum and Slaivix pastilles may be helpful for some residents.

For residents who are close to death, perceptions of mouth comfort and appearance matter to relatives, and although the outcomes of oral hygiene are different and less determined approaches may be used, care of the mouth remains an important marker of the overall quality of nursing home care.

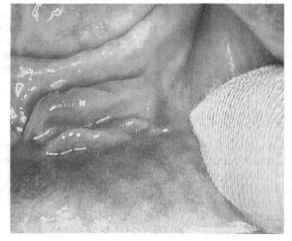
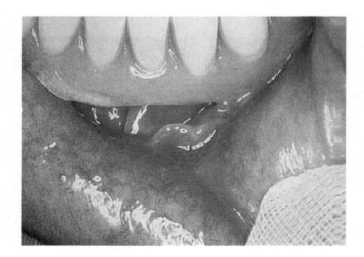

Figure 21–3. Denture-induced ulceration and hyperplasia.

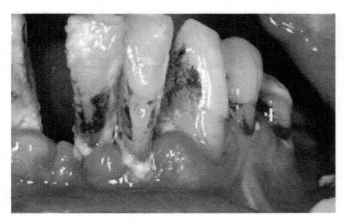

Figure 21–4. Periodontal disease.

Table 21–5.	CONDITIONS FAVORING OVERGROWTH OF *CANDIDA*

- Xerostomia
- Human immunodeficiency virus
- Infections
- Malnutrition
- Age-related immunity reduction
- Leukemia
- Denture use
- Drugs
  - Steroid inhaler use
  - Corticosteroids
  - Antibiotics
  - Chemotherapy
- Radiation therapy causes xerostomia

ORAL LESIONS

Numerous lesions can be found in the mouths of nursing home residents. The most common are candidiasis, aphthous stomatitis, and erythema migrans. Oral lesions have been linked to a variety of systemic disease, including diabetes, myocardial infarction, pneumonia, rheumatologic conditions, and dementia.

Candidiasis

Oral thrush (candidiasis) is commonly seen in nursing home residents. *Candida* is a part of the normal oral flora, and overgrowth leads to disease when any of a number of factors favoring *Candida* overgrowth is present (Table 21–5). *Candida* infection can present with burning in the mouth or may be asymptomatic. Oral candidiasis presents in three different forms:

- **Pseudomembranous:** An adherent white plaque that can be removed by scraping with a tongue blade or wiping with gauze
- **Erythematous glossitis**, which occurs on the hard palate associated with denture use (not removing dentures for sufficient time during course of day usually recommended over night; inadequate denture hygiene also implicated)
- **Angular cheilitis (perlèche)**, which consists of red scaling lesions at the corner of the mouth; this can also be caused by *Staphylococcus aureus*

The treatment is topical regimens (e.g., nystatin or clotrimazole; it is important that the regimen is sugar free; amphotericin is recommended because it is sugar free) or, if these fail, systemic antifungals (fluconazole, ketoconazole, and itraconazole). Systemic antifungals need to be used when the person develops esophageal candidiasis or topical treatments fail. For denture-related stomatitis, both the mucosa and the dentures need to be treated with a topical antifungal. The dentures need to be cleaned daily by brushing with soap and water and then allowing them to soak in sodium hypochonte solutions (1 part bleach and 10 parts water) overnight, which gives the oral mucosa time to recover.

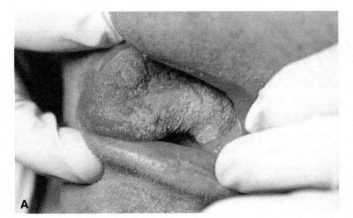
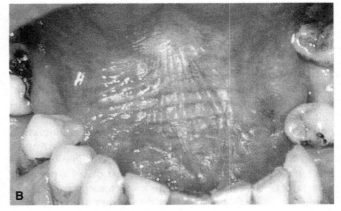

Figure 21–5. Dry mouth associated with radiotherapy (**A**) and drug induced (**B**).

OTHER SUPERFICIAL LESIONS

"Canker sores" (aphthous stomatitis) are painful ulcers covered by a yellowish membrane. Chlorhexidine mouthwash and Amlexanox paste may both play a role in treatment. Steroid gels have also been used. Severe cases need to be referred to a dermatologist.

Erythema migrans (geographic tongue) is an inflammatory condition. These lesions have erythema in the center, are elevated, and have a yellowish border. They tend to migrate on the tongue.

Lichen planus is an immunologic condition that occurs in older persons and is slightly more common in women. It can either present as white lines on the buccal mucosa (reticular form) or painful redness or ulcers (erosive form). If the lesions are painful, topical corticosteroids can be used.

When the tongue is painful, as if it has been burnt each day but appears normal, it is called a burning tongue. It can be caused by variety of conditions such as diminished salivation, nutritional deficiency, infections, and allergic reactions. Both α-lipoic acid and clonazepam may be helpful.

A smooth, shiny tongue with a pinkish background is called atrophic glossitis. It has numerous causes, including vitamin deficiencies (especially vitamin B_{12}), iron deficiency and folic acid. Other causes include oral lesions and infection. These include celiac disease, drugs, sarcoid, Sjogren's syndrome, pemphigoid pemphigus vulgaris, and candidiasis. Hairy tongue is associated in heavy smokers with poor oral hygiene. The keratin strands can be removed with a toothbrush.

Benign Oral Masses

Bony protuberances (Tori), which are seen in the midline of the roof of the palate or mandibular can be confused with malignancy. They occur in up to one third of the population. They require no treatment.

Local irritation can cause red, rapidly growing masses that bleed easily. These are called pyogenic granuloma. They occur most commonly on the gingiva.

Fibroma occur on the buccal mucosa due to chewing trauma. They are smooth nodules or polyps. They are treated by excision.

Premalignant Lesions

The potentially malignant lesions in the mouth are listed in Table 21–6.

Leukoplakia is defined by the World Health Organization as "a keratotic white patch or plaque that cannot be scraped off and cannot be characterized clinically or pathologically as any other disease." These adherent patches occur in about 2.5% of the world's population but with a major higher prevalence in India. They are associated with tobacco use and chewing guthka. The transformation to malignancy is at the rate of just over 1% per year. The factors that increase the risk of cancer are given in Table 21–7. Leukoplakia often disappears after a person stops smoking.

Table 21–6.   WORLD HEALTH ORGANIZATION'S ORAL CANCER GROUP'S POTENTIALLY MALIGNANT CONDITIONS
• Leukoplakia
• Erythroplakia
• Oral lichen planus
• Oral submucous fibrosis
• Discoid lupus erythematosus
• Palate lesions from reverse cigarette smoking
• Actinic keratosis

Erythroplakia is a "furry red patch or a bright red velvety plaque." It occurs in only one area, helping differentiate it from more diffuse lesions. On biopsy, it often is seen as "carcinoma in situ" or even invasive cancer. Three quarters of erythroplakia transform to a malignancy within 10 years.

Observation is appropriate for small premalignant lesions that do not appear malignant. If they continue to grow, surgical excision is the appropriate treatment.

Oral Cancer

Oral cancers account for 2% to 3% of all cancers in the United States. Oral cancer is much more common in older persons. Ninety percent of oral cancers are squamous cancers. The most common sites are the tongue, mouth floor, and lower lip (Figure 21–6). Screening can be done using a VELscope, which is a portable device that uses a blue light to detect abnormal tissue. Treatment is excision, often coupled with either radiation or chemotherapy. About half of persons treated for oral cancer are still alive 5 years later. Oral cancer has a high mortality rate compared with many other cancers and is relatively preventable.

ORAL HYGIENE

Given the importance of oral health and the limited capacity that many nursing home residents have in terms of self-care, it is essential that staff provide effective mouth care.

Table 21–7.   FACTORS THAT INCREASE THE RISK THAT LEUKOPLAKIA WILL BECOME CANCEROUS
• Large size
• Female
• Presence for a long time
• Nonhomogeneous kind
• Presence in nonsmoker
• Found on floor of mouth or tongue
• Epithelial dysplasia
• Concomitant candidiasis

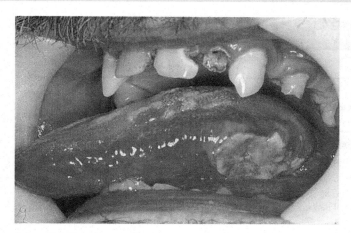

Figure 21–6. Tongue with oral cancer.

The impact of neglecting a resident's oral health and failure clean the mouth is shown in Figure 21–7.

The National Health Service Quality Improvement Scotland's (NQIS) Best Practice Statement (2005) acknowledges that nursing staff may perceive caring for a person's mouth as difficult, distressing, and intrusive. It can also be tempting in a busy shift to pay superficial attention to the mouth or delegate mouth care to the least skilled members of the care home team. However, it is important that nurses pay attention to the condition of the mouth, promptly identify changes, and take action to prevent deterioration. Furthermore, staff should know when to seek medical or specialist dental review. Nursing staff should be aware of common fungal infections and treatments and know about other common problems and the signs of oral cancer. A person with a history of smoking and heavy alcohol use is particularly at risk.

Initial assessment of the resident's mouth should include an inspection of the lips, mouth, and teeth; a good light is required, and a pen light is particularly useful. The condition of natural teeth or their absence, including loose teeth that might become dislodged and cause choking, should be noted on the resident's record. A prompt dental referral should be made because it may be safer to extract a loose tooth that can be hazardous and will impede cleaning of the mouth. If

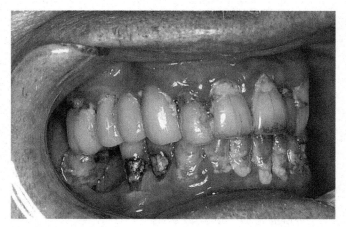

Figure 21–7. Poor oral hygiene and caries.

dentures are worn, the condition and reported comfort of the dentures should be recorded. It is wise to label dentures using a denture labeling kit because lost dentures cause no end of problems to nursing home staff! The moisture or dryness of the mouth should be inspected alongside the condition of the soft tissue, including the tongue. Abnormalities should be investigated promptly.

There is a lack of evidence and consensus on the frequency of oral care in older nursing home residents; however, in healthy younger gums, it takes just 2 days for plaque to build up and gingivitis to occur on the discontinuation of oral hygiene. Table 21–8 shows an evidence-based daily care regimen that is recommended in the United Kingdom, and is part of a Best Practice Statement on working with dependent older people to achieve good oral health (NHSQIS, 2005; available at http://www.geronurse.com/en/best-practice-statements/oral-health-best-practice-statement.asp).

Brushing with a soft toothbrush can remove plaque and debris from the surfaces and crevices of teeth. A fluoride-based toothpaste helps to prevent caries and protects gums (a full toothbrush head is recommended). For residents able to do self-care, it may be helpful to provide advice on effective techniques for toothbrushing; the bass technique, also known as the sulcular vibration technique, is recommended and requires a systematic approach. Toothbrushing should be observed, and if the resident is not able to do it effectively, then it should be carried out by a nursing aide or nurse. For residents with dexterity problems, an occupational therapist can advise on assistive devices, and sometimes simply creating a larger grip–handled toothbrush using rubber bands can be a cheap, temporary solution. The handle must be cleaned regularly and bands replaced as required.

Interdental cleaning is important for gum health, so it is important that nursing aides are skilled in using floss and other devices such as TePe brushes. Further information on interproximal cleaning techniques and devices are available at http://www.tepe.com/products/interdental-brushes/.

Flossing another person's teeth is not the easiest of procedures and can be impossible if the resident resists. Alternative regimens are often required for confused residents and those who do not find flossing acceptable.

Sometimes the presence of a relative or friend can help residents cooperate with inspections of their mouth, and some may accept mouth care by a nurse that they would otherwise refuse. Just as natural teeth need cleaning, so do dentures to reduce yeast infections such as *Candida*. Once daily (recommended at night) brushing of dentures is the minimum recommended frequency along with overnight soaking.

When brushing is impossible or for certain mouth conditions, it might be appropriate to use a mouth wash such as chlorhexidine, but the decision to use this should be made with the physician and when possible with referral to a dental specialist.

Dentures should be cleaned with liquid soap because toothpaste has abrasives added to increase cleaning power; although this is good on natural teeth, if used frequently on dentures, it will wear away the dentures, ruining their fit. Ill-fitting dentures cause mucosal problems from frictional forces as the dentures move and can create a choking hazard.

Table 21–8. EVIDENCE-BASED DAILY ORAL CARE PROTOCOL FOR DEPENDENT OLDER PEOPLE	
Care	**Rationale for Care**
Care of the Lips • Clean with water-moistened gauze and protect with a lubricant (e.g., Oralbalance gel)	To minimize the risk of dry, cracked, uncomfortable lips
Care of a Person Who Is Edentulous (No Natural Teeth) with Dentures • Ensure that dentures are marked with the person's name (using a Denture Marking Kit). • Leave dentures out at night if acceptable to the individual. • Soak plastic dentures in dilute sodium hypochlorite (e.g., 1 part Milton to 80 parts water) or chlorhexidine solution (e.g., Corsodyl 0.2%wv) for dentures with metal parts. • Clean dentures with individual brush under running water. • Rinse dentures after meals. • Use small quantity of cream or powder fixative if required. Clean off and replace before meals and clean off last thing at night.	To enable continued comfortable wearing of dentures and maintain mucosal and denture cleanliness
Care of Natural Teeth • Clean twice daily and after meals with fluoridated toothpaste and a soft toothbrush. • Provide additional plaque control if required using Corsodyl mouthwash or spray or gel. • Enable residents who use a powered toothbrush to continue with it. (Appropriate training is essential before staff use powered toothbrushes for others.)	To prevent dental decay and gum disease To maintain oral comfort To reduce risk of damage to gums and oral mucosa
Care of Oral Mucosa • Inspect in a good light. • Report any unusual appearances. • Clean with water-moistened gauzed fingers, water-moistened sponge sticks, a TePe special care toothbrush, or a baby toothbrush.	To provide a moist, comfortable, fresh environment and reduce the risk of infection
Care of a Person with Xerostomia (Dry Mouth) • Provide oral lubrication in the form of sips of water or spray or use mucin-based artificial saliva and use high-dose fluoride toothpaste supplied by dental services.	To ensure regular removal of debris and moistening of the oral soft tissues To prevent rapid development of dental caries

Reproduced with permission of Health Improvement Scotland (formerly Quality Improvement Scotland).

KEY POINTS

1. Oral candidiasis is a common, treatable condition in nursing homes, and all staff should be taught to recognize it.
2. Premalignant lesions (e.g., leukoplakia and erythroplakia) need to be examined for and carefully watched in nursing home residents.
3. Oral cancer occurs in 2% to 3% of older persons and can be successfully treated with surgery if diagnosed early.
4. Adequate oral hygiene is important to the overall health of older nursing home residents through the prevention of opportunistic and commensal infection.
5. Denture hygiene is as important as natural teeth hygiene; dentures should be scrupulously cleaned.

SUGGESTED READINGS

Gonsalves WC, Chi AC, Neville BW. Common oral lesions: part I. Superficial mucosal lesions. *Am Fam Physician.* 2007;75:501-507.

Gonsalves WC, Chi AC, Neville BW. Common oral lesions: part II. Masses and neoplasia. *Am Fam Physician.* 2007;75:509-512.

Gonsalves WC, Wrightson AS, Henry RG. Common oral conditions in older persons. *Am Fam Physician.* 2008;78:845-852.

Haumschild MS, Haumschild RJ. The importance of oral health in long-term care. *J Am Med Dir Assoc.* 2009;10(9):667-671.

Donnelly LR, MacEntee MI. Social interactions, body image and oral health among institutionalised frail elders: an unexplored relationship. *Gerodontology.* 2012;29:e28-e33.

Lin K. Cochrane briefs: screening for the early detection and prevention of oral cancer. *Am Fam Physician.* 2011;83(9):1047.

Matear DW, Locker D, Stephens M, Lawrence HP. Associations between xerostomia and health status indicators in the elderly. *J R Soc Health.* 2006;126:79-85.

Nair DR, Pruthy R, Pawar U, Chaturvedi P. Oral cancer: premalignant conditions and screening—an update. *J Cancer Res Ther.* 2012;8:57-66.

Müller F, Schimmel M. Tooth loss and dental prostheses in the oldest old. *Eur Geriatr Med.* 2010;1(4):239-243.

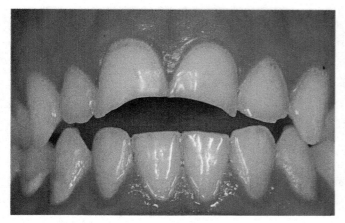

Plate 1. Tooth wear and erosion.

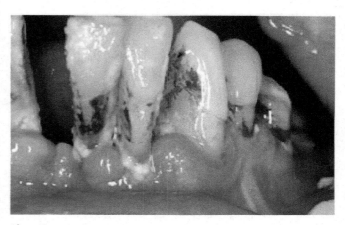

Plate 3. Periodontal disease.

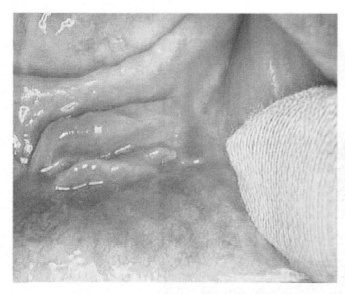

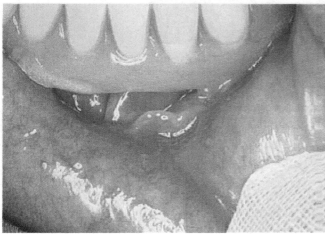

Plate 2. Denture-induced ulceration and hyperplasia.

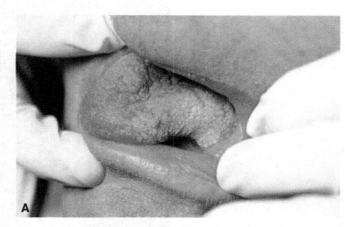

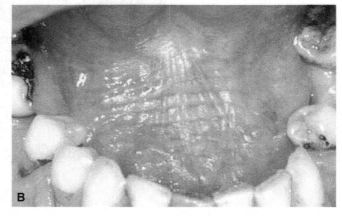

Plate 4. Dry mouth associated with radiotherapy (**A**) and drug induced (**B**).

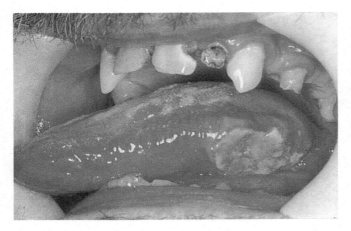

Plate 5. Tongue with oral cancer.

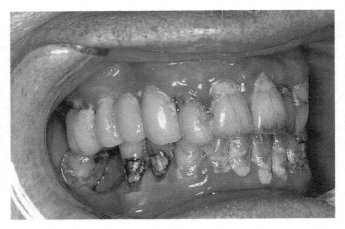

Plate 6. Poor oral hygiene and caries.

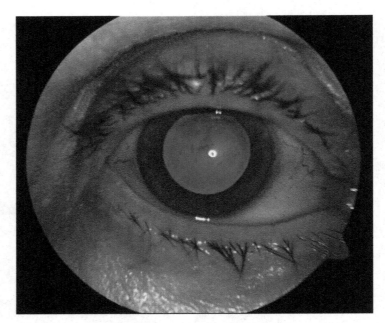

Plate 7. View of a 1+ nuclear sclerotic cataract. In cataract-free people, the lens is equally optically clear in all areas. With cataract, you will see what appears to be a circle in the lens, and the lens is slightly more opaque within the circle. That is the edge of the lens nucleus. As the nucleus becomes more sclerotic, the light diffracts differently through it, allowing one to see the nuclear edge.

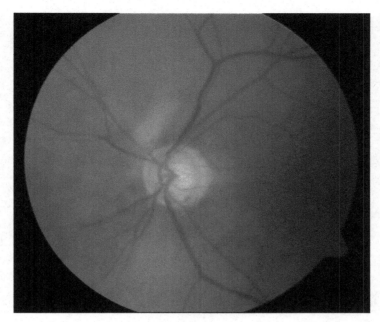

Plate 8. Glaucoma. This is a photo of the left optic nerve where about 60% of the nerve has been "cupped" by glaucoma. To the untrained eye, the pale area in the center of the nerve is the area of concern. The experienced examiner would note that the area where the vessels enter is also involved. The key point is that the pale area is the sclera. It should not be visible because the nerve should be filled with nerve fibers. The upper limit of normal for the size of that pale area in the human eye is about 30% of the size of the optic nerve. Chronic elevated eye pressure (glaucoma) has crushed the nerve fibers, leaving this enlarged cup.

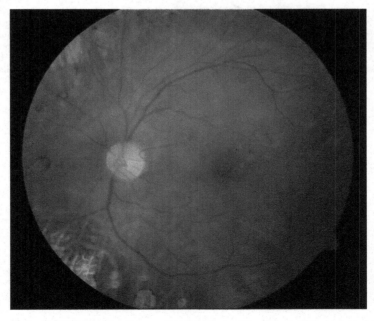

Plate 9. Diabetic retina 1 year after diabetic laser treatment. The pigmented areas at the edge of the photo represent the laser treatment scars. There may be some residual abnormal vessels within the optic nerve at its 9:00 o'clock margin, but without angiography, it would be difficult to confirm their presence.

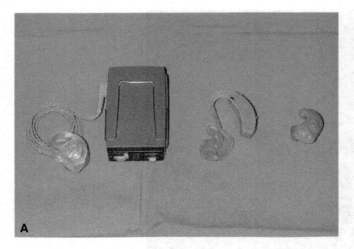

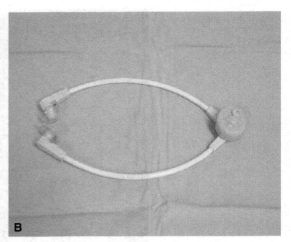

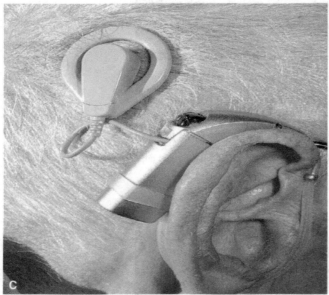

Plate 10. Hearing aids and other amplification devices. (**A**) From left to right. Body-worn hearing aid with ear mold, behind-the-ear analogue hearing aid, and in-the-ear analogue hearing aid. (**B**) A simple communicator (pocket talker) with central amplifier and volume control. (**C**) Cochlear implant. (Permission granted by patient. Photo courtesy of the MRC Institute of Hearing Research, Glasgow, UK.)

Nicol R, Petrina Sweeney M, McHugh S, Bagg J. Effectiveness of health care worker training on the oral health of elderly residents of nursing homes. *Community Dent Oral Epidemiol.* 2005;33:115-124.

Pearson L, Hutton J. A controlled trial to compare the ability of foam swabs and toothbrushes to remove dental plaque. *J Adv Nurs.* 2002; 39(5):489-489.

Porter SR, Scully C, Hegarty AM. An update of the etiology and management of xerostomia. *Oral Surg Oral Med Oral Pathol Oral Radiol Endod.* 2004;97(1):28-46.

Reamy BV, Derby R, Bunt CW. Common tongue conditions in primary care. *Am Fam Physician.* 2010;81:627-634.

Scottish Department of Health. *Caring for Smiles Guide for Trainers: Better Oral Health for Dependent Older People*. Scottish Department of Health. http://www.healthscotland.com/documents/4169.aspx. Published 2010. Accessed September 9, 2012.

Ship JA, Fischer DJ. The relationship between dehydration and parotid salivary gland function in young and older healthy adults. *J Gerontol A Biol Sci Med Sci.* 1997;52(5):310-319.

Singh K S, Brennan D. Chewing disability in older adults attributable to tooth loss and other oral conditions. *Gerodontology.* 2012;29: 106-110.

Sjogren P, Nilsson E, Forsell M, et al. A systematic review of the preventive effect of oral hygiene on pneumonia and respiratory tract infection in elderly people in hospitals and nursing homes: effect estimates and methodological quality of randomized controlled trials. *J Am Geriatr Soc.* 2008;56:2124–30.

Sreebny LM, Schwartz SS. A reference guide to drugs and dry mouth, 2nd edition, *Gerodontology.* 1997;14:33–47.

Sweeney MP, Williams C, Kennedy C, et al. Oral health care and status of elderly care home residents in Glasgow. *Community Dent Health.* 2007;24:37-42.

Yoneyama T, Yshida M, Ohrui T, et al. Oral care reduces pneumonia in older patients in nursing homes. *J Am Geriatr Soc.* 2002;50: 430-433.

MULTIPLE CHOICE QUESTIONS

21.1   Which oral lesion has a red center with a yellow border and migrates on the tongue?

a. Aphthous stomatitis
b. Lichen planus
c. Candidiasis
d. Erythema migrans
e. Erythroplakia

21.2   Which of these is *not* a premalignant lesion in the mouth?

a. Actinic keratosis
b. Erythroplakia
c. Erythema migrans
d. Discoid lupus erythematosus
e. Leukoplakia

21.3   Which of the following is true concerning oral cancers?

a. Most oral cancers are adenocarcinomas.
b. The 5-year survival rate for oral cancers is more than 70%.
c. The tongue is the most common site for oral cancer.
d. Oral cancers account for 10% of all cancers in the developed world.
e. Chemotherapy is not used to treat oral cancers.

21.4   Which of the following is not an age-related change?

a. Loss of mass and strength of orofacial muscles (jaw muscles)
b. Decrease in pulp of vital teeth
c. Teeth grinding
d. Increase in secondary dentine deposits
e. Loss of bone support around the teeth
f. Erosion of other tooth surfaces

21.5   Programs of effective oral hygiene in nursing homes could prevent one in 10 deaths from pneumonia in nursing homes.

a. True
b. False

21.6   Which of the following approaches to dentures care is a recommended practice?

a. Daily brushing with a fluoride toothpaste
b. Nightly soaking in chlorhexidine solution (e.g., Corsodyl 0.2%wv)
c. Soaking in dilute sodium hypochlorite
d. Rinse under running water after meals

21.7   Which of the following is the key reason to explain why an older nursing home resident with intact cognition may not report toothache when he or she has dental carries?

a. Fear of the dentist
b. Other more important things to complain about
c. Dental carries are not painful
d. Secondary dentine growth forms a protective coating
e. Dry mouth alters pain reception

Chapter 22

COMMUNICATION CHALLENGES: VISION, HEARING, AND SPEECH

Losses of visual and auditory acuity are common age-related experiences, and the consequences for an individual range from that of mild nuisance to severely disabling conditions that restrict communication, independence in activities of living, mobilization, and quality of life. There is also a spectrum of speech and language disorders arising from long-term conditions such as stroke and dementia that are relatively common in the nursing home population. For nursing home practitioners intent on delivering resident-centered care and promoting resident well-being, strategies to ameliorate the impact of communication disorders must be high on the agenda. To do so requires a basic understanding of communication theory, an ability to identify and manage underlying causes, access to specialist services, and a commitment to maximizing effective communication. This requires a range of knowledge and competencies, reciprocity, knowing the resident as an individual, and good humor. It is not unusual for one or two members of the staff to be able to communicate well with a particular resident when other members of the team fail. Reasons for this vary, and often it is the nursing aide or team member who spends most time in direct caregiving who has the greatest opportunity to become a skilled communication partner for an individual. In these situations, it is worth noting details within the care plan and observing how this staff member communicates with the resident to assist others to replicate approaches.

Communication is a complex process that involves sending, receiving, interpreting, and responding to signals. Effective communication requires sensory, motor, cognitive, psychological, and social functional integrity. Human communication serves many functions, and for older people with diminishing opportunities for self-realization, the ability to communicate with staff, family and friends, and fellow residents is a prerequisite for well-being. Figure 22–1 shows a range of resident communication needs extending from comfort and reassurance through information and advice.

Conceptual models remind us that the opportunity and desire to communicate are critical within the communication chain. It therefore follows that having something or someone that attracts the resident's attention is the starting point of the cycle of communication, coupled with the resident's desire to engage with the stimulus. There is nothing more disengaging than sitting in the same chair every day seeing the same people around you falling asleep because of lack of meaningful activity. Lack of purpose and absence of people to talk to and who have something interesting to say, unfortunately, typifies daily life for many nursing home residents.

There are a number of barriers that impede nursing home residents' opportunity to communication as shown in Table 22–1.

In addition to the barriers listed in Table 22–1, long-term conditions such as stroke and Parkinson's disease are associated with speech and language impairments.

The three most common speech and language disorders affecting older nursing home residents are:

- Disorders of reception
- Disorders of perception
- Disorders of articulation

Problems of reception are exacerbated by sensory impairments (vision and hearing), anxiety, and alterations in conscious level. Perceptual difficulties arise from conditions such as stroke, dementia, and delirium. Articulation is compounded by neurologic conditions such as stroke and Parkinson's disease and advanced chronic respiratory conditions such as chronic obstructive airways disease and asthma.

Aphasia (fluent and nonfluent) and dysphasia, which are common after stroke, have a profound impact on communication and psychological well-being. The extent of the impairment depends on the location and severity of the stroke. The effects of aphasia range from an inability to speak coherently to difficulties interpreting and comprehending spoken words or writing. Whereas persons with nonfluent aphasia speak slowly and require effort to find words, persons with fluent aphasia talk without problem, but their language has no meaning. Wernicke's aphasia is a fluent aphasia together with problems with auditory comprehension.

Persons with memory or attention deficits develop cognitive-communicative disorders. These persons have disorganized conversation, may speak in a monotone, confabulate, fail to impart appropriate emotional tone and gestures to their speech, focus on irrelevant details, or have tangential conversations.

Damage to Broca's area results in apraxia of speech. These persons can produce words but cannot appropriately create words. Thus, they may ask for a cup of "toffee"

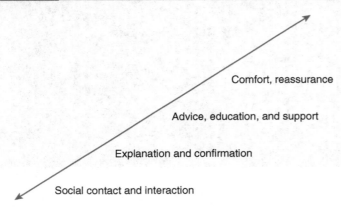

Figure 22–1. Range of resident communication needs.

instead of a cup of "coffee." Other conditions that alter the ability to speak clearly include breathing disorders, damage to the vocal cords, tracheotomy, tumors, damage to the recurrent laryngeal nerves, and conversion voice impairment caused by psychological disorders. Hoarseness occurs from excessive screaming or inappropriately clearing one's throat.

Dysarthria compromises the intelligibility of speech by poor muscle coordination and difficulties in articulation, phonation, and resonance (the quality of sounds produced, including loudness). Residents with voice tremors or slow or hesitant speech should be referred to speech and language therapists for assessment and management.

Talking Mats (http://www.talkingmats.com/) is a deceptively simple communication framework based on easily recognizable images and symbols that enable people to express themselves. The resident sorts a small number of cards to indicate things he or she likes or dislikes and so on. This research-based framework has been developed for use with people with communication difficulties arising through stroke, dementia, learning disability, and motor neuron disease. Following training practitioners can use the Talking Mat kits to work with older residents to discuss and discover their views and choices in subjects such as eating and food preferences and other complex

Table 22–1.	EXAMPLES OF COMMUNICATION BARRIERS WITHIN NURSING HOMES

- Culture that creates an impoverished communication environment
- Lack of active management of communication problems
- Physical environment: background noise, poor acoustics, inadequate lighting, lack of communication aids, seating arrangements that impede conversation between residents
- Nonuse or failure to maintain hearing aids
- Nonuse of glasses or dirty glasses
- Lack of skilled communication partners (staff, visitors, residents)
- Lack of community engagement
- Lack of meaningful activity

topics that would otherwise be too difficult for the person with impaired communication to express their views. Photographs of the "mats" can be captured and pasted into a resident's record and assist in the creation of person centered care planning.

The availability of iPads with appropriate communication programs is greatly improving the ability of persons with speech problems to communicate.

Nurses and nursing aides may be among the first to identify speech and language problems in residents and to witness changes; deterioration should be reported promptly to senior practitioners, who will collaboratively determine the need for urgent physician review. Speech and language problems are frustrating, embarrassing, and demoralizing, and specialist referrals should be made soon after admission to commence or continue rehabilitative interventions and to optimize communication opportunities and reduce disabilities when no further improvement is anticipated.

Thankfully for many nursing home residents with age-related hearing and visual problems, there are effective ways to reduce disability and maximize communication opportunity. Corrective glasses and sound amplification devices are well-known technologies that are tolerated by many nursing home residents but may be rejected by people with advanced dementia. Although some ocular conditions have potential serious consequences, it is still possible to treat some of the most serious eye conditions if treatment is initiated early.

Regardless of the cause, visual impairment is likely to have some impact on communication, for example:

- Difficulties in finding one's way
- Reduced ability to read or write
- Reduced ability to independently use a telephone
- Reduced confidence interacting with others, particularly strangers
- Reduced ability to interpret nonverbal audio cues.
- Exaggerates problems following conversations in people with impaired hearing

In different ways, hearing impairments also restrict communication:

- Restriction of functional communication and ability to follow conversation
- Difficulty locating noises and "alert sounds"
- Listening requires increased effort "listening fatigue"
- Slower auditory processing and delayed responses
- Difficulties with phone calls

All of these communication impacts make it difficult for the nursing home resident to build relationships with staff, to fully participate in shared decision making about their care, and to express their identity and character. These difficulties make it challenging to deliver resident-centered care and frustrate opportunities for personal autonomy. Apart from the relational impacts and associated frustrations and isolation, such sensory declines limit enjoyment of recreational activities and entertainments such as reading, watching television, and listening to music. These impacts have wide-reaching psychosocial

Table 22–2. COMMUNICATION STRATEGIES FOR RESIDENTS WITH HEARING AND VISUAL DISABILITIES	
Visual Problems	**Hearing Problems**
Ensure spectacles are of a current prescription and are appropriate (distance or readers) and that they are clean and belong to the resident who is wearing them.	Ensure personal hearing aids are of a current prescription and that they are clean and belong to the resident who is wearing them.
Provide glare-free or adequate-strength lighting.	Check that hearing aids are working properly, are switched on, and are correctly inserted into the ear. If the hearing aid is whistling, it is due to feedback of amplified sound into the microphone, and its cause needs to be identified and rectified. Common causes are wax in the ear canal, preventing a snug fit, or split tubing, which require replacement.
Reduce potentially confusing moving visual stimuli, including shadows, or move to a calmer, low-stimuli area.	Reduce background noise, turn off radios and TVs, close doors, or move to quiet surroundings.
Provide color contrast signs and large, clear signage.	Ensure your mouth can be seen to enable lip reading when speaking and do not shout because this distorts mouth shape during word formation. Make sure there is sufficient light on your face.
Orientate the person to his or her environment and remove clutter and trip hazards.	Use nonverbal cues, facial expressions, and gestures to reinforce meaning.
Stand or sit within the resident's visual field.	Pause between sentences to allow time for slower auditory processing and stop to check understanding. If misunderstood, rephrase.
Identify yourself on arrival and make it clear when you are leaving.	Supplement spoken with written information.
Attract the person's attention when you wish to talk and use touch within communication in accord with cultural sensitivities.	Gain the person's attention before speaking but be aware that you may surprise residents who do not hear your arrival or see you. Use touch within communication as appropriate.

consequences, increasing the sense of dependency, loneliness, and low mood. There is little research-based evidence on the personal impacts of hearing and visual disabilities on the lives of nursing home residents, but the small studies that exist concur that the impacts are detrimental, hinder resident-to-resident interactions, lower self-esteem, and reduce quality of life. Strategies to communicate with residents with hearing and visual disabilities are shown in Table 22–2.

AGE-RELATED EYE CHANGES

Decline in visual acuity is a common age-related change associated with pupillary miosis (pupil contraction), reduced lens transparency, decreased corneal transparency, and loss of retinal cones. Although refractive errors associated with presbyopia are improved with corrective lenses, eye glasses do not remedy all of the age-related ocular conditions.

Studies indicate that the normal visual field decreases by approximately 1 to 3 degrees per decade, the cumulative result for someone in their seventies and eighties is between 20 to 30 degrees visual field reduction. Visual field reduction is a major cause of accidents in older people along with slower adaptation to dark–light contrasts, which can be a particular problem for residents with nocturia. It has also been estimated that older people require as much as three times more light to see clearly compared with younger adults, yet many older people develop sensitivity to glare and delayed glare recovery. Other age-related changes include floaters, flashing lights, and dry eyes. Several studies have demonstrated that the levels of lighting in both European and U.S. nursing homes are inadequate, and this is thought to be associated with a higher risk of residents falling (see Chapter 18).

Visual impairment is variably defined as best corrected vision worse than 20/40 or worse than 20/50 but better than 20/200, the threshold for legal blindness. Prevalence of vision impairment increases with age and ranges from 1% in persons from 65 to 69 years of age to 17% in persons older than 80 years.

For many nursing home residents, visual impairment coexists with other disabilities. The prevalence of dual visual and hearing impairments in older people has been estimated at 5.5% in the 70- to 79-year age group and 24.8% in the 80 years and older age group. Some commentators believe this to be an underestimation because of a lack of robust studies. Dual vision and hearing impairments are common in residents who fall and in older people with hip fracture. Some evidence suggests that visual impairment and memory impairment are closely linked because of the role played by the cerebral cortex in attention, memory, and processing of visual images. Several studies have found that older people with visual impairment are three times more likely to be depressed than those without sight problems.

Screening for Visual Problems

A recent systematic review reveals that 20% to 50% of older people have undetected reduced vision, but the majority of these visual problems (refractive errors or cataract) are correctable.

Visual function in older people is not fully described by high-contrast visual acuity (e.g., the conventional letter chart test) or by self-reports of visual difficulties. Other tests that may be relevant include visual field testing, low-contrast visual acuity, contrast sensitivity, and stereoacuity. The literature suggests that quite basic tests may be useful to detect uncorrected refractive errors and cataracts. However, there is a dearth of robust research with dependent older people and nursing home populations. Screening questions can be used to elicit self-perceived problems with vision. However, compared with a visual acuity test or ophthalmologic examination, they are not accurate for identifying residents with vision impairment. A visual acuity test (e.g., the Snellen eye chart) is the usual method for visual acuity screening in older adults. In the United States and Europe, a standardized test of visual acuity is the usual test for identifying the presence of vision impairment. It assesses a person's ability to recognize, from a prespecified distance (typically 20 feet), letters of different sizes arranged in rows. Compared with a detailed ophthalmologic examination, visual acuity screening tests are not accurate in the diagnosis of any underlying visual condition. Because of the high prevalence of eye problems in later life, we recommend that nursing home residents are screened on admission using self-reported methods that include discussion and observation of the resident's visual function with corrective spectacles, have access to professional eye care, and are offered annual screenings by a qualified ophthalmologist. In some countries, eye services provide an outreach service, visiting nursing homes to assess resident and prescribe corrective lenses. Alternatively, arrangements should be made to enable residents to visit opticians and eye clinics as appropriate.

Common Eye Conditions

Presbyopia, literally "old eyes," is the most common age-related ocular condition. It arises through normal aging changes in the crystalline lens that reduce the ability of the eye to focus at near distances. It is easily corrected by the prescription of reading glasses.

Dry eye is a common problem with increasing age. It can be caused by reduced tear production, poor tear quality, or rapid tear evaporation. It is frequently associated with rheumatoid arthritis and is one of the triumvirate of signs in Sjögren's syndrome. A variety of medications can cause dry eyes (Table 22–3). Treatment is normally by the use of artificial tear solution. Preservative-free artificial tears are of use in persons who need them more than five times a day. Lipid-containing tears are useful in persons with meibomian gland dysfunction. Hypotonic tears or those with compatible solutes should be used for persons with a hypertonic tear film. A major component of dry eye syndrome when it becomes a moderate problem is caused by inflammation. This should be treated with 0.05%

Table 22–3.   MEDICATIONS THAT CAUSE DRY EYES
• Antidepressants
• Antihistamines
• Antihypertensives
• Oxybutynin or tolterodine
• Opiates
• Diuretics
• Antipsychotics

cyclosporine drops. Oral omega-3-fatty acids can be helpful in evaporative eye disease. For some with very severe dry eyes, punctate plugs can be put in the lacrimal puncti of the lower eyelids.

Table 22–4 provides an overview of dry eye in terms of resident-reported or observed outcomes and management options. Residents may complain that corrective glasses are no use because of blurring of vision: they may rub their eyes or have a tendency to close their eyes. Moreover, in residents who appear withdrawn or apathetic, the possibility of dry eye should be investigated. In nursing homes with air conditioning or with a warm and dry internal atmosphere, dry eye can be exaggerated, and strategies to humidify the air can be helpful. A bowl of fresh water placed daily on a shelf in a resident's room can be sufficient to alleviate mild forms of dry eye that are irritated by dry air conditions.

Ectropion (outward turning of the eyelid) or *entropion* (inward turning of the eyelid) are problems that occur because of age-related deterioration of the connective tissue in the eyelids and can cause exposure and mechanical damage to the ocular surface. Surgical intervention is indicated in severe cases of either ectropion or entropion.

Cataract is a common age-related change in the eye and a major global cause of blindness (Figure 22–2). Bilateral cataracts are common, but sometimes asymmetry occurs. In a cataract, the lens material becomes opaque, preventing the formation of a clear image and causing blurred vision. Cataract development is painless, development is often

Table 22–4.   THE EXPERIENCE AND MANAGEMENT OF DRY EYE IN NURSING HOMES
• **Experience:** Resident reports eye discomfort (feels gritty, stabbing sensations, redness, irritation, photophobia, tired eyes) and has mild to severe blurred vision.
• **Response:** Resident closes eyes, has sleepiness or fatigue, and shows apathetic and withdrawn behaviors.
• **Assessment:** Self-report, tear deficiency, ocular surface health
• **Treatment**   ▪ Artificial tears   ▪ 0.05% Cyclosporine eye drops   ▪ Punctate plugs   ▪ Oral omega-3-fatty acids
• **Environmental:** Adjust humidity.

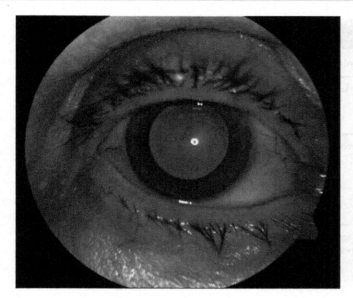

Figure 22–2. View of a 1+ nuclear sclerotic cataract. In cataract-free people, the lens is equally optically clear in all areas. With cataract, you will see what appears to be a circle in the lens, and the lens is slightly more opaque within the circle. That is the edge of the lens nucleus. As the nucleus becomes more sclerotic, the light diffracts differently through it, allowing one to see the nuclear edge. (Courtesy of Dr. Stephen Feman, MD, Department of Ophthalmology, Saint Louis University, with permission.)

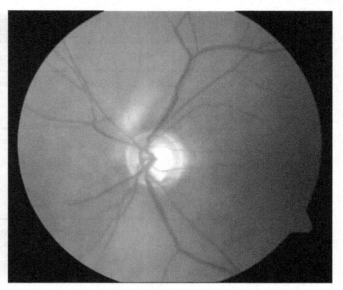

Figure 22–3. Glaucoma. This is a photo of the left optic nerve where about 60% of the nerve has been "cupped" by glaucoma. To the untrained eye, the pale area in the center of the nerve is the area of concern. The experienced examiner would note that the area where the vessels enter is also involved. The key point is that the pale area is the sclera. It should not be visible because the nerve should be filled with nerve fibers. The upper limit of normal for the size of that pale area in the human eye is about 30% of the size of the optic nerve. Chronic elevated eye pressure (glaucoma) has crushed the nerve fibers, leaving this enlarged cup. (Courtesy of Dr. Stephen Feman, MD, Department of Ophthalmology, Saint Louis University, with permission.)

insidious, and older people may not report symptoms until the cataract is fairly advanced or "ripe." Surgical removal is the only treatment option but is straightforward, and 90% of patients experience visual improvement, achieving visual acuity greater than 20/40. Results from studies in adults older than 85 years are mixed, but best practice guidance suggests that cataract surgery is beneficial for all older persons.

Primary open-angle glaucoma is an insidious disease that causes irreversible damage to the optic nerve head, which is asymptomatic until significant visual loss has occurred (Figure 22–3). The disease becomes increasingly prevalent with age but can in most cases be treated successfully with prostaglandin or β-blocker eye drops (or both). Residents with suspected glaucoma should be referred to a specialist eye clinic for assessment and treatment. A resident with an acute painful red eye with decreasing vision has an ophthalmologic emergency suggesting acute closed-angle glaucoma. Table 22–5 provides the medications used to treat glaucoma. Prostaglandin analogs are mostly the first choice. Unfortunately, there is a tendency for optometrists and ophthalmologists to use multiple different eye drops rather than optimizing one drug. This leads to polypharmacy. A clinical pathway detailing evidence-based diagnostics and treatment options for glaucoma is available at http://pathways.nice.org.uk/pathways/glaucoma.

People with diabetes are at increased risk for developing glaucoma and cataracts. *Diabetic retinopathy* is the third leading cause of adult blindness (Figure 22–4). It is estimated that individuals with diabetes are 25 times more likely than the general population to lose their sight. High glucose levels weaken blood vessels in the retina, resulting in leakage of fluid and capillary occlusion. This results in

swelling of the retina in the hypoperfusion of retinal areas; this is called nonproliferative diabetic retinopathy. The retinal hypoperfusion leads to the secretion of vascular growth factors and retinal neovascularization; this stage is called proliferative diabetic retinopathy. Complications related to proliferative diabetic retinopathy are vitreous hemorrhage, retinal detachment, and neovascular glaucoma, which is a very poor prognosis. Retinopathy results in poor visual acuity, changes in color perception, scotomas, glare disability, and problems with contrast sensitivity and dark–light adaptation. Glucose control with a HbA1C of 7% reduces the development of retinopathy. All residents with diabetes should have a dilated eye examination yearly. Treatments of diabetic retinopathy consists firstly in the treatment of systemic factors (glucose control and treatment of arterial hypertension) and secondly in peripheral or central retinal laser, intravitreal injections of antibodies directed against vascular growth factor, and vitreoretinal surgery.

Red eyes that are itchy or painful are a common problem in the nursing home. The major causes are listed in Table 22–6.

Aging can also affect the neural components of the eye. Apoptosis of photoreceptor cells at the fovea, caused by the action of free radicals, leads to *age-related macular degeneration* (AMD) and a reduction in detailed vision. This disease is progressive and currently untreatable, although lifestyle factors such as stopping smoking and dietary supplements are thought to slow the progression of the condition. There are two forms of AMD, dry and wet. The acute form of the disease (wet AMD) is aggressive and causes a

Table 22–5.   DRUGS USED TO TREAT GLAUCOMA[a]

Class	Drugs	Mechanism of Action	Side Effects
Prostaglandin analogs	Latanoprost Bimatoprost Travoprost	Increase uveoscleral outflow	Darkening of iris Increased growth of eyelashes
Topical β-adrenergic blockers	Timolol Levobunolol Carteolol Betaxolol Metipranolol	Lower production of aqueous humor	Bradycardia Hypotension Bronchospasm
Topical α_2-adrenergic agonists	Apraclonidine Brimonidine	Reduce aqueous humor secretion and increase uveoscleral outflow	Dry nose Dry mouth Allergies Red conjunctiva Visual disturbances
Carbonic anhydrase inhibitors	Brinzolamide Dorzolamide	Lower production of aqueous humor	Eye discomfort Altered taste Headache Anorexia Urolithiasis
Cholinergic agonists	Pilocarpine Carbachol	Increase uveoscleral outflow	Myopia Impaired night vision Multiple daily dosing

[a]To reduce systemic absorption, the finger should press gently on the inside corner of the eyelid to produce nasolacrimal occlusion, and the eyelids should be kept closed for 30 seconds after instillation of the drop.

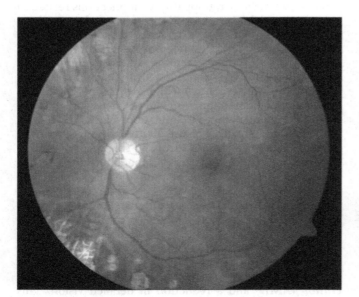

Figure 22–4. Diabetic retina 1 year after diabetic laser treatment. The pigmented areas at the edge of the photo represent the laser treatment scars. There may be some residual abnormal vessels within the optic nerve at its 9:00 o'clock margin, but without angiography, it would be difficult to confirm their presence. (Courtesy of Dr. Stephen Feman, MD, Department of Ophthalmology, Saint Louis University, with permission.)

rapid reduction of vision over a period of weeks and needs urgent investigation and treatment by an ophthalmologist within 1 to 2 weeks after the onset of symptoms. Exudative (wet) AMD accounts for 90% of blindness associated with macular degeneration. Treatments for exudative (or wet) AMD include intravitreal injections of vascular endothelial growth factor inhibitors and other treatments such as laser photocoagulation and verteporfin photodynamic therapy. Antioxidant vitamins and minerals are treatments for dry AMD, but evidence about their effectiveness is limited.

Table 22–6.   CAUSES OF A RED EYE

Conjunctivitis (viral or bacterial)

Scleritis

Corneal ulcers

Uveitis

Allergic conjunctivitis

Foreign bodies

Subconjunctival hemorrhage

Glaucoma (acute closed angle)

Other changes with age include reduced *contrast sensitivity*, poor *dark–light adaptation*, and *reductions in visual field*. These increase the risk of falls and may lead to inactivity through fear in older people.

Strategies to Enhance Low Vision

Visual performance can be enhanced through use of contrast, color, light, and size. Task illumination is generally recommended for older people because the decreased light reaching the retina is thought to cause poorer performance, It is important, however, to avoid glare. For nursing home residents, it is helpful to determine the activities that are bothersome to the individual and personalize solutions. The use of colored plates on a contrasting table cloth can assist people to locate their meals. Use of light decor on walls and contrasting floor colors and door frames can assist visually impaired resident to mobilize independently. It is important to avoid glossy floor surfaces because reflected light can make it difficult for people to judge changes in depth or steps.

Low-vision optical strategies include spectacles with corrective lens and handheld or stand magnifiers with or without internal illumination. For some residents, a variety of technologies that display magnified text or images on a screen can be useful, and these can be connected to a TV magnifier or computer. Low-vision services are provided by many eye clinics, and when appropriate, low-vision experts should assess the residents with severe problems within the environment of the nursing home to advise on the most appropriate adaptations and devices. For older persons who are registered blind, a nursing home specializing in the care of residents who partially sighted or blind might be a preferred option.

HEARING AND LISTENING

Hearing and listening are integral to communication that involves speech or other sounds, and it is important that nursing home staff appreciate the reasons why a resident may sometimes appear to hear and other times do not. In the specialist literature, the term "patchy auditory performance" may be used. In the nursing home staff room, this translates into such statements as "he hears you when he wants to hear." Interestingly, staff rarely comment that a blind resident is someone who sees you when they want to do so! There is much stigma associated with hearing problems, and many older people incorrectly link hearing changes with senility.

Hearing is a passive activity in that an individual's ability to hear is a given; listening, on the other hand, is an active and dynamic process. It is important for nursing home staff to appreciate the difference between hearing and listening (Table 22–7) and create the conditions to enhance a resident's capacity to listen and engage in conversation.

A nursing home resident's capacity to listen and his or her motivation to engage in the act of listening depend on a number of factors. Sound perception depends on lower level sensory as well as higher level cognitive processes, slower neural conduction time, and the presence of competing noise stimuli reduce the ability to discriminate

Table 22–7.	A COMPARISON OF HEARING AND LISTENING
Hearing	**Listening**
• Hearing is a passive activity	• Listening is active; there is an element of choice
• Minimal control	• Requires concentration, effort, and energy
	• Effort related to ability to hear

words and auditory cues, and difficulties are exaggerated with declining memory and cognitive deterioration.

Attentiveness and apathy, for example, influence how alert and responsive a resident is to sounds and how he or she tunes in and focuses on interesting ones and dismiss sounds that have become dull and monotonous stimuli. Disinterest in the activities or people around them, tiredness, distractions, and low mood all make residents disinclined to listen. Similarly, if a resident feels excluded from a conversation, he or she may appear not to listen as he or she exercises choice over intentional listening.

There are many occasions in nursing homes when levels of background noise create disabling listening circumstances for residents with hearing impairment; this means that greater effort is required to understand what is being said, and the work of listening becomes harder. A common complaint of older residents is that sometimes people, including nurses and physicians, exclude them from conversations or expect them to communicate in a disabling listening environment. It is important for all nursing home practitioners to recognize the disabling effects of the listening environment and consider simple interventions that will assist residents to participate in conversations, particularly when it is about their own treatment and care plans.

Optimal Listening Environments

The environment in which we exist and communicate has important implications for both our ability to hear and desire to listen. It is important to appreciate the complexity of the listening environment and the considerations necessary to create an enabling environment for residents with age-related hearing problems. For example, the intentional sounds that are directed to an individual such as talking with staff often compete with auditory signals from unintentional sound or background noise such as radios, air conditioning, groups of staff chatting, and external traffic noise. Unless background noise is low or absent, a listener with presbycusis will struggle to follow the conversation.

Staff and visitors need to be aware of the disabling impact of background noise and take steps to reduce it or when this cannot be achieved to move to a quieter area in the nursing home. Nurses who turn off radios and televisions and close windows in high traffic areas during visits from families and health professionals are promoting an enabling listening environment.

A balance is required between quiet times and access to sounds that provide stimulation and enjoyment such as music. However, rather than simply providing background music for residents' entertainment, attention should be paid to enabling residents to hear their choice of music with clarity, such as may be achieved using induction loops and personal earphones. There is some evidence to suggest that if a person can control the noise level and type of noise that he or she is exposed to, it will facilitate a positive listening experience. Observational studies have reported that inappropriate radio channels and television programs are either playing to themselves or seem to be turned on for the benefit of staff rather for resident entertainment.

Physical environments with hard sound-reflective surfaces give rise to high levels of reverberation. Reverberation increases difficulties with word discrimination and the ability to understand speech. The provision of soft furnishings and wall coverings not only creates a homely ambience but also serves to dampen room reverberation and improves the listening environment within a nursing home.

The behaviors that a hearing impaired person develops to improve communication in various listening situations are collectively described as hearing tactics. Popular hearing tactics used by older nursing home residents include turning their better hearing ear toward the speaker, avoiding communal areas with background noise, taking cues from facial expressions and gestures, requesting repetition, and explaining to staff what they can do to make it easier (e.g., speaking up but not shouting or exaggerating lip movements). Many hearing impaired residents rely heavily on lip reading. This requires that the person speaking to them is looking at them and their face is clearly lighted. Persons with foreign accents move their lips differently and can make lip reading very difficult. Staff who are familiar with a resident's hearing tactics are more likely to be able create positive listening conditions and promote effective

communication. Experienced nurses and staff who have the opportunity to get to know an individual over time will find it relatively easy to identify such adaptive behaviors. An interesting exercise is to casually observe an older person during communication from a little distance and watch for such tactics. By understanding, raising awareness, reinforcing successful strategies, and skill building, a nurse can enable the listener and speaker to maximize communication potential.

Age-Related Hearing Loss

Hearing loss is the third most common chronic condition reported by older people. Age-related hearing problems affects the ability to understand speech in both quiet conditions and particularly in the presence of background noise and reverberation (caused by hard surfaces in the environment). Age-related sensorineural hearing loss (presbycusis) is compounded by a history of industrial or leisure noise exposure, previous otologic disease, and ototoxicity. The prevalence of presbycusis rises exponentially with increasing age as illustrated in the international trends shown in Figure 22–5.

Overall about 12% of people age 55 to 74 years have a hearing loss that causes moderate or severe worry and frustrates communication. General population studies for people older than the age of 85 years suggest that 80% have hearing problems that limit communication. Small studies of dependent older people in long-term care facilities suggests figures of 90% and above, although these studies recognize that not all residents are suitable candidates for hearing aids. It therefore follows that auditory rehabilitation is an important component of nursing home care and

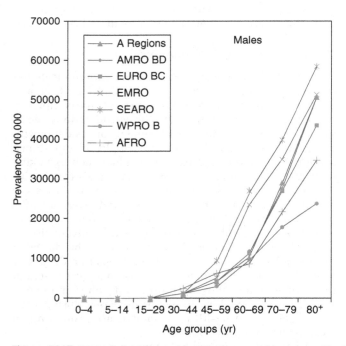
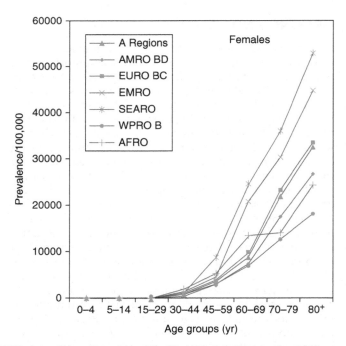

Figure 22–5. Estimated adult-onset hearing loss prevalence rates, 41+ dBHTL, by region and sex. (From the World Health Organization. Mathers C, Smith A, Concha M. Global Burden of Disease: Global burden of hearing loss in the year 2000. Page 21. www.who.int/healthinfo/statistics/bod_hearingloss.pdf.)

Table 22–8.	KEY FEATURES OF PRESBYCUSIS (AGE-RELATED SENSORINEURAL HEARING LOSS)

- Loss of hearing acuity and central changes
- Internally generated distortion of sound
- Slower auditory processing
- Reduced ability to hear high frequencies
- Difficulties with speech discrimination, particularly in noise

that attention should be paid to create an optimal listening environment to reduce the disabling impacts of age-related hearing problems for all residents, not just those who are fitted with hearing aids. A recent Japanese study showed that hearing loss not only affects nursing home residents' communication but also has negative impacts on social and emotional well-being. The stigma associated with age-related hearing problems is well known, and the Japanese study highlighted that communication misunderstanding led to feelings of shame and withdrawn behaviors in residents. The effects of presbycusis on communication are outlined in Table 22–8.

Assessment of Hearing

There are a number of well-known simple screening tests that can be used with nursing home residents, including self-report and the finger rub test. However, the accuracy of such approaches can be challenged. Self-report is fallible because many older people either do not recognize that they have a problem or they know they have a problem but claim otherwise because of stigma or reluctance to accept a hearing aid. Interestingly, it is not unusual for admission screening practices such as the Minimum Data Set to rely on self-report of hearing problems, which may account for the notorious underreporting and failure to manage hearing disability in many nursing homes. Tuning fork tests are not appropriate for older nursing home residents with presbycusis because this is characterized by high-frequency loss. In contrast, a number of national guidelines, including those in the United Kingdom and Australia, recommend the use of Whispered Voice Testing (WVT). Sensitivity of the WVT has been estimated between 90% and 100% with a specificity of 80% to 87%. This implies that a positive test result is good at ruling in a hearing impairment and that when the test result is negative, it is very unlikely that a person does not has a hearing impairment. Because it requires no equipment, it is a cheap and useful method to screen nursing home residents.

Free-field, live voice tests such as the WVT offer inexpensive forms of screening that with a little training and supervised practice can be undertaken by nursing home practitioners with nonconfused residents. The WVT involves whispering as loudly as you can combinations of three numbers such as five, three, seven, or letters—for example, "a," "s," and "m" and asking the resident to repeat. The task should be explained carefully and practiced before completion. Each ear should be tested, and the nontest ear

should be masked so that you know in which ear the sound is being heard. The best way to mask the nontest ear is to press on the tragus (the flap of cartilage immediately in front of the ear canal) with your finger so as to occlude the ear canal and then rub gently. With one hand masking the nontest ear, you should stand to the side of the test ear as far away from the ear as your arm will allow and without the patient seeing your lips. It is not necessary for the resident to hear every number or letter, but if the person can correctly repeat at least 50% of the numbers, then he or she passes the test. More than 90% of individuals with a pure-tone hearing average above 30 dBHL will be unable to repeat more than 50% of the numbers and letters whispered at arm's length from the test ear. Residents who fail the WVT in both ears should be considered candidates for a hearing aid or other form of hearing management, and specialist advice should be sought. Live-voice testing by competent examiners has been demonstrated to be reliable, but it must be emphasized that poorly trained assessors who fail to perform voice tests in quiet environments render the test meaningless and unreliable. It is therefore important for nursing home practitioners who wish to use this method to receive appropriate brief training and clinical supervision from experts.

Measuring Hearing Impairment: Audiometry

Pure-tone audiometry is the gold standard test that assesses hearing thresholds over a range of frequencies for each ear. The audiogram displays the volume required for a person to hear pure notes across frequencies used in normal human speech. Figure 22–6 shows an audiogram for a older person with typical sensorineural hearing impairment.

Audiometric testing is ideally performed by an audiologist in a soundproofed room or booth. Tones through a range of frequencies are played into each ear, and the individual reports when he or she hears them. The scale is designed so that normal hearing thresholds are between 0 and 20 dBHL. Rather than reporting audiometry as numerical thresholds that mean relatively little to nonspecialists, it is usually reported in terms that convey the hearing disability the individual with those thresholds is likely to have. Portable audiometers and handheld testing devices

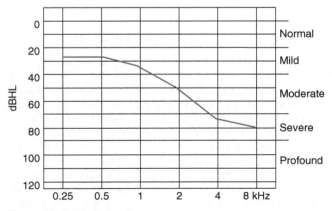

Figure 22–6. Typical audiogram.

do exist, and when they are used, it is essential that the test environment is quiet, that masking is used within the test procedures, and that masking is accounted for in the determination of a hearing aid prescription.

Measuring Hearing Disability

The aim of understanding a resident's hearing disability is to facilitate care planning and as far as possible adapt the environment. A number of person-centered questionnaires exist, some of which combine scales with open-ended questions; these are often used before and after the provision of a hearing aid or other assistive listening devices. The Glasgow Hearing Aid Benefit Profile (GHABP) is a client-centered outcome measure designed to evaluate the effectiveness of hearing aid provision. It is a valid, easy, self-complete questionnaire that is popular in the United Kingdom as a tool for clinicians to use to assess hearing aid benefit over time. Although it is not specifically developed for nursing home residents, it has been used in a number of studies of dependent older people, and the context items can be easily adapted to common listening situations experienced by nursing home residents. The GHABP examines six dimensions of outcome, including disability, handicap, hearing aid use, benefit, satisfaction, and residual disability. It consists of four predetermined and four patient-nominated items, so that residents an identify listening situations that are important to them. Examples of resident-defined situations might include:

- Hearing what my daughter is saying when she visits me
- Listening to the radio in my room at a volume that does not annoy the lady in the next room
- Speaking with the doctors and nurses about my care

If no benefit is evident or an individual is dissatisfied, it may indicate that a different hearing aid is required, that the existing aid is not working properly or requires fine adjustments, or perhaps that other aspects of auditory rehabilitation require attention such as the listening environment. Nurses and nursing aides can facilitate completion of the GHABP or comparable scales to problem solve and in collaboration with audiologic experts support residents as they acclimatize to listening with a hearing aid. The tools and instructions for administration are available at http://www.mrchear.info/cms/Resource.aspx?ResourceID=308.

Hearing Aids and Other Amplification Devices

There are a variety of analogue and digital hearing aids, including those worn in the ear, behind the ear, and on the body. Selection of most suitable devices should be undertaken mindful of the individual's diagnosis, self-care capacity, and manual dexterity. Most hearing aid manufacturers offer a limited choice of colors in flesh tones, and many new hearing aid wearers, irrespective of aid, prefer discrete devices. At its most basic, a hearing aid consists of a microphone, an amplifier, an ear piece, and a battery to power it. Controls vary, but there will be an on–off switch and usually a choice a settings that allow for the normal microphone or usage within a induction loop system. Choosing

the induction loop means that only auditory signals and sounds produced within the field of the loop system are heard; thus, loop systems exclude other sounds. The advantage of focusing on discrete sounds means that in public places a micro enabling listening environment is created for that person; the downside is forgetting to switch back to the normal listening function when leaving the loop area. Hearings aids need to be maintained and like all electrical equipments should not be warn in the shower! Hearing aids should not whistle; if they do, there is a problem causing acoustic feedback, which can often be simply resolved. A poorly fitting mold may require replacement, a spilt in the tubing can be replaced, and ear wax can be removed. A simple way to tell that a hearing aid battery is working is to hold it your hand, switch it on, turn the volume up, and cup your other hand around it. If the battery is working, then you create acoustic feedback (discussed earlier), and it will whistle.

Older people with profound hearing impairment may not benefit from standard hearing aids, and for these individuals, consideration may be given to a cochlear implant. A cochlear implant is a speech processor connected to a row of electrodes that directly feed into the cochlear to stimulate the auditory nerve. Several small studies have shown that people older than the age of 65 years can adapt well to cochlear implants, but careful selection of candidates is required because adaptation to use can be challenging.

A useful environmental listening device for use in nursing homes is an induction hearing loop. These can be installed around the periphery of a room such as a small cinema or chapel. It radiates electromagnetic signals that can be used by a receiver in most hearing aids and cochlear implants. By selecting the "T" function, the receiver connects to the "T Loop" and amplifies sounds coming from the speaker's microphone or electronic device such as a television set located within the area of the induction loop. An advantage of using a loop system is that it excludes background noise. It is important to adjust the setting on the resident's hearing device back to normal listening when the person moves out of the area of the loop system because when it outside of the induction loop, it will act as an earplug and it will not amplify other sounds.

Many residents benefit from a "pocket talker" (communicators), which can be used by the nurse to communicate with the resident by increasing the nurse or doctor's voice amplification.

Communicators (see example in Figure 22–7) are simple sound amplification devices designed to assist short conversational exchanges. Many physicians and nurses carry these small devices with them, cleaning the ear pieces with alcohol wipes between usage, to facilitate brief consultations with older nursing home residents. Unlike personal hearing aids, it is not possible to make fine adjustments for an individual other than a basic volume control function, but the immediacy and simplicity of use can enable a relatively private conversation to take place that would otherwise be impossible.

Evidence demonstrates that new hearing aid users require a period of time to adapt before they can derive maximum benefit in listening with amplified sound. Regardless of the age and ability of the individual, all new

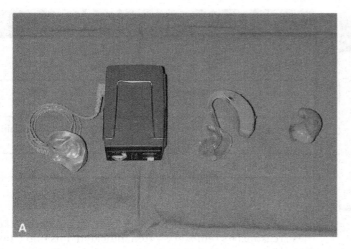

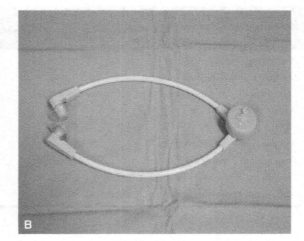

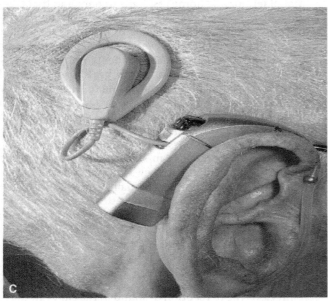

Figure 22–7. Hearing aids and other amplification devices. (**A**) From left to right. Body-worn hearing aid with ear mold, behind-the-ear analogue hearing aid, and in-the-ear analogue hearing aid. (**B**) A simple communicator (pocket talker) with central amplifier and volume control. (**C**) Cochlear implant. (Permission granted by patient. Photo courtesy of the MRC Institute of Hearing Research, Glasgow, UK.)

hearing aid users are advised to begin using the aid within quiet situations before they attempt to listen in situations of competing noise.

Hearing aids are designed to amplify speech, but they do not restore normal hearing, so it is not unusual for residents to sometimes feel disappointed with their new hearing aid. A period of acclimatization, up to 3 months, if often necessary as the brain has adjusted to hearing sounds at low volume, particularly at some frequencies at which the impairment is most marked. At first, the resident may describe the sound as "tinny" because it is different than the sound that he or she has become used to; it is important to encourage the person to persevere and gradually build up the length the time that a new aid is worn each day. Many hearing aids are rejected because of unrealistic expectations, failure of staff to provide suitable quiet listening conditions, absence of skilled communication partners, and unfamiliarity with how the aids work and should be maintained. The multifactorial barriers for the use of hearing aids in nursing homes are listed in Table 22–9.

Nurses can support older residents by reinforcing information about how hearing aids work; how to insert them and use the controls; and maintenance, including battery replacement and cleaning (Table 22–10). An equally important role is to develop the skills of communication partners who are unfamiliar with talking to people who use hearing aids.

Ear Care and Wax

Cerumen (waxy-type substance) that is found in normal ears is produced by two types of secretory glands located in the outer third of the external ear canal. Cerumen acts as a protective substance to prevent dirt entering the ear canal; it lubricates and also repels water. Ear wax plays a role in bacterial defense but can become a medium for bacterial growth, especially when water remains in the ear canal.

Ear wax contains desquamated skin cells, loose hairs, and gland secretions; it slowly migrates out of the ear canal

Table 22–9.	BARRIERS TO USE OF HEARING AIDS IN NURSING HOMES

No hearing evaluation

Staff not aware of hearing problem

Staff do not know why resident does not have a hearing aid

Aid inconvenient to use

Aid fits poorly

Aid does not function properly

Help needed in using aid

Staff do not know how to use aid

Staff do not know how to clean or maintain hearing aid

| Table 22–11. | CERUMEN-SOFTENING AGENTS |

Oil Based	Water Based	Nonwater or Oil Based
Arachis oil	Docusate sodium	Carbamide peroxide (Debrox)
Olive oil	3% Hydrogen peroxide	50% Choline salicylate and glyceride
Almond oil		

in minute amounts and can be wiped away. As people age, the proportion of sebum (which is under the control of testosterone) within ear wax declines, making the ear wax harder and heavier, which slows migration out of the ear canal. Ear wax composition reflects ethnicity with 80% of whites having a wet, sticky type and East Asians having a dry grey, brittle, "rice bran" wax.

If wax is impacted against the tympanic membrane or if it totally occludes the ear canal, it may cause a conductive hearing impairment. When impaction has occurred, removal can improve a person's perception of their ability to hear. However, many older people incorrectly assume that wax removal will significantly improve their hearing and are left disappointed. Wax obstruction can feel

Table 22–10.	HEARING AID MAINTENANCE

- When removing hearing aid, turn it off, turn down the volume, and open the battery door to allow air to enter.
- Removing the battery when the hearing aid is not in use prolongs battery use and stops corrosion of the hearing aid.
- For in-the-ear aids, dry with soft cloth or tissue.
- If wax has accumulated, remove it with the brush or wire pick that comes with the aid or a toothbrush. Wire picks can push ear wax deeper into the plastic tube.
- For behind-the-ear aids, detach the ear mold from the hearing aid and soak it in mild soap and water. Do not use alcohol or oil.
- Blow water out of the ear mold tubing.
- Replace tubing every 3 to 6 months.
- Store hearing aids away from heat and moisture.
- Be careful not to drop the hearing aid on a hard surface.
- Do not leave the hearing aid in while using hairsprays, creams, or gels.
- If volume is low:
  - Check if the volume is turned up.
  - Make sure there is not ear wax in the ear mold.
  - Check the battery by listening for whistling sound when the volume is high.
  - Check that the batteries are in proper positions.
  - Check for wax in ear canal.

uncomfortable and interferes with hearing aid fitting. For these reasons, its removal is often indicated. It is important that older nursing home residents understand that they are unlikely to notice a marked improvement in their ability to hear given the high prevalence of acquired sensorineural hearing impairment. However, in our experience, removal of ear wax in nursing home residents improves the Mini Mental Status Examination score by 1.5 points, which is better than seen with drugs available to treat dementia.

When wax has become impacted, there are three options. The most desirable is to use softening ear drops (Table 22–11). If ear drops fail, ear syringing can be performed by a skilled nurse or physician. Although this is a relatively safe procedure in skilled hands, some residents dislike it, particularly if they experience the unpleasant sensation of vertigo, most usually caused by the water being too cold or too hot. Ear curettes or picks can be used to remove wax by health professionals. This is much easier to do in Asian populations. Cotton swabs (Q-Tips) must *not* be used.

Tinnitus

Tinnitus is the perception of sound in the ear or in the head that does not arise from the external environment. Sounds such as vascular bruits are not tinnitus, and neither are auditory hallucinations such as hearing voices. Sounds are most often described as ringing (38% of patients), buzzing (11%), like a cricket (9%), hissing (8%), whistling (7%), and humming (5%). The nature of the perceived sound is of little relevance in management. Around 20% of older people have tinnitus. Many people with tinnitus also have depression, although it is unclear which comes first.

The most important aspect of management of tinnitus is reassurance, and it is helpful for residents to understand that tinnitus is a symptom, not a disease and not, as some may fear, associated with a brain tumor. Tinnitus is usually associated with hearing impairment and is uncommon in people with normal hearing, and awareness heightens when surrounding are quiet such as when residents are going to bed at night. Although unhelpful when residents want to hear and participate in conversation, background noise such as radio is helpful because it serves to distract from troublesome tinnitus.

Residents who are bothered by tinnitus may not realize that selective use of background noise can be helpful; a radio or television provides noise that masks the tinnitus. Some find loudly ticking clocks helpful. Those who have significant hearing impairment should be fitted with a hearing aid. In severe cases, tinnitus maskers are sometimes provided. These are small devices similar to hearing aids that create a high-frequency noise in the ear to conceal the tinnitus. There are few evidence-based management options, but it is important that nursing staff take the problem seriously, particularly when tinnitus disturbs sleep, and staff should be alert for other signs of low mood and take steps to prevent depression (see Chapter 12). Cognitive behavioral therapy (relaxation, restructuring of the thoughts and reactions to exacerbating situations), although it does not decrease the loudness of the tinnitus, improves quality of life of the resident and improves underlying dysphoria.

Anticholinergic antidepressants, such as nortriptyline or desipramine, improve tinnitus in some persons. Recently, some studies have suggested that low-frequency repetitive transmagnetic stimulation may decrease the loudness of tinnitus.

KEY POINTS

1. Communication is key to resident-centered care, and there are many communication barriers within nursing homes that compound age- and condition-related problems.
2. Human communication serves many functions, and for older people with diminishing opportunities for self-realization, the ability to communicate with staff, family and friends, and fellow residents is a prerequisite for well-being.
3. Speech and language problems require thorough investigation if the underlying cause is not known, and specialist referrals should be made soon after admission to commence or continue rehabilitative interventions.
4. Dual vision and hearing impairments are common in residents that fall and in older people with hip fracture.
5. About 20% to 50% of older people have undetected reduced vision, and the majority of these visual problems (refractive errors or cataract) are correctable.
6. Older people with visual impairment are three times more likely to be depressed than those without sight problems.
7. A severely painful red eye is an ophthalmologic emergency.
8. Pocket talkers can be used to help communicate with hearing impaired resident.
9. Ear wax removal can improve functioning of the resident.
10. Barriers to hearing aid use include staff not being aware of hearing problems, problems with the hearing aid, and staff poorly trained to maintain the hearing aid.
11. Tinnitus is often associated with depression.

SUGGESTED READINGS

Adams-Wendling L, Pimple C, Adams S, Titler MG. Nursing management of impairment in nursing facility residents. *J Gerontol Nurs.* 2008;34:9-17.

Chia EM, Mitchell P, Rochtchina E, et al. Association between vision and hearing impairments and their combined effects on quality of life. *Arch Ophthalmol.* 2006;124:1465-1470.

Clegg AJ, Loveman E, Gospodarevskaya E, et al. The safety and effectiveness of different methods of earwax removal: a systematic review and economic evaluation. *Health Technol Assess.* 2010;14(28):1-192.

Cohen-Mansfield J, Taylor JW. Hearing aid use in nursing homes. Part 2: barriers to effective utilization of hearing aids. *J Am Med Dir Assoc.* 2004;5:289-296.

Cook G, Brown-Wilson C, Forte D. The impact of sensory impairment on social interaction between residents in care homes. *Int J Older People Nurs.* 2006;1:216-224.

Davis A, Smith P, Ferguson M, et al. Acceptability, benefit and costs of early screening for hearing disability: a study of potential screening tests and models. *Health Technol Assess.* 2007;11:42.

De Lepeleire J, Bouwen A, De Coninck L, Buntix F. Insufficient lighting in nursing homes. *J Am Med Dir Assoc.* 2007;8(5):314-317.

Distelhorst JS, Hughes GM. Open-angle glaucoma. *Am Fam Physician.* 2003;67:1937-1944.

Evans BJW, Rowlands G. Correctable visual impairment in older people: a major unmet need [review]. *Ophthalmol Physiol Opt.* 2004;24:161-180.

Gatehouse S. A self-report outcome measure for the evaluation of hearing aid fittings and services. *Health Bull (Edinb).* 1999;57:424-436.

Grue EV, Kirkevold M, Ranhoff AH. Prevalence of vision, hearing and combined vision and hearing impairments in patients with hip fractures. *J Clin Nurs.* 2009;18:3037-3049.

Jessa Z, Evans B, Thomson D, Rowlands G. Vision screening of older people. *Ophthalmol Physiol Opt.* 2007;27:527-546.

Jung S, Coleman A, Weintraub NT. Vision screening in the elderly *J Am Med Dir Assoc.* 2007;8(6):355-362.

Latkany R. Dry eyes: etiology and management. *Curr Opin Ophthalmol.* 2008;19:287-291.

Lethbridge-Cejku M, Schiller JS, Bernadel L. Summary health statistics for US adults; National Health Interview Survey 2002. *Vital Health Stat.* 2004;10(222):1-151.

Martinez-Devesa P, Perera R, Theodoulou M, Waddell A. Cognitive behavioural therapy for tinnitus. *Cochrane Database Syst Rev.* 2010;(9):CD005233.

McCarter DF, Courtney AU, Pollart SM. Cerumen impaction. *Am Fam Physician.* 2007;75:1523-1528.

Medical Research Council Institute for Hearing Research (MRC-IHR) (2006) Protocol - Glasgow Hearing Aid Benefit Profile. MRC-IHR Glasgow, UK. Available at http://www.mrchear.info/cms/Resource.aspx?ResourceID=308. Accessed April 10, 2013.

Meng Z, Liu S, Zheng Y, Phillips JS. Repetitive transcranial magnetic stimulation for tinnitus. *Cochrane Database Syst Rev.* 2011;(10):CD007946.

National Institute for Health and Helathcare Excellence. (NICE) (2011) Glaucoma Pathway Overview. NICE Pathways. NICE. Manchester, UK. Available at http://pathways.nice.org.uk/pathways/glaucoma. Accessed April 10, 2013.

Pirozzo S, Papinczak T, Glasziou P. Whispered voice test for screening for hearing impairment in adults and children: systematic review. *BMJ.* 2003;327:967-971.

Rosenberg EA, Sperazza LC. The visually impaired patient. *Am Fam Physician.* 2008;77:1431-1436.

Sharts-Hopko NC, Glynn-Milley C. Primary open-angle glaucoma. *Am J Nurs.* 2009;109:40-47.

Smeeth L, Fletcher AE, Siu Woon Ng E et al. Reduced hearing, ownership and use of hearing aids in elderly people in the UK the MRC trial of the assessment and management of older people in the community: a cross sectional survey. *Lancet.* 2002;359:1466-1470.

Tolson D, Swan IRC. Hearing. In Redfern S, Ross F (eds). *Nursing Older People.* 3rd ed. London, UK: Churchill Livingstone Elsevier; 2006.

Tolson D, Swan I. Gentle persuasion. *Nurs Times.* 1991;87(23):29-31.

Tolson D, Swan IRC, McIntosh J. Auditory rehabilitation: needs and realities on long-stay wards for elderly people. *Br J Clin Pract.* 1995;49(4):243-245.

Tsuruoka H, Masuda S, Ukai K, et al. Hearing impairment and quality of life for the elderly in nursing homes. *Auris Nasus Larynx.*
2001;28:45-54.
U.S. Preventive Services Task Force. Screening for impaired visual acuity
in older adults: U.S. Preventive Services Task Force recommendation statement. Ann Intern Med. 2009;151(1):37-43.
Waddell A, Canter R. Clinical evidence concise: a publication of BMJ
Publishing group. *Am Fam Physician.* 2004;69:591-592.
Yao Q, Davidson RS, Durairaj VD, Gelston CD. Dry eye syndrome: an
update in office management. *Am J Med.* 2011;124:1016-1018.

MULTIPLE CHOICE QUESTIONS

22.1   Visual screening questions are as reliable as visual
acuity tests for older nursing home residents.

a. True
b. False?

22.2   What percentage of older nursing home residents
are likely to have age-related hearing loss that
hinders functional communication?

a. 80% to 90%
b. 60% to 70%
c. 40% to 50%
d. Less than 40%

22.3   Acute onset of a very painful red eye with
decreased vision may be caused by:

a. Open-angle glaucoma
b. Closed-angle glaucoma
c. Age-related macular degeneration
d. Dry eye

22.4   Which of the following is a water-based cerumen-
softening agent?

a. Arachis oil
b. Carbamide peroxide
c. 50% Choline salicylate
d. Almond oil
e. 3% Hydrogen peroxide

22.5   Cognitive behavioral therapy for tinnitus has been
shown to:

a. Decrease loudness
b. Alter quality of the sounds
c. Improve quality of life
d. Be ineffective
e. Mask the tinnitus sound

Part 4

DISEASE MANAGEMENT

Chapter 23

HYPERTENSION, HYPOTENSION, AND HEART FAILURE

In the United States, 18% of men and 21% of women in nursing homes have congestive heart failure with a worldwide prevalence of between 15% and 40%. Hypertension is the most common medical condition, occurring in 53% of men and 56% of women. Atrial fibrillation occurs in 11% of women and 14% of men.

HYPERTENSION

High blood pressure damages multiple organs, including the heart, peripheral vascular system, kidneys, eyes, and brain. It is now well accepted that systolic hypertension is more damaging in older persons than is diastolic hypertension. In addition, a wider pulse pressure increases the risk of cardiac disease. Epidemiologic studies in persons older than 80 years of age suggest that high systolic blood pressures are much less harmful than they are in the young old. At present, controlled treatment trials show that lowering systolic blood pressure below 160 mm Hg decreases stroke risk and, in some cases, mortality rate. The Hypertension in the Very Elderly Study (HYVET) showed lowering blood pressure below 160 mm Hg in highly healthy community-dwelling persons 80 years and older decreased stroke, heart failure, and mortality. Antihypertensive treatment in this group did not alter the rate of cognitive decline. The Cochrane collaboration showed that lowering blood pressure below 160 mm Hg in persons 60 to 80 years of age decreased cardiovascular disease and total mortality. However, in persons 80 years and older, although there was a decrease in cardiovascular disease, there was no improvement in total mortality and a significant increase in adverse events. These data argue that blood pressure in most nursing home residents should only be treated to below 160 mm Hg. "On Target" found that even in middle-aged persons, reducing the blood pressure below 130 mm Hg was associated with an increased mortality rate.

Blood pressure is often poorly measured in nursing homes. Ambulatory blood pressure measurements have shown that nurses' measurements are often spuriously elevated, a form of "white coat" hypertension. On admission, blood pressure should be measured in both arms and thereafter measured in the arm with the higher blood pressure. Orthostasis occurs in at least 30% of persons in nursing homes. As such, all blood pressures should be measured standing. Orthostasis is more common in the morning, and as such, blood pressure should be measured in the morning. It needs to be recognized that orthostasis is only present about half the time.

Postprandial hypotension occurs in 26% of nursing home residents. Similar to orthostasis, its occurrence is variable and is more common in the morning. Postprandial hypotension is associated with falls, syncope, stroke, and myocardial infarction. In nursing homes, it has been shown to be associated with an increase in all-cause mortality. Measurement of blood pressure before and 1 hour after breakfast can identify postprandial hypotension. Ambulatory blood pressure monitoring is the gold standard for diagnosing postprandial hypotension. Postprandial hypotension can be treated by taking an α_1-glucosidase inhibitor (acarbose or miglitol) taken with the first bite of the meal. These agents increase glucagon-like peptide I and slow gastric emptying, thus reducing food-induced hypotension.

Pseudohypertension caused by severe arteriosclerosis can result in spuriously high blood pressures in older persons. Although the "Osler maneuver" (the artery remains palpable after the sphygmomanometer pressure is increased above the systolic pressure) may suggest pseudohypertension, it has poor sensitivity and specificity.

From the treatment viewpoint, it is important to realize that although reducing salt intake and weight loss reduces blood pressure, these approaches in older persons increase mortality rates and decrease quality of life. A regular salt diet with no added salt is now the recommendation for all older nursing home residents.

For treatment of high blood pressure, the first-line drugs should be a thiazide diuretic or an angiotensin-converting enzyme (ACE) inhibitor. β-Blockers can be added to these treatments but have higher mortality rates when used alone. In all cases, the literature supports the use of the cheapest available ACE inhibitors or β-blockers. If a nursing home resident develops hypokalemia, the diuretic should be replaced with spironolactone because hyporenin hyperaldosteronism (either Conn tumor or syndrome) is not rare in older persons. ACE inhibitors should not be used together with angiotensin receptor blockers (ARBs). Nitrendipine is the only calcium channel antagonist for which there is evidence that it can be used as first-line therapy for hypertension.

Table 23–1.   CAUSES OF THERAPY FAILURES IN NURSING HOMES

- Taking antihypertensive medications with calcium or iron because they are malabsorbed
- Use of NSAIDs
- Use of glucocorticoids
- Depression (increases cortisol)
- Medication pocketing
- Hypovitaminosis D
- Pain
- Nocturnal hypoglycemia
- Sleep apnea (common)
- Pheochromocytoma (rare)
- Hyporenin hyperaldosteronism (common)

NSAID, nonsteroidal antiinflammatory drug.

The most common causes of therapy failure in nursing homes are given in Table 23–1. In some cases, resistant isolated systolic hypertension responds to a nitric oxide donor (e.g., isosorbide dinitrate).

Because of weight loss in nursing home residents and a target level of 160 mm Hg systolic blood pressure, many nursing home residents do not need antihypertensives, resulting in a marked decrease in polypharmacy.

HEART FAILURE

The clinical symptoms of heart failure are dyspnea, orthopnea, paroxysmal nocturnal dyspnea, fatigue, and swollen ankles. The clinical signs are ankle or sacral edema (if the resident spends all his or her time in bed), jugular venous distension (JVD), basal crepitations, and a third heart sound. Peripheral edema in older persons has many causes, making it a poor sign to use to diagnose heart failure (Table 23–2). Basal crepitations are present in 5% to 10% of older persons without heart failure.

When examined at 45 or 90 degrees, JVD is a more accurate sign of right-sided heart failure: The classical signs of heart failure on chest radiographs are given in Table 23–3.

Table 23–2.   CAUSES OF EDEMA IN AN OLDER PERSON

- Venous insufficiency
- Low albumin (low oncotic pressure)
- Poor muscle tone
- Local disease
- Anemia
- Liver and kidney disease
- Heart failure
- Pooling of fluid from sitting all day

Table 23–3.   SIGNS OF HEART FAILURE ON CHEST RADIOGRAPHS

	Pulmonary Capillary Wedge Pressure (mm Hg)
Increased vascular pedicle Prominent pulmonary vessels Enlarged heart	13–18
Peribronchial cuffing Kerley lines Thickened interlobar fissure	18–25
Pleural effusion Air bronchogram Cotton wool appearance	>25

PCWP, pulmonary capillary wedge pressure.

The New York Heart Association (NYHA) has created a functional classification for heart failure (Table 23–4). For persons with NYHA stage III or IV heart failure, the average survival rate is 14% within 30 days of hospital admission and 53% within 1 year. The readmission rates to hospital are 27% in the first month and 76% within 1 year. Heart failure is on the whole a disease of older person with a high dependence in activities of daily living and instrumental activities of daily living. At least 70% of patients with heart failure have more than three comorbidities.

There are two types of heart failure, left ventricular systolic dysfunction (systolic heart failure) and heart failure with preserved ejection fraction (diastolic heart failure with ejection fraction >50%). Coronary artery disease is the most common cause of systolic heart failure, and uncontrolled hypertension the most common cause of diastolic heart failure. Table 23–5 compares the two types of heart failure.

Table 23–4.   NEW YORK HEART ASSOCIATION CLASSIFICATION OF HEART FAILURE

Class	Description
I	No problems with physical activity
II	No limitations at rest, but normal activity causes fatigue, tachycardia, or dyspnea
III	Minimal activity results in fatigue, palpitations, or dyspnea
IV	Symptoms at rest; cannot carry out any physical activity without discomfort

Table 23–5. COMPARISONS OF SYSTOLIC AND DIASTOLIC HEART FAILURE

	Systolic Heart Failure	Diastolic Heart Failure
Symptoms	Similar in both conditions	
Brain natriuretic peptide	Elevated in both conditions	
Ejection fraction	<50%	>50%
Left ventricular mass	Markedly increased	Increased
Left ventricle		
End-diastolic volume	Increased	Normal
Exercise capacity	Decreased in both conditions	

Brain natriuretic peptide or N-terminal proBNP can be useful in recognizing residents with heart failure in whom the clinical situation is uncertain. It must be recognized that the decreased renal function in older persons can lead to markedly elevated natriuretic peptide levels without heart failure. Although two-dimensional echocardiograms are the gold standard for diagnosis, large variations in laboratories occur, and a difference of at least 11% is required to be certain that a change in left ventricular ejection function is real.

Diuretics are useful for rapid symptom relief but should be avoided or used in minimal doses for long-term care. ACE inhibitors (or if not tolerated ARBs) are the first line of treatment. All patients should also receive a β-blocker. If symptoms persist, spironolactone should be added to the treatment. A supervised group exercise-based rehabilitation program improves quality of life and will decrease heart failure–associated readmissions. N-3 polyunsaturated fatty acids reduce complications and death, but statins do not. In residents with a tachycardia or atrial fibrillation, digoxin can be helpful. Amlodipine has been shown to increase heart failure and should be avoided. Nonsteroidal antiinflammatory drugs should be avoided in patients with heart failure. The treatment of patients with diastolic heart failure is similar, but blood pressure should be lowered to a systolic pressure below 140 mm Hg. Natriuretic peptides should not be used to monitor treatment responses in persons older than 75 years of age.

Although low-salt diets have been classically used in patients with heart failure, therapeutic diets in nursing homes are no longer recommended. A diet of 3 to 4 g/day of salt is a very reasonable approach. Cardiac cachexia is a poor prognostic factor, and persons with body mass indexes above 30 have lower levels of mortality. Thus, loss of weight needs to be avoided when possible.

Implantable cardioverter defibrillators have not been shown to be useful in persons older than 75 years. If the resident has a QRS greater than 120 msec, cardiac resynchronization therapy has been shown to maintain 6-minute walk distance and quality of life with more than 7 years of follow-up.

Persons with heart failure should be considered for hospice care if they have two of the following criteria:

- Blood urea nitrogen >30 mg/dL (10.71 mmol/L)
- Systolic blood pressure <120 mm Hg
- Peripheral arterial disease
- Sodium <135 mEq/L or mmol/L

Community specialist heart failure nurses have been shown to reduce rehospitalizations in the United States, the United Kingdom, and Switzerland.

ATRIAL FIBRILLATION

Atrial fibrillation occurs in 8% to 10% of persons 80 years of age or older. Atrial fibrillation increases the risk of a stroke by about sevenfold. It can present with palpitations, angina, fatigue, dizziness, or dyspnea. The pulse is irregularly irregular. In many persons, it can be asymptomatic. Persons with sleep apnea are particularly likely to have atrial fibrillation. The electrocardiogram shows absence of P waves and irregular R-R intervals.

The management of atrial fibrillation requires either rate or rhythm control and antithrombotic therapy. Rate or rhythm control produce similar benefits. Because antiarrhythmic agents have more toxicity in older persons, rate control is the preferred approach. In general, rate control can be obtained with β-blockers. Nondihydropyridine calcium channel blockers are second-line agents. In heart failure, digoxin used with another agent, but not alone, can improve rate control when it cannot be obtained with a single agent. A randomized controlled trial has suggested that keeping the heart rate below 110 beats/min is as efficacious as when it is kept below 80 beats/min, and it results in less bradyarrhythmias. In general, antiarrhythmic drugs increase mortality rates and should be avoided in older persons unless rhythm control fails to control symptoms. The multiple side effects of amiodarone and dronedarone have suggested their use is inappropriate in nursing home residents. Surgical or catheter ablation of the electrical activity in the atria can be appropriate for some elderly adults. Removal of the atrial appendage can decrease thrombotic formation.

Anticoagulation with warfarin to prevent thromboembolic events has been a key treatment for older persons with atrial fibrillation. Even in persons with multiple falls outcomes, using warfarin are better than in those not receiving warfarin. Warfarin is superior to the combination of aspirin together with clopidogrel. Anyone with a $CHADS_2$ score of a 2 or greater should be anticoagulated (Table 23–6). The $CHADS_2VAS_c$ score is more accurate using the same cutoff of 2.

Deciding the appropriate starting dose of warfarin should use the guidelines at WarfarinDosing.org (http://www.warfarindosing.org). When possible, the person's genotype for the vitamin K epoxide reductase

Table 23–6. CHADS₂ SCORE[a]

- Congestive heart failure (1 point)
- Hypertension: >140/90 mm Hg (1 point)
- Age older than 75 years (1 point)
- Diabetes mellitus (1 point)
- Prior stroke or transient ischemic attack (2 points)

[a]The CHADS$_2$VAS$_c$ score is more accurate. It includes 1 point each for vascular disease, age 65 years 74 years, and female sex.

Table 23–7. DOSE REDUCTION OF WARFARIN WHEN THE INTERNATIONAL NORMALIZED RATIO IS ELEVATED

International Normalized Ratio	Approach
>9	Stop warfarin and give 2.5–5 mg of vitamin K orally or 1 mg parenterally
7–9	Hold warfarin
5–7	Give 25% of dose; check INR daily
3–5	Halve warfarin dose; check INR in 48 hours

INR, international normalized ratio.

and the cytochrome P450 2C9 genes should be known because it greatly improves the ability to get the appropriate warfarin dose. A total of 722 drugs have been shown to interact with warfarin, which requires great care to be taken when adding a drug in a person taking warfarin. A variety of foods rich in vitamin K (beef liver, broccoli, Brussels sprouts, soybeans, and spinach and other green leafy vegetables) can antagonize the effects of warfarin. Influenza vaccination also interacts with Coumadin. These factors make it difficult to control the international normalized ratio (INR) in the nursing home. Blood transport to a distant site on a hot day can further lead to spurious INR values. For these reasons, point-of-contact INR testing in the nursing home is preferred. All persons taking warfarin should have a simple flow sheet clearly displayed in the medical record (see Toolkit). Because warfarin has a prolonged half-life when a person has an elevated INR up to 7, the next warfarin dose should not be withheld but rather reduced if there is no bleeding

(Table 23–7). In nursing homes, warfarin should not be given with aspirin or other antiplatelet agents.

A number of drugs directly inhibit either coagulation factor II–thrombin (dabigatran) or factor Xa (rivaroxaban, apixaban, and endoxaban). Most studies suggest that these drugs are slightly more effective than warfarin in reducing stroke risk. These drugs have both advantages and disadvantages compared with warfarin (Table 23–8). Dabigatran was placed on the new "Beers list of potentially inappropriate drugs" because of its renal clearance, poor reversibility, and possibly worse outcomes in older persons. On the whole, however, it does not appear more dangerous than warfarin.

Table 23–8. COMPARISON OF WARFARIN AND NEW ORAL ANTICOAGULANTS

	Warfarin	Dabigatran	Rivaroxaban
Administration	Daily	Twice daily	Daily
Effect on mortality	Good	Better	Better
Half-life (hr)	40	12–14	7–11
Interactions	Multiple	P-glycoprotein transporter	CYP3A and P-glycoprotein transporter
Renal clearance (%)	0	80	35
INR monitoring	Yes	No	No
Reversal	Vitamin K	None	None
Convenience	Low	High	High
Major bleeding	High	Less	Less
Efficacy (stroke prevention)	Good	Better	Better
Dose titration	Yes	No	No
Cost	Low (excluding hospitalization)	High	High

INR, international normalized ratio.

KEY POINTS

1. In nursing home residents, the systolic blood pressure should be kept below 160 mm Hg.
2. Standing blood pressure needs to be measured in all nursing home residents regularly.
3. Persons with low potassium levels often have hyporenin hyperaldosteronism and respond to spironolactone.
4. Sleep apnea elevates blood pressure.
5. There are many causes, besides heart failure, of edema.
6. Treatment of heart failure is ACE inhibitors and β-blockers. Diuretics are mainly for symptom relief.
7. Very-low-salt diets need to be avoided in patients with heart failure.
8. Anticoagulation improves outcome in persons older than 70 years of age even if they are recurrent fallers.
9. Unless the INR is greater than 7, the warfarin dose should be reduced, and warfarin should still be given.
10. The place of newer anticoagulants for atrial fibrillation is evolving.

TOOLKIT

Warfarin Flow Chart

Date Warfarin Started: ___/___/___   Diagnosis: _____

Date	Warfarin Dose	INR

SUGGESTED READINGS

Allen LA, Hernandez AF, Peterson ED, et al. Discharge to a skilled nursing facility and subsequent clinical outcomes among older patients hospitalized for heart failure. *Circ Heart Fail.* 2011;4:293-300.

Ansell J. Should newer oral anticoagulants be used as first-line agents to prevent thromboembolism in patients with atrial fibrillation and risk factors for stroke or thromboembolism? New oral anticoagulants should not be used as first-line agents to prevent thromboembolism in patients with atrial fibrillation. *Circulation.* 2012;125:165-170.

Aurigemma GP, Gaasch WH. Diastolic heart failure. *N Engl J Med.* 2004;351:1097-105.

Case R, Haynes D, Holaday B, Parker VG. Evidence-based nursing: the role of the advanced practice registered nurse in the management of heart failure patients in the outpatient setting. *Dimens Crit Care Nurs.* 2010;29:57-62.

Chen J, Ross JS, Carlson MD, et al. Skilled nursing facility referral and hospital readmission rates after heart failure or myocardial infarction. *Am J Med.* 2012;125:100.e1-9.

Curtis AB, Rich MW. Atrial fibrillation in the elderly: mechanisms and management. *Heart Rhythm.* 2007;4:1577-1579.

Daamen MA, Schols JM, Jaarsma T, Hamers JP. Prevalence of heart failure in nursing homes: a systematic literature review. *Scand J Caring Sci.* 2010;24:202-208.

Darby AE, DiMarco JP. Management of atrial fibrillation in patients with structural heart disease. *Circulation.* 2012;125:945-957.

Granger CB, Armaganijan LV. Should newer oral anticoagulants be used as first-line agents to prevent thromboembolism in patients with atrial fibrillation and risk factors for stroke or thromboembolism? Newer oral anticoagulants should be used as first-line agents to prevent thromboembolism in patients with atrial fibrillation and risk factors for stroke or thromboembolism. *Circulation.* 2012;125: 159-164.

Gutierrez C, Blanchard DG. Atrial fibrillation: diagnosis and treatment. *Am Fam Physician.* 2011;83:61-68.

Hernandez AF, Greiner MA, Fonarow GC, et al. Relationship between early physician follow-up and 30-day readmission among Medicare beneficiaries hospitalized for heart failure. *JAMA.* 2010;303: 1716-1722.

Leventhal ME, Denhaerynck K, Brunner-La Rocca HP, et al. Swiss Interdisciplinary Management Programme for Heart Failure (SWIM-HF): a randomised controlled trial study of an outpatient inter-professional management programme for heart failure patients in Switzerland. *Swiss Med Wkly.* 2011;141:w13171.

McMurray JJV. Systolic heart failure. *N Engl J Med.* 2010;362:228-238.

Moore KL, Boscardin WJ, Steinman MA, Schwartz JB. Age and sex variation in prevalence of chronic medical conditions in older residents of U.S. nursing homes. *J Am Geriatr Soc* 2012;60(4): 756-764.

Morley JE. Hypertension: is it overtreated in the elderly? *J Am Med Dir Assoc.* 2010;11:147-152.

Mossello E, Pieraccioli MC, Zanieri S, et al. Ambulatory blood pressure monitoring in older nursing home residents: diagnostic and prognostic role. *J Am Med Dir Assoc.* 2012;13:760.e1-e5.

Pihl E, Cider A, Stromberg A, et al. Exercise in elderly patients with chronic heart failure in primary care: effects on physical capacity and health-related quality of life. *Eur J Cardiovasc Nurs.* 2011;10: 150-158.

Shah SM, Carey IM, Harris T, et al. Quality of chronic disease care for older people in care homes and the community in a primary care pay for performance system: retrospective study. *BMJ.* 2011; 342:d912.

Whittingham K, Pearce DE. Carer support from a community-based heart specialist nurse service. *Br J Nurs.* 2011;20:1388-1393.

MULTIPLE CHOICE QUESTIONS

23.1 In persons older than 80 years of age, treating blood pressure has been shown to decrease heart failure when the systolic blood pressure is greater than:

    a. 120 mm Hg
    b. 140 mm Hg
    c. 150 mm Hg
    d. 160 mm Hg
    e. There is no evidence.

23.2 Which of the following is true concerning blood pressure measurements in nursing home residents?

    a. Measurements by nurses are often lower than real blood pressure.
    b. Orthostasis is uncommon in nursing home residents.
    c. Postprandial hypotension is present in a quarter of nursing home residents.
    d. Pseudohypertension causes a lower blood pressure to be measured.

23.3   Which of the following is *not* a cause of failure to control hypertension in nursing home resident?

a. NSAIDs
b. Weight loss
c. Sleep apnea
d. Hyporenin hypoaldosteronism
e. Glucocorticoids

23.4   A 90-year-old woman has peripheral edema and a cough. She has sinusitis. She can only walk a few steps and has basal crepitations. Jugular venous distension is not noted. She does not have varicose veins. Her laboratory values are normal. Which of the following is the most likely reason for her pedal edema?

a. Heart failure
b. Renal failure
c. Venous insufficiency
d. Sitting most of the day
e. Anemia

23.5   Which of the following is not a component of the criteria for referring someone with congestive heart failure for hospice care?

a. Blood urea nitrogen >30 mg/dL (10.71 mmol/L)
b. Systolic blood pressure less than 120 mm Hg
c. Peripheral arterial disease
d. Sodium less than 135 mEq/L or mmol/L

23.6   A 67-year-old woman with atrial fibrillation is admitted to a nursing home. She has congestive heart failure. She had one fall in the past month. According to the $CHADS_2VAS_c$ score, she should *not* be treated with anticoagulation.

a. True
b. False

23.7   Which of the following does not alter the INR?

a. Broccoli
b. Spinach
c. Blood transportation on a cold day
d. Influenza vaccination
e. Beef liver

Chapter 24

NEUROLOGIC DISORDERS

Persons with neurologic disorders often need to go to nursing facilities either for rehabilitation or because of the heavy functional burden these conditions often place on the caregiver.

STROKE

Strokes cause 10% of deaths worldwide. Disability is present in 60% of stroke survivors. Approximately 90% of strokes are ischemic in origin, and the rest are caused by hemorrhage. After a stroke, optimal outcomes depend on an early multidisciplinary approach using a wealth of evidence-based medicine. To prevent a second stroke, all persons who have had a stroke should receive antiplatelet medicine with aspirin, and those with atrial fibrillation should be anticoagulated with warfarin. There is no evidence to support the use of aspirin and Coumadin together. The newer anticoagulants should be used with caution in persons older than 80 years of age or with impaired renal function.

Recovery from stroke involves both neuronal regeneration and developing adaptive changes to overcome disability. Although recovery occurs quickly in the first few weeks, it then continues slowly for a number of years. About 60% of stroke survivors are independent in self-care by 3 months. Transmagnetic cranial stimulation coupled with functional magnetic resonance imaging can be used to predict long-term potential for improvement from stroke.

Stroke rehabilitation works on focusing on minimizing the limitation of activities the person has and modifying the environment to decrease the ability of the person to participate in activities. Minimization of learned dependence is a key component of therapy. The components of modern stroke rehabilitation are:

- Early mobilization
- Restoration of motor function
- Neuromuscular stimulation
- Motor imagery
- Reduction in deficits in attention

Motor function is improved by focusing on exercising basic movements, gait training, and balance exercises. Treadmill training can improve gait and walking speeds. Constraint-induced movement therapy consists of limiting function in the good hand by wearing a soft mitten and thus forcing the person to use the affected limb. Whether this is better than intensive exercises of the affected limb has been questioned. There are both harms and frustration associated with constraint-induced movement therapy. Robotic devices to assist with limb movements are now becoming available.

Neuromuscular stimulation can be applied peripherally. More recently, this has been coupled with repetitive transcranial magnetic stimulation.

Mental practice and mental imagery can be used to help enhance upper limb therapy. These techniques can be used outside of the formal therapy sessions. The use of virtual reality environments can be helpful to enhance the person's ability to do mental imagery. Mirror therapy, in which the person performs tasks with the unaffected limb in front of a mirror while the affected arm is not in view. This creates an illusory belief that the affected arm is functioning and increases activation of the affected brain hemisphere.

Training in attention activities in a generalized way appears to be as useful as focusing specifically on areas of spatial neglect.

Numerous syndromes occur in persons who have had a stroke, and each of these requires special attention (Table 24–1).

PARKINSON DISEASE

Parkinson disease occurs in 1% of persons 65 years of age and older and up to 10% of persons in long-term care. Persons with Parkinson disease have five times the chance of being in a nursing home compared with other older persons. In Norway, persons with Parkinson disease in the nursing home cost four times as much to care for compared with other residents.

Parkinson disease is a progressive neurologic disease caused by a lack of dopamine in the substantia nigra. The disease is characterized by a difficulty in initiating (akinesia) and a slowness (bradykinesia) of movement and tremulousness (Figure 24–1). The clinical features are described in Table 24–2.

Medications are the cornerstone of treatment for Parkinson disease. L-Dopa together with a peripheral dopamine decarboxylase inhibitor (carbidopa or benserazide) is the most effective therapy. Direct dopamine agonists (pramipexole, piribedil, ropinirole, or rotigotine) can also

Table 24–1.	MANAGEMENT OF COMMON PROBLEMS IN PERSONS WITH STROKE

Syndrome	Management
Dysphagia	Speech pathologist
	Appropriate diet
	Focus on mouth hygiene (to prevent aspiration)
	Pharyngeal stimulation
	Cortical stimulation (rTMS)
	Drugs (ACE inhibitors, capsaicin, dopamine agonists)
	Laryngeal electrical pacemakers
	Enteral tube feeding
Speech problems • Dysphasia • Dysarthria	Speech pathologist Communication groups Alternative communication methods
Hemineglect	Occupational therapy Attention training Prism correction
Apraxia • Inability to carry out learned sequences	Recognition and training (poor outcomes)
Agnosias • Inability to interpret sensory or visual data from environment	Practice with the stimulus (good outcomes)
Shoulder subluxation or pain	Hot packs or ultrasonography Analgesics Proper positioning Avoidance of abnormal movements Sling Steroid injections
Depression	Cognitive behavioral therapy Consider antidepressant
Reduced attention span	Shorter therapy sessions

ACE, angiotensin-converting enzyme; rTMS, repetitive transcranial magnetic stimulation.

be used but tend to have more side effects and be less effective. Amantadine can be used in some individuals. Selegiline and rasagiline (selective monoamine oxidase B inhibitors) are less effective. These drugs together with catechol-O-methyl transferase inhibitors (entacapone or tolcapone) can be used to treat persons who have early wearing off effects when given L-dopa alone. Subcutaneous apomorphine penject can rescue refractory periods. An apomorphine pump can treat motor fluctuations but requires

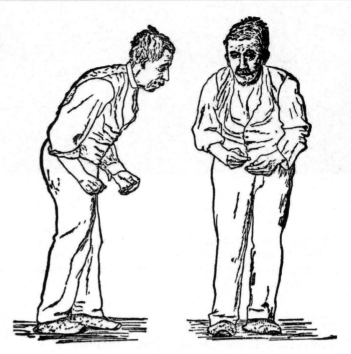

Figure 24–1. Difficulty in initiating movement with Parkinson disease (bradykinesia).

careful management of emesis, care with skin hygiene, and nursing support. The side effects of these drugs are given in Table 24–3. Drugs to be avoided in persons with Parkinson are listed in Table 24–4.

Table 24–2.	SIGNS AND SYMPTOMS OF PARKINSON DISEASE

- Akinesia (difficulty in initiating movements)
- Bradykinesia (slow movements)
- Tremor (pill rolling; 4–6 Hz at rest)
- Muscular rigidity (cogwheeling or lead piping)
- Stooped posture with flexed limbs
- Postural instability
- Hallucinations
- Asymmetrical
- Micrographia
- Dysphoria (soft spoken; monotonous tone)
- Dysphagia
- Cognitive problems
- Fatigue
- Frozen face
- Disability
- Depression
- Falls
- Weight loss
- Constipation
- Urge incontinence
- Pedal edema

Table 24–3. SIDE EFFECTS OF DRUGS FOR PERSONS WITH PARKINSON DISEASE

L-Dopa–Carbidopa	Direct Dopamine Agonists	Monoamine Oxidase β Inhibitors	Catechol-O-Methyl Transferase Inhibitors
Nausea	Gastrointestinal effects	Constipation	Dyskinesia
Anorexia	Psychiatric effects	Diarrhea	Sleep disorders
Syncope	Edema	Drowsiness	Orthostasis
Orthostasis	Sleep attacks	Flu-like illness	Confusion
Hypomania	Impulse control disorders	Skin rash	Neuroleptic malignant syndrome
Depression		Orthostasis	
Delirium		Bleeding	Diarrhea
Hallucinations		Hallucinations	Agitation
Hemolytic anemia			

Physical therapy has three roles for patients with Parkinson disease:

1. Strategy training
   - Compensatory strategies to bypass the defective basal ganglia and use the frontal cortex (e.g., focusing on taking long steps, avoiding dual tasking, stepping over objects, visualization)
   - Improve performance through daily practice, which may need to be divided into multiple 5- to 10-minute periods
2. Management of deconditioned musculoskeletal and cardiorespiratory systems
3. Promotion of physical exercise (together with restorative nurse) and falls prevention

Specific exercise training includes resistance exercise, treadmill training, tai chi (for balance), whole-body vibration, training for dual tasking, cycling, and axial range of motion and flexibility exercises. Wheeled walking may enhance walking speed for persons with Parkinson disease. A speech therapist should be involved in treating dysphonia.

Deep brain stimulation is a useful treatment for persons with medication-refractory Parkinson treatment. It should be performed before the resident develops contractures. It improves medication refractory tremor, but with other conditions, it may only allow medication dosage to be reduced. The FLASQ-PD (Florida Surgical Questionnaire for Parkinson Disease) can be used to determine if the referral to a specialist is appropriate.

A number of nonmotor symptoms of Parkinson disease might benefit from therapy (Table 24–5).

Table 24–4. DRUGS TO BE AVOIDED IN PERSONS WITH PARKINSON DISEASE

- Antipsychotics
- Metoclopramide
- Chlorpromazine
- Monoamine oxidase inhibitors
- Anticholinergics (in presence of cognitive dysfunction)

Table 24–5. MANAGEMENT OF NONMOTOR SYMPTOMS FOR PARKINSON DISEASE

Symptom	Management
Excessive daytime somnolence	Modafinil
Fatigue	Amantadine / Methylphenidate
Periodic limb movements of sleep	L-dopa–carbidopa / Atropine eye drops
Drooling	Botulinum toxin
Constipation	Polyethylene glycol, lactulose, sorbitol
Orthostatic hypotension	Midodrine, fludrocortisone
REM sleep behavior disorder	Clonazepam
Insomnia	Sleep hygiene / Melatonin
Depression	Cognitive behavioral therapy
Excessive sweating	Propantheline / Propanol / Topical aluminum creams

REM, rapid eye movement.

Table 24–6.   APPROACHES TO MAINTAINING NUTRITIONAL STATUS

- Avoid excess long-chained branch amino acids because they interfere with transport of L-dopa into the brain.
- Use energy-dense foods and caloric supplements.
- Medicines should be given so they are maximally effective at mealtimes.
- Extra time is necessary for eating.
- Provide aids to allow independent eating in persons with severe tremor.
- Food can go cold, so plate warmers are useful.
- Provide privacy while eating if requested by the resident.
- Ensure adequate fluid intake.

Table 24–7.   DISEASE-MODIFYING DRUGS USED FOR MULTIPLE SCLEROSIS

Fingolimod (oral sphingosine-1-phosphate)

Interferon β-1a and 1b

Glatiramer (non-interferon, nonsteroid immunomodulator)

Mitoxantrone (immunosuppressant)

Natalizumab (a humanized monoclonal antibody)

Cladribine (purine nucleoside analog)

Residents in nursing homes with Parkinson disease require extra support of nursing staff, including help with personal hygiene, encouragement to remain mobile and care against falling during transfers, improved communication (requiring extra time), constipation (with toileting after a meal and holding a pillow against the stomach on the toilet), and psychological support. Special help is required to maintain nutritional support (Table 24–6).

MULTIPLE SCLEROSIS

Multiple sclerosis (MS) is a demyelinating disease that leads to mobility problems, spasticity, fatigue, pain, speech disorders, cognitive problems, dysphagia, fatigue, and bowel and bladder incontinence. About 20% to 25% of persons with MS will need long-term care with a variable number needing to go to a nursing home depending on available community services. Ten years after diagnosis, half will need to use a cane and 15% will be in a wheelchair. The majority of residents with MS in nursing homes are younger than 60 years of age. In nursing homes, three quarters of people with MS use a wheelchair. Persons with MS are admitted to nursing homes because of bowel dysfunction, poorer health, functional decline, and caregiver burden. Over the first year in a nursing home, residents with MS show a decline in motor ability, cognition, communication skills, and bowel and bladder function and are more likely to be depressed.

Infections or elevated ambient temperature tend to produce disease exacerbations. Spasticity can be treated with baclofen or diazepam. Botulinum toxin can help in some cases in combination with physical therapy. Fatigue is common and can be treated with dextroamphetamine, modafinil, methylphenidate, or pemoline. Detrusor hyperactivity (urge incontinence) and detrusor sphincter dyssynergy need careful treatment and are often associated with recurrent urinary tract infections. Intermittent catheterization is preferred to indwelling catheters. Bowel incontinence and diarrhea can occur, but severe constipation can be a major problem.

Paroxysmal neurologic symptoms are common. These include sensory syndrome such as trigeminal or tongue neuralgia and paresthesias that can be painful and be associated with burning, itching, or thermal sensations. In some cases, episodic dystonias responds to membrane-stabilizing anticonvulsant medications.

All residents with MS should receive 1000 IU of vitamin D daily. Male residents with MS are often hypogonadal and may benefit from testosterone replacement.

During acute attacks, high-dose corticosteroids may be helpful. Table 24–7 provides the presently available disease-modifying drugs. The injectable agents can all cause local skin irritation and, on occasion, muscle necrosis. Persons who have antibodies to the JC virus cannot receive natalizumab because it increases the risk of multifocal leukoencephalopathy.

EPILEPSY

Epilepsy is common in nursing homes with from 5% to 9% of residents receiving antiepileptic drugs in the United States and Germany, although some of these drugs are being used inappropriately for behavior modification. The diagnosis of epilepsy can take up to 2 years to make in older persons. This is because more than half have partial complex seizures and 5% have absence seizures. Many residents are prescribed long-term antiepileptic therapy after a single seizure associated with hypoxia, stroke, or neurosurgery. These can be stopped 6 weeks after the event. Table 24–8

Table 24–8.   DRUGS USED TO TREAT EPILEPSY

First Line
  Phenytoin
  Carbamazepine
  Sodium valproate
  Lamotrigine
  Levetiracetam
  Benzodiazepines (for acute seizures)

Second Line
  Gabapentin–pregabalin
  Topiramate
  Zonisamide
  Lacosamide
  Tiagabine

provides a list of the medicines commonly used to treat seizures. Barbiturates should not be used. With phenytoin, it is difficult to maintain levels, and levels need to be corrected for albumin level. There is no need to monitor blood levels for the newer antiepileptics. Sodium valproate concentrations fluctuate widely during the day, making the value of blood levels questionable. Topiramate can cause severe weight loss. Common side effects of the other drugs include dizziness, ataxia, sedation, rash, edema, osteoporosis, and cardiac conduction problems. A number of therapeutic devices for treating drug-resistant epilepsy are now appearing in nursing homes. These include vagal nerve stimulation, deep brain stimulation of the anterior thalamus, and responsive neurostimulation.

HUNTINGTON DISEASE

Huntington disease is a hereditable disorder that presents with involuntary writhing movements (chorea). The age of onset is between 35 and 44 years of age. Many of these persons will spend 10 to 20 years in a nursing home. With progression of the disease, the person has problems eating, chewing, swallowing, and speaking. Severe weight loss and protein energy undernutrition are not rare. Problems with executive function occur fairly early in the disorder with memory problems occurring later. A variety of neuropsychiatric symptoms (irritability, apathy, anxiety, depression, and psychosis) are common, which make caring for the person difficult. Suicide risk is higher than average. The Unified Huntington's Disease Rating Scale can be used to follow progression of the disease.

Tetrabenazine has been approved for treatment of chorea by the Food and Drug Administration in the United States. Very high doses of neuroleptics and benzodiazepines are often needed to control involuntary movements. Amantadine and remacemide have had some success. Valproic acid can be used for myoclonic hyperkinesia.

Nursing home residents need to be reminded to eat slowly and eat small pieces of food to avoid choking. Aspiration pneumonia is common in these residents. A percutaneous endoscopic gastrostomy may be necessary to maintain nutritional status. When the resident is anxious, the flailing movement worsens, and he or she may injure staff. Persons with Huntington disease often have good understanding, and staff need to be aware of this. Sensory stimulation needs to be provided for the resident. Support for the family is an important component of care. Guidelines for physical therapy in Huntington disease are available from the European Huntington's Disease Network (http://www.euro-hd.net/html/network/groups/physio/physiotherapy-guidance-doc-2009.pdf).

TREMORS

Tremors become more common with aging. Essential tremor is the most common tremor. Some essential tremors progress from the hands to the head and the legs. Essential tremors can interfere with eating and other activities of daily living. Drug treatments include β-blockers, primidone, and methazolamide. Asymmetrical tremors

Table 24–9. DRUGS ASSOCIATED WITH TREMOR

L-Thyroxine	Caffeine	Lithium
Amiodarone	Albuterol	Fluoxetine
Theophylline	Methylphenidate	Terbutaline
Valproic acid	Carbamazepine	Antipsychotic drugs

at rest are most commonly caused by Parkinson disease. Cerebellar disease presents with an intention tremor with dysmetria. Psychogenic tremors are common in anxious persons or after a stressful event. Tremors occurring in younger persons include dystonic tremor (irregular and jerky tremor) and Wilson disease ("wing-beating" tremor). If Wilson disease is suspected, a serum ceruloplasmin and a 24-hour urine copper level should be obtained. Numerous drugs can cause or exacerbate tremors (Table 24–9). Hyperthyroidism causes a fine tremor.

KEY POINTS

1. Persons with stroke can show rehabilitation potential more than 1 year after the stroke.
2. Rehabilitation of stroke includes mobilization; a focus on motor function, including using a treadmill and robotics; neuromuscular stimulation; motor imagery; reduction in attention deficits; and psychosocial rehabilitation.
3. A focus on the syndromes associated with stroke can improve quality of life.
4. Multiple drugs can cause tremors.
5. L-Dopa–carbidopa is the primary medicine for Parkinson disease. Other medications and deep brain stimulation can help to moderate the "on–off" reactions and dyskinesias.
6. Physical therapy, vibration exercise, and resistance exercise can slow mobility deterioration in Parkinson disease.
7. Nutritional management for Parkinson disease involves avoidance of long-branch chain amino acids, high-calorie foods, and special attention to eating and swallowing.
8. Persons with MS are younger and often deteriorate after admission to a nursing home.
9. Persons with MS have a decline in function after admission to a nursing home.
10. The diagnosis of epilepsy, especially when presenting with partial complex seizures, is difficult to make in nursing home residents.
11. Most persons with Huntington disease in nursing homes are younger, and despite their involuntary writhing movements and difficulty in speaking, have good understanding.
12. Essential tremor is the most common cause of tremor in nursing homes.

TOOLKIT

UF | UNIVERSITY of FLORIDA

DBS Fast Track Network of Referring Physicians

"Every Parkinson's Patient Who Needs DBS Should Have DBS"

*Please take 3-5 minutes and fill out this questionnaire and fax it to us at 352-273-5575 c/o Dr. Okun

We will review the consult within 24 hours and schedule the patient for an appointment in 1-6 weeks (as soon as insurance is verified if the patient has insurance).

Patient Name: _____

Patient Home Contact Phone Number(s):

_____

Patient Insurance:

_____

Referring Physician Name:

_____

Referring Physician Address/City:

Referring Physician/Health Care Provider Phone Number:

Referring Physician Fax Number:

_____

Appendix for article: Okun et. al. Development and initial validation of a screening tool for parkinson's disease surgical candidates. *Neurology*. 2004.

UF | UNIVERSITY *of* FLORIDA

DBS Fast Track Network of Referring Physicians

Florida **S**urgical **Q**uestionnaire for **P**arkinson **D**isease **(FLASQ-PD)**
© Okun and Foote 2003

Date of Evaluation: _____

Please verify a diagnosis of idiopathic PD by assuring your patient meets the UK Brain Bank Criteria (Hughs et al.):

A. Diagnosis of Idiopathic Parkinson's Disease

Diagnosis 1: Is bradykinesia present? Yes/No (Please circle response)

Diagnosis 2: *(check if present):*

____ Rigidity (stiffness in arms, leg, or neck)
____ 4-6 Hz resting tremor
____ Postural instability not caused by primary visual, vestibular, cerebellar, proprioceptive dysfunction

Does your patient have at least 2 of the above? Yes/No (Please circle response)

Diagnosis 3: *(check if present):*

____ Unilateral onset
____ Rest tremor present
____ Progressive disorder
____ Persistent asymmetry affecting side of onset most
____ Excellent response (70-100%) to levodopa
____ Severe levodopa-induced dyskinesia
____ Levodopa response for 5 years or more
____ Clinical course of 5 years or more

Does your patient have at least 3 of the above? Yes/No (Please circle response)

("Yes" answers to all 3 questions above suggest the diagnosis of idiopathic PD)
B. Findings Suggestive of Parkinsonism Due to a Process Other Than Idiopathic PD

Primitive reflexes
1- RED FLAG – presence of a grasp, snout, root, suck, or Myerson's sign
N/A – not done/unknown

Presence of supranuclear gaze palsy
 1- RED FLAG – supranuclear gaze palsy present
N/A – not done/unknown

Presence of ideomotor apraxia
 1- RED FLAG – ideomotor apraxia present
N/A – not done/unknown

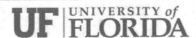

DBS Fast Track Network of Referring Physicians

Presence of autonomic dysfunction
1- RED FLAG – presence of new severe orthostatic hypotension not due to medications, erectile dysfunction, or other autonomic disturbance within the first year or two of disease onset
N/A – not done/unknown

Presence of a wide-based gait
 1- RED FLAG – wide-based gait present
 N/A – not done/unknown

Presence of more than mild dementia
1- RED FLAG – frequently disoriented or severe cognitive difficulties or severe memory problems, or anomia
 N/A – not done, not known

Presence of severe psychosis
 1- RED FLAG – presence of severe psychosis, refractory to medications
 N/A – not done, not known

History of unresponsiveness to levodopa
1- RED FLAG – Parkinsonism is clearly not responsive to levodopa, or patient is dopamine naïve, or patient has not had a trial of levodopa
 N/A – not done, not known

(Any of the "FLAGs" above may be contraindications to surgery)

C. Patient Characteristics *(Circle the one best answer that characterizes your Parkinson's disease surgical candidate):*

1. Age:
    0 – >80
    1 – 71-80
    2 – 61-70
    3 – <61

2. Duration of Parkinson's symptoms:
    0 – <3 years
    1 – 4-5 years
    2 – >5 years

3. On-off fluctuations (medications wear-off, fluctuate with dyskinesia and akinesia)?
    0 – no
    1 – yes

4. Dyskinesias
    0 – none
    1 – <50% of the time
    2 – >50% of the time

5. Dystonia
    0 – none
    1 – <50% of the time
    2 – >50% of the time
General Patient Characteristics Subscore ____

UF | UNIVERSITY of FLORIDA

DBS Fast Track Network of Referring Physicians

D. Favorable/Unfavorable Characteristics

6. Gait freezing
   0 – not responsive to levodopa during the best "on"
   1 – responsive to levodopa during the best "on"
   NA – not applicable

7. Postural instability
   0 – not responsive to levodopa during the best "on"
   1 – responsive to levodopa during the best "on"
   NA – not applicable

8. Warfarin or other blood thinners
   0 – on warfarin or another blood thinner besides antiplatelet therapy
   1 – not on warfarin or another blood thinner besides antiplatelet therapy

9. Cognitive function
   0 – memory difficulties or frontal deficits
   1 – no signs or symptoms of cognitive dysfunction

10. Swallowing function
    0 – frequent choking or aspiration
    1 – occasional choking
    2 – rare choking
    3 – no swallowing difficulties

11. Continence
    0 – incontinent of bowel and bladder
    1 – incontinent of bladder only
    2 – no incontinence

12. Depression
    0 – severe depression with vegetative symptoms
    1 – treated, moderate depression
    2 – mild depressive symptoms
    3 – no depression
13. Psychosis
    0 – frequent hallucinations
    1 – occasional hallucinations – probable medication-related
    2 – no hallucinations

Favorable/Unfavorable Characteristics Subscore ____

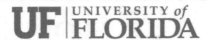

DBS Fast Track Network of Referring Physicians

E. Medication Trials *(circle the best answer)*

14. Historical response to levodopa:
    0 – uncertain historical response to levodopa, or no trial of levodopa
    1 – history of modest improvement with levodopa
    2 – history of marked improvement with levodopa
15. Trial of Sinemet (carbidopa/levodopa or Madopar or equivalent):
    0 – no trial or less than three times a day
    1 – Sinemet three times a day
    2 – Sinemet four times a day
    3 – Sinemet greater than four times a day
16. Trial of dopamine agonist:
    0 – no trial or less than three times a day
    1 – Dopamine agonist three times a day
    2 – Dopamine agonist four times a day
    3 – Dopamine agonist greater than four times a day
17. Trial of Sinemet extender
    0 – no trial
    1 – Trial of either tolcapone or entacapone
18. Trial of a combination of sinemet or equivalent wit h a dopamine agonist
    0 – no trial
    1 – Trial of sinemet or equivalent with a dopamine agonist

Medication Trial Subscore: _____

FLASQ-PD Scoring:

A. Met Diagnostic Criteria of Idiopathic PD: Yes/No
B. Contraindications (FLAGS) Subscore: _____ (8 possible – any flags = likely not a good candidate)
C. General Characteristics Subscore _____ (10 possible)
D. Favorable/Unfavorable Characteristics Subscore: _____ (14 possible)
E. Medication Trial Subscore _____ (10 possible)

Total Scale Score (C+D+E): _____ (34 possible)

Presence of Refractory Tremor:

Yes/No (Presence of moderate-to-severe tremor that is refractory to high doses and combinations of levodopa, dopamine agonists, and anticholinergics may be an indication for surgery in some candidates, independent of their score on the remainder of the questionnaire)

SUGGESTED READINGS

Birnbaum AK. Pharmacokinetics of antiepileptic drugs in elderly nursing home residents. *Int Rev Neurobiol.* 2007;81:211-220.

Buchanan RJ, Martin RA, Wang S, Ju H. Analyses of nursing home residents with multiple sclerosis at admission and one year after admission. *Mult Scler.* 2004;10:74-79.

Buchanan RJ, Martin RA, Zuniga M, et al. Nursing home residents with multiple sclerosis: comparisons of African American residents to white residents at admission. *Mult Scler.* 2004;10:660-667.

Buchanan RJ, Radin D, Huang C, Zhu L. Caregiver perceptions associated with risk of nursing home admission for people with multiple sclerosis. *Disabil Health J.* 2010;3:117-124.

Courtney AM, Treadaway K, Remington G, Frohman E. Multiple sclerosis. *Med Clin North Am.* 2009;93:451-476.

Crawford P, Zimmerman EE. Differentiation and diagnosis of tremor. *Am Fam Physician.* 2011;83:697-702.

Crayton H, Heyman RA, Rossman HS. A multimodal approach to managing the symptoms of multiple sclerosis. *Neurology.* 2004; 63(suppl 5):S12-S18.

Earhart GM, Williams AJ. Treadmill training for individuals with Parkinson disease. *Phys Ther.* 2012;92(7):893-897 April 26.

Fisher RS. Therapeutic devices for epilepsy. *Ann Neurol.* 2012;71:157-168.

Green T, Kelloway L, Davies-Schinkel, et al. Nurses' accountability for stroke quality of care: part one: review of the literature on nursing-sensitive patient outcomes. *Can J Neurosci Nurs.* 2011;33:13-15.

Hardie NA, Garrard J, Gross CR, et al. The validity of epilepsy or seizure documentation in nursing homes. *Epilepsy Res.* 2007;74:171-175.

Huying F, Klimpe S, Werhahn KJ. Antiepileptic drug use in nursing home residents: a cross-sectional, regional study. *Seizure.* 2006;15:194-197.

Lau RW, Teo T, Yu F, et al. Effects of whole-body vibration on sensorimotor performance in people with Parkinson disease: a systematic review. *Phys Ther.* 2011;91:198-209.

Lees AJ, Hardy J, Revesz T. Parkinson's disease. *Lancet.* 2009;373:2055-2066.

Lindsay MP, Kelloway L, McConnell H. Research to practice: nursing stroke assessment guidelines link to clinical performance indicators. *AXON.* 2005;26:22-25.

Miravalle A, Corboy JR. Therapeutic options in multiple sclerosis. *Neurol Clin Pract.* 2010;75(suppl I):S22-S27.

Morris ME, Martin CL, Schenkman ML. Striding out with Parkinson disease: evidence-based physical therapy for gait disorders. *Phys Ther.* 2010;90:280-288.

Pelletier D, Hafler DA. Fingolimod for multiple sclerosis. *N Engl J Med.* 2012;366:339-347.

Reddy MP, Reddy V. Stroke rehabilitation. *Am Fam Physician.* 1997;55:1742-1748.

Rodriguez RL, Fernandez HH, Haq I, Okun MS. Pearls in patient selection for deep brain stimulation. *Neurologist.* 2007;13:253-260.

Stein MS, Liu Y, Gray OM, et al. A randomized trial of high-dose vitamin D2 in relapsing-remitting multiple sclerosis. *Neurology.* 2011;77:1611-1618.

The European Huntington's Disease Network. http://www.euro-hd.net/html/network/groups/physio/physiotherapy-guidance-doc-2009.pdf. Accessed April 15, 2013.

Thomas S, MacMahon D. Managing Parkinson's disease in long-term care. *Nurs Older People.* 2002;14:23-29.

Voxxius C, Nilsen OB, Larsen JP. Parkinson's disease and nursing home placement: the economic impact of the need for care. *Eur J Neurol.* 2009;16:194-200.

MULTIPLE CHOICE QUESTIONS

24.1 Which of the following is true concerning mirror therapy for stroke?

a. The task is performed with the affected arm in front of a mirror.
b. It increases activation of the affected brain hemisphere.
c. The unaffected arm is hidden from view.
d. It requires some function in the affected arm.

24.2 Which is true concerning Parkinson disease?

a. Fewer than 1% of nursing home residents have Parkinson disease.
b. Residents with Parkinson disease cost the same to treat as other residents.
c. Persons with Parkinson disease have five times the chance of being in a nursing home compared with other older persons.
d. Parkinson residents have no difficulty in initiating movement.

24.3 Which of these drugs should be avoided in persons with Parkinson disease?

a. Antipsychotics
b. Digoxin
c. Ropinirole
d. Amantadine
e. Rasagiline

24.4 Which of the following drugs can be used to treat drooling in Parkinson disease?

a. Modafinil
b. Amantadine
c. Propantheline
d. Midodrine
e. Botulinum toxin

Chapter 25

MUSCULOSKELETAL DISORDERS

A total of 35% of women and 26% of men in nursing homes in the United States have arthritis. Arthritis is the major cause of pain in nursing home residents and is an independent risk factor for falls. In one nursing home study, arthritis was responsible for 70% of pain complaints. Arthritic pain is undertreated in persons with dementia. Persons with arthritis use wheelchairs and walking aids and require assistance with transferring and walking to a greater extent that those without arthritis.

OSTEOARTHRITIS

Osteoarthritis is a degenerative disorder of joints caused by damage to the cartilage and overgrowth of bone. Joint pain that is worse with activity leading to loss of function is the classical presenting features. The signs and symptoms of osteoarthritis are given in Table 25–1.

The first component of treatment for osteoarthritis is an exercise program that strengthens the muscles and maintains range of motion around the joint. Both land- and water-based exercises decrease pain and improve function. Ultrasound does not appear to provide clinically significant improvement. Unstable joints can be braced, and a cane or walker can be used to relieve weight on the joint. Residents should be given pain medicine before they have to do relatively long walks (e.g., to the dining room, before exercise sessions in the nursing home).

Acetaminophen (paracetamol; 1000 mg four times a day) is the most effective treatment of osteoarthritis. Nonsteroidal antiinflammatory drugs (NSAIDs) can be added to acetaminophen when acetaminophen alone does not produce pain relief, although there is a marked increase in side effects (see Chapter 11). Celecoxib produces less gastrointestinal bleeding but increases cardiovascular risk and is expensive. NSAIDs should be avoided in patients with hypertension and heart failure. Opioids are added only when acetaminophen and NSAIDs have failed to control pain.

Intraarticular injections of corticosteroids or hyaluronic acid can provide relief for 8 to 16 weeks. They should not be done more than four times a year.

Complementary treatments include the use of glucosamine and chondroitin therapy and capsaicin cream, which is a topical anesthetic that reduces osteoarthritic pain. The supplement S-adenosylmethionine can reduce functional limitations to the same extent as NSAIDs, with fewer side effects.

Joint replacement is an excellent option for persons with severe pain nonresponsive to other treatments that is leading to functional limitation. The comorbidities of most nursing home residents, however, limit this option (Figure 25–1).

RHEUMATOID ARTHRITIS

Rheumatoid arthritis most commonly develops in persons age 30 to 50 years. Approximately 2% of persons older than 60 years of age have rheumatoid arthritis. A subset of persons develop rheumatoid arthritis after the age of 60 years, and this is referred to as elderly-onset rheumatoid arthritis (EORA). Disability is a common occurrence in rheumatoid arthritis.

The classical presentation of rheumatoid arthritis is pain with morning stiffness lasting more than 1 hour. The joints most commonly involved are the wrists, proximal interphalangeal joints, and metacarpophalangeal joints. Boggy swelling (synovitis) over the joints is not rare. Fever, malaise, and weight loss can occur. Rheumatoid nodules may also be present. Rheumatoid factor and anticitrullinated protein antibody are present in about 80% of persons.

EORA has an abrupt onset with large joint involvement predominating. These patients have a higher level of disease activity. Sjögren's disease is a common concomitant. Patients are more likely to have fever, weight loss, fatigue, and a high erythrocyte sedimentation rate. Bone erosions advance rapidly. They are less likely to be rheumatoid factor positive. The disease is as likely to occur in men as in women. The differential diagnosis of rheumatoid arthritis is given in Table 25–2.

Rheumatoid arthritis has a variety of extraarticular manifestations (Table 25–3).

Similar to osteoarthritis, exercise, physical therapy, and occupational therapy to limit disabilities are a cornerstone of long-term therapy. Pain and acute inflammation can be treated with NSAIDs and corticosteroids. Complementary therapies that have demonstrated limited evidence for efficacy are γ-linoleic acid (evening primrose or black currant seed oil) and *Tripterygium wilfordii* (thundergod vine).

Disease-modifying antirheumatic drugs, including biologicals, are the mainstays of treatment (Table 25–4). Hydroxychloroquine is safe and does not require monthly blood tests, making it an attractive option for nursing home residents.

Table 25–1.	SIGNS AND SYMPTOMS OF OSTEOARTHRITIS

- Pain worse on movement
- Movement after rest aggravates pain ("gelling phenomenon")
- Morning stiff for less than 30 minutes
- Swelling around hand joints (Heberden nodes)
- Limitation of range of motion
- Crepitus during range of motion
- Valgus deformities
- Buttock pain (hip osteoarthritis)
- Pseudoclaudication (spinal stenosis)
- Leg weakness and sensory loss (spinal stenosis)
- Pain worse on standing (spinal stenosis)

Table 25–2.	DIFFERENTIAL DIAGNOSIS OF RHEUMATOID ARTHRITIS IN OLDER PERSONS

- Polymyalgia rheumatica
- Remitting seronegative symmetrical synovitis with pitting edema
- Osteoarthritis
- Gout
- Pseudogout
- Autoimmune arthritis (e.g., psoriatic, ankylosing spondylitis)
- Neoplastic-related arthritis
- Sarcoidosis
- Infectious (e.g., hepatitis)

Table 25–3.	EXTRAARTICULAR MANIFESTATIONS OF RHEUMATOID ARTHRITIS

- Rheumatoid nodules
- Pleural effusion
- Lung nodules
- Interstitial lung disease
- Pericarditis
- Episcleritis or ulcerative keratitis
- Keratoconjunctivitis sicca
- Amyloidosis
- Peripheral neuropathy
- Depression
- Infection
- Lymphoma

PSEUDOGOUT (CHONDROCALLINOSIS)

Approximately half of persons older than age 85 years have calcium pyrophosphate dehydrate disease. Acutely, it presents with red, tender, swollen joints of the knees, wrists, or hips. Radiographs show calcified masses in the joint capsule or ligament flavum. Synovial fluid shows calcium pyrophosphate crystals. Treatment consists of corticosteroids, NSAIDs, or both during the acute attack.

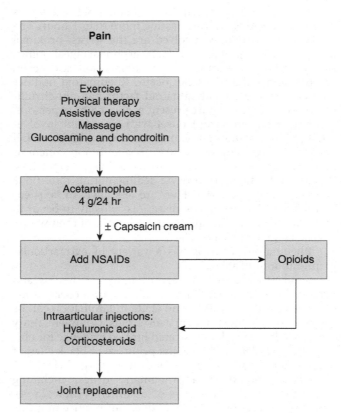

Figure 25–1. A schema for management of osteoarthritic pain. NSAID, nonsteroidal antiinflammatory drug.

Table 25–4.	DISEASE-MODIFYING ANTIRHEUMATIC DRUGS	
Drug	**Adverse Effects**	
Hydroxychloroquine	Ocular toxicity	
Methotrexate	Liver disease, anemia, oral lesions	
Leflunomide	Liver disease, GI distress	
Sulfasalazine	Anemia, I effects	
Anti-TNF agents[a]	Tuberculosis, opportunistic infection, lymphoma, malignancies	
Abatacept	Infection	
Anakinra	Infection, pain at injection site	
Tocilizumab	Infection	
Rituximab	Infusion reaction, progressive multifocal leukoencephalopathy, infection	

[a]Adalimumab, certolizumab pegol, etanercept, golimumab, infliximab.
GI, gastrointestinal; TFN, tumor necrosis factor.

CONTRACTURES

Contractures are caused by a combination of muscle shortening and joint fixation. The major cause is immobility caused by bed rest, strokes, or pain. Contractures occur in nearly one third of residents in U.S. nursing homes and 55% of residents in Scottish care homes. Contractures are even more common in persons with end-stage Alzheimer disease. The effects of contractures are shown in Table 25–5.

Stretching of contractures is the most commonly used management of contractures. Unfortunately, systematic reviews found no evidence demonstrating effectiveness of stretch as a therapy. Similarly, little evidence supports the use of splinting devices to prevent upper extremity contractures. Prevention of contractures requires using the upper extremities in normal activities on a regular basis. Restorative care nursing follows this model both in prevention and in attempting to maintain gains. Walking residents to the dining room instead of pushing them in wheelchairs represents an example of restorative preventive care.

Botulinum neurotoxin type A (Botox) therapy for spasticity and contractures is gaining popularity. Botox has been shown to reduce limb spasticity and reduce the need for bracing. Gait speed may be improved. A study of intramuscular injections of Botox for contractures in long-term care decreased caregiver burden. Botox also improved patients' range of motion.

GOUT

Gout usually presents as pain, redness, and swelling in one joint (or at times more) in the legs. Swelling of the first metatarsal joint (podagra) is classical. The attacks last about 5 to 7 days. Gout attacks may resemble cellulitis or septic arthritis. It is caused by deposition of monosodium urate crystals in the joint. Recurrent gout attacks can lead to the deposition of urate crystals in soft tissues (tophi). These can occur over the joints or in the helix of the ear. Fever and fatigue can be associated with the acute attacks. Most gout attacks occur in persons with uric acid levels greater than 9 mg/dL (535 µmol/L). However, values above 7 mg/dL (415 µmol/L) can also trigger attacks.

Table 25–5.	NEGATIVE EFFECTS OF CONTRACTURES
Pain	
Cannot self-feed	
Cannot dress	
Limited personal hygiene	
Interfere with walking	
Problems with toileting	
Pressure ulcers	
Depression	
Cannot sit comfortably	
Falls	
Fractures	

Table 25–6. RENAL DOSING FOR ALLOPURINOL	
Creatinine Clearance (mL/min)	**Allopurinol Dose**
60–90	200 mg
30–59	100 mg
10–29	50 mg
<10	Consider febuxostat

Treatment of acute attacks involves NSAIDs, corticosteroids, or colchicine. Colchicine should be used in a dosage of 0.6 mg three times a day. Doses need to reduced in persons with renal disease (<50 mL/min glomerular filtration rate [GFR] 0.6 mg twice daily; 35–50 mL/min GFR 0.6 mg/day; <10 mL/min GFR 0.6 mg every second or third day). Side effects include bone marrow suppression and neurologic and muscle damage.

Chronic treatment should attempt to lower uric acid to below 6 mg/dL (355 µmol/L) and should not be begun until 4 to 6 weeks after the acute attack to avoid a flare-up. Concurrent therapy with 0.6 mg of colchicine may reduce flare-ups. Allopurinol (300 mg/day) is the treatment of choice. The dosage should be reduced in persons with low creatine clearance (Table 25–6). Probenecid, losartan, and fenofibrate are uricosuric agents that can be used if the resident cannot tolerate allopurinol. An alternative to allopurinol is febuxostat. It is not more effective than allopurinol.

POLYMYALGIA RHEUMATICA

Polymyalgia rheumatica (PMR) is an inflammatory disorder characterized by muscle pain and morning stiffness in the proximal muscles. Persons with PMR may also have weight loss, fatigue, low-grade fever, peripheral arteritis, and distal swelling of limbs. It can be associated with giant cell arteritis (GCA), an inflammatory, vascular disorder that can lead to vision loss. Symptoms of GCA include headaches, jaw claudication, and fever. The temporal artery may be palpable. In both conditions, elevated erythrocyte sedimentation rate or C-reactive protein is highly suggestive of the disorder in the presence of suspicious symptoms. In Minnesota, PMR occurs in about one in 200 persons older than 50 years of age and in Spain in about one in 1000 persons.

In PMR, magnetic resonance imaging will show vasculitis in one third of patients. The vasculitis may lead to ischemic complications. Ultrasonography may demonstrate subdeltoid or subacromial bursitis. In persons suspected of having CGA, the diagnosis needs to be confirmed with a temporal artery biopsy. The differential diagnosis of PMR is given on Table 25–7.

Treatment of PMR requires initially 15 to 20 mg/day of prednisone for 4 weeks and then a slow taper to 10 mg/day. Corticosteroids can result in a steroid myopathy, so all residents should receive physical therapy to strengthen muscles and improve balance. Vitamin D should also be prescribed to all patients.

Table 25–7.	DIFFERENTIAL DIAGNOSIS OF POLYMYALGIA RHEUMATICA

Rheumatoid arthritis

Pseudogout

Remitting seronegative symmetrical synovitis with pitting edema

Infections

Lymphoma

Hypothyroidism

Amyloidosis

Inclusion body myositis

KEY POINTS

1. Patients with osteoarthritis should first be treated with acetaminophen (4 g/24 hr) before NSAIDs are added.
2. Strengthening muscles and maintaining range of motion around the joint improve symptoms associated with osteoarthritis.
3. EORA tends to be more aggressive than classical rheumatoid arthritis.
4. Treatment of rheumatoid arthritis involves disease-modifying antirheumatic drugs, which can be nonbiologics or biologics.
5. Allopurinol should not be given for 4 to 6 weeks after an acute gout flare.
6. The doses of colchicine and allopurinol need to be reduced in persons with renal failure.
7. Stretching is ineffective for contractures. Some evidence supports the use of Botox.
8. Proximal muscle weakness with painful muscles suggests the diagnosis of polymyalgia rheumatica.

SUGGESTED READINGS

Abell JE, Hootman JM, Helmick CG. Prevalence and impact of arthritis among nursing home residents. *Ann Rheum Dis*. 2004;63:591-594.

Chen XL, Liu YH, Chan DK, et al. Characteristics associated with falls among the elderly within aged care wards in a tertiary hospital: a retrospective. *Chin Med J (Engl)*. 2010;123:1668-1672.

Eggebeen AT. Gout: an update. *Am Fam Physician*. 2007;76:801-808.

Ernst ME, Fravel MA. Febuxostat: a selective xanthine-oxidase/xanthine-dehydrogenase inhibitor for the management of hyperuricemia in adults with gout. *Clin Ther*. 2009;31:2503-2518.

Katalinic OM, Harvey LA, Herbert RD, et al. Stretch for the treatment and prevention of contractures. *Cochrane Database Syst Rev*. 2010;(9): CD007455.

Katalinic OM, Harvey LA, Herbert RD. Effectiveness of stretch for the treatment of prevention of contractures in people with neurological conditions: a systematic review. *Phys Ther*. 2011;91:11-24.

Lam K, Lau KK, So KK, et al. Can botulinum toxin decrease carer burden in long-term care residents with upper limb spasticity? A randomized controlled study. *J Am Med Dir Assoc*. 2012;13:477-484.

Lapane KL, Quilliam BJ, Chow W, Kim M. The association between pain and measures of well-being among nursing home residents. *J Am Med Dir Assoc*. 2012:13:344-349.

Oliver J, Esquenazi A, Fung VSC, et al. Botulinum toxin assessment, intervention and aftercare for lower limb disorders of movement and muscle tone in adults: International consensus statement. *Eur J Neurol*. 2010;17(suppl 2):57-73.

Schmidt J, Warrington KJ. Polymyalgia rheumatica and giant cell arteritis in older patients. *Drugs Aging*. 2011;28:661-666.

Sinusas K. Osteoarthritis: diagnosis and treatment. *Am Fam Physician*. 2012;85:49-56.

Soriano A, Landolfi R, Manna R. Polymyalgia rheumatica in 2011. *Best Pract Res Clin Rheumatol*. 2012;26:91-104.

Souren LE, Franssen EH, Reisberg B. Contractures and loss of function in patients with Alzheimer's disease. *J Am Geriatr Soc*. 1995;43: 650-655.

Villa-Blanco JI, Calfo-Alén. Elderly onset rheumatoid arthritis: differential diagnosis and choice of first-line and subsequent therapy. *Drugs Aging*. 2009;26:739-750.

Wagner LM, Capezuti E, Brush BL, et al. Contractures in Frail nursing home residents. *Geriatr Nurs*. 2008;29:259-266.

Wasserman AM. Diagnosis and management of rheumatoid arthritis. *Am Fam Physician*. 2011;84:1245-1252.

Yip B, Stewart DA, Roberts MA. The prevalence of joint contractures in residents in NHS continuing care. *Health Bull (Edinb)*. 1996;54: 338-343.

MULTIPLE CHOICE QUESTIONS

25.1   What is the treatment of choice for osteoarthritis?

   a. NSAIDs
   b. Celecoxib
   c. Capsaicin cream
   d. Paracetamol (acetaminophen)
   e. Opioids

25.2   Which of the following is true concerning rheumatoid arthritis?

   a. EORA is more aggressive than classical rheumatoid arthritis.
   b. Rheumatoid arthritis occurs in 10% of persons older than 60 years of age.
   c. EORA involves mainly small joints.
   d. Anticitrullinated protein antibody is present in 100%.
   e. Rheumatoid factor is present in 100%.

25.3   Evidence-based treatment of contractures in nursing homes includes:

   a. Splinting devices
   b. Stretching of contractures
   c. Botox
   d. All of the above

25.4   Which of the following is *not* true concerning gout?

   a. Gout classically occurs in the first metatarsal joint.
   b. Gout is caused by deposition of monosodium urate crystals in the joint.
   c. Doses of allopurinol need to be reduced in persons with renal failure.
   d. Colchicine is not cleared by the kidney, so there is no need to reduce doses in persons with renal failure.
   e. Febuxostat is not more effective than allopurinol.

25.5   An 85-year-old woman presents with progressive proximal weakness associated with morning stiffness and muscle pain, which is exacerbated when the muscles are squeezed. Her ESR is 75 mm/hr. She has lost 5% of her weight in the past year. Ultrasonography shows subacromial bursitis. She has headaches and intermittent jaw claudication. An MRI of the temporal artery shows no vasculitis. Which of the following is the most likely diagnosis?

a. Remitting seronegative symmetrical synovitis with pitting edema
b. Polymyalgia rheumatica
c. Polymyalgia rheumatica with giant cell arteritis
d. Pseudogout
e. Inclusion body myositis

25.6   A 74-year-old woman has an abrupt onset of pain in the knees and elbows. She has a dry mouth. She loses 5% of her weight over a few months. She has fatigue and fevers. Her erythrocyte sedimentation rate (ESR) is elevated. She had rapidly advancing bone erosions. She is rheumatoid factor negative. She has rapid functional deterioration. What is the most likely diagnosis?

a. Rheumatoid arthritis
b. Elderly-onset rheumatoid arthritis
c. Polymyalgia rheumatica
d. Sarcoidosis
e. Psoriatic arthritis

Chapter 26

INFECTIONS AND THEIR CONTROL

Infections are very common in nursing homes with a point prevalence of 5.4 to 32.7 per 100 residents. These studies tend to overestimate chronic infections. The incident rates of infections are 10 to 20 infections for every 100 residents per month. Overall the precision of infection rates reported in nursing homes appears to be questionable. Several studies have shown that there is no documentation of justifiable indications for antibiotics prescribed for many of these infections. Although this may in part reflect poor documentation practices after antibiotics are prescribed by telephone by on-call clinicians, inappropriate prescribing results in adverse effects, a high incidence of *Clostridium-difficile* associated diarrhea, unnecessary expenditures, and the potential for antibiotic resistance. Unnecessary antibiotic prescribing is, in fact, a major care quality issue in U.S. nursing homes. Improving antibiotic stewardship is a major opportunity for medical directors and other leaders in nursing homes.

Nursing home residents' propensity to develop infections is increased because of age-related changes in immunity, poor functional status, an increased tendency to aspirate, physiological alterations leading to retention of urine and fecal incontinence, and a high level of comorbidities such as diabetes and chronic pulmonary disease that predispose to infection. The most common infections in nursing homes are urinary tract infections (UTIs), respiratory infections, skin and soft tissue infections, and gastroenteritis.

Infections often present atypically. Fever may be absent, and there may even be hypothermia. Delirium with falls, decreased functional status, apathy, or agitation are commonly seen. A decrease in food or fluid intake associated with tachypnea can rapidly lead to dehydration. Hypotension may occur with septicemia. New onset of or worsening urinary incontinence may occur.

A decision of whether or not to admit a resident to an acute care facility is often difficult. Guidelines to help make this decision are given in Table 26–1. INTERACT, a quality improvement program designed to improve the management of acute changes in condition in vulnerable elderly long-term and post-cute care patients, has Care Paths that provide specific guidance on the identification, evaluation, and management of fever; symptoms of lower respiratory illness; and UTI. These Care Paths are consistent with practice guidelines produced by the American Medical Directors Association and can be downloaded at http://interact2.net.

PNEUMONIA

Pneumonia has been reported to occur in between 3.3% and 11.4% of residents in nursing homes every year. More than half of these residents may die during an episode. The most common symptoms associated with pneumonia are listed in Table 26–2. The typical triad of cough, fever, and shortness of breath is present in only about half of the residents.

The most common pathogens isolated in nursing home–acquired pneumonia are summarized in Table 26–3. *Chlamydia pneumoniae* infection presents with a nonproductive cough often associated with hoarseness or pharyngitis. It can be chronic, lasting for months if not treated. Identification requires polymerase chain reaction (PCR) of nasopharyngeal swabs or direct fluorescent antibody staining. The diagnosis can be made by following serologic titer changes, but this should be retrospective. *Legionella* infection presents with sudden onset of headaches, myalgia, malaise, bradycardia, diarrhea, hyponatremia, and hepatic dysfunction. Urine antigen testing for *Legionella pneumophila* serotype I can be used. Rapid antigen tests of nasopharyngeal or throat swabs are used to diagnose influenza and respiratory syncytial virus should be considered to identify outbreaks that require rapid intervention with isolation and other secondary preventive measures.

Older persons with pneumonia can have either a leukocytosis or a leukopenia with an increase in band forms. A normal C-reactive protein level makes the diagnosis of pneumonia extremely unlikely. Procalcitonin is a poor diagnostic test for respiratory infection in older persons. Adequate sputum specimens are difficult to obtain in the nursing home population with samples of good quality being obtained in fewer than 20% of nursing home residents. Thus, chest radiography represents the key investigation to identify pneumonia in nursing home residents. If the pulse oximetry is below 94%, arterial blood gases may be useful to exclude hypercapnia in patients with chronic obstructive lung disease and asthma, especially in the presence of tachypnea or accessory respiratory muscle use.

Table 26–1.	CRITERIA FOR ADMISSION OF NURSING HOME RESIDENT TO AN ACUTE CARE FACILITY

- Clinical instability or severe illness
  - Tachypnea >28 breaths/min
  - Pulse >120 beats/min
  - Systolic blood pressure <100 mm Hg
  - Severe dehydration
  - Anuria
  - Delirium that cannot be treated in nursing home
- Consideration of code status (e.g., hospice patients should be treated in nursing homes as can many others when residents or family have requested less aggressive intervention)
- Lack of essential diagnostic tests in the nursing home
- Inability to perform therapy or to monitor the patient in the facility
- Inability to provide adequate infection control with the resident in the building (extremely rare)
- Facility cannot provide comfort measures

Table 26–2.	COMMON SYMPTOMS OF PNEUMONIA IN NURSING HOME RESIDENTS

Symptom	Frequency (%)
Dyspnea	40–80
Delirium	50–80
Tachycardia	66
Fever	60–75
Sputum production	35
Chills	25
Pleuritic pain	5–25
Incontinence	5

Recommended treatment for pneumonia in persons older than 65 years both in Britain and the United States is currently an antipneumococcal fluoroquinolone (e.g., levofloxacin or moxifloxacin) or a second- or third-generation cephalosporin (e.g., cefuroxime, ceftriaxone, cefpodoxime) together with azithromycin. For mild and moderate pneumonia, oral therapy should be used. Intramuscular therapy with cefepime or aftriaxone has been successfully used with a 65% to 80% response rate. These injections need to be given with lidocaine to decrease the pain. In some cases, using intramuscular therapy initially for 3 to 5 days and then switching to oral therapy is effective and can reduce cost and discomfort. For residents with a severe infection requiring hospitalization, guidelines suggest the following:

- An antipseudomonal cephalosporin or carbapenem or an extended-spectrum β-lactam/β-lactamase inhibitor

Together with

- An antipseudomonal fluoroquinolone or aminoglycoside

Together with

- An anti–methicillin-resistant *Staphylococcus aureus* (MRSA) drug (e.g., vancomycin or an aminoglycoside)

Older persons with pneumonia are very prone to develop dehydration, and treatment for moderate or severe pneumonia requires fluid replacement either intravenously or subcutaneously. One study found that in persons at end of life in a nursing home, antibiotics did not alter mortality rate nor did they have a significant effect on mortality rate. Recurrent episodes of pneumonia in residents with end-stage dementia or other severe comorbidities are an indication to consider palliative or hospice care.

TUBERCULOSIS

Tuberculosis is four times more common in residents living in nursing homes than in the community. This may be even higher in developing countries. Employees in long-term care are also at high risk for tuberculosis. Congregate

Table 26–3.	COMMON PATHOGENS FOR NURSING HOME–ACQUIRED PNEUMONIA

Bacteria	Frequency (%)
Streptococcus pneumoniae	30–50
Staphylococcus aureus	17–33
Haemophilus influenzae	22
Pseudomonas aeruginosa	7
Klebsiella pneumoniae	6
Moraxella catarrhalis	3
Escherichia coli	2
Atypical Bacteria	
Chlamydia pneumoniae	18
Legionella pneumophila	1–6
Mycoplasma pneumoniae	1
Viruses	
Influenza A	4
Respiratory syncytial virus	4
Parainfluenza	2
Adenovirus	<1

Table 26–4.   FACTORS PRODUCING FALSE-POSITIVE AND FALSE-NEGATIVE TUBERCULIN SKIN TEST RESULTS

False-Positive Results	False-Negative Results
"Boost phenomenon"	Age-related immune dysfunction
Previous bacille Calmette-Guerin (BCG) vaccination	Undernutrition
Cross-reaction with other antigens	Acquired immunodeficiency syndrome
Error in test administration	Live virus vaccinations injected up to 2 months before testing
	Sarcoidosis
	Corticosteroids
	Zinc deficiency
	Error in test reading

Table 26–5.   SPUTUM COLLECTION TECHNIQUE FOR SUSPECTED TUBERCULOSIS

- Wear respiratory protection.
- Maintain isolation protocol.
- Collect on awakening in morning.
- Remove dentures and rinse mouth.
- Use an inhaled saline mist to stimulate cough.
- Inspect the specimen to see it contains sputum, not saliva.
- Consider nasotracheal suction if unsuccessful.

living in nursing homes increases the risk of person to person transmission because six air exchanges per hour are needed to adequately remove and dilute the tuberculosis bacillus from the ambient air. The need to keep doors and windows shut in nursing homes for patient safety means a need for pressure airflow systems, which are rarely found in nursing homes.

The classical screening test for tuberculosis is the targeted tuberculin skin test (Mantoux) test. An intradermal injection of 0.1 mL of purified protein derivative is placed on the forearm. A positive reaction is a 10-mm induration in diameter at 48 hours. All persons with negative test results should undergo two-step testing with a second test 2 to 3 weeks later (i.e., booster testing after the first time they are tested, or the "booster phenomenon"). All new nursing home residents should receive this two-step testing on admission, and then the single test should be repeated yearly in all residents with negative test results. There are a number of causes of both false-positive and false-negative results (Table 26–4). Using a control antigen (mumps or *Candida*) or the other arm can help to identify persons with immune deficiency.

Screening for tuberculosis can also be done with in vitro interferon-γ release assays. In the United States, the only approved test is the QuantiFERON TB Gold Test. They are less affected by bacille Calmette-Guerin (BCG) vaccinations, differentiate nontuberculosis reactions, and do not require the two-step test.

All persons with a positive screening test result require a chest radiography, and if those results are normal, they are treated for latent tuberculosis infection. If chest radiography has abnormal findings or the resident has a cough, fever, or weight loss, the diagnosis of active tuberculosis needs to be ruled out (i.e., sputum for fluorescence microscopy [auramine-rhodamine]) (Table 26–5) and culture or for *Mycobacterium tuberculosis*. If the smear result is positive, PCR can be done to differentiate different types of mycobacteria. Figure 26–1 gives the approach

to diagnosis and treatment of tuberculosis. Side effects of drugs given for tuberculosis chemotherapy are listed in Table 26–6. Isoniazid should always be given with pyridoxine (vitamin B$_6$).

URINARY TRACT INFECTIONS

Urinary tract infections are common in long-term care, occurring in 0.6 residents per 1000 bed days. Asymptomatic bacteriuria is extraordinarily common with a prevalence of 15% to 50%. Persons with a chronic urinary catheter are more than six times likely to develop a UTI, and almost 100% have asymptomatic bacteriuria. Asymptomatic bacteriuria should not be treated in nursing home residents.

Asymptomatic bacteriuria is defined as occurring in a person who has no signs or symptoms of UTI and 100,000 CFU/mL or greater of one bacterial species in the urine. In men, a single voided specimen is sufficient to make the diagnosis, but in women, two specimens are required. White blood cells (WBCs) are present in the urine up to 30% of nursing home residents, making this a poor test to confirm an infection. This has led to substantial overtreatment of presumed UTI.

Urine dipstick testing for leukocyte esterase and nitrites has little value in the nursing home. If both test results are negative, the likelihood of bacteriuria is extremely rare. If only one of the test results is negative, then between 10% and 20% of individuals may still be bacteriuric.

The diagnosis of a UTI requires dysuria or a change in the character of the urine (odor, color, or turbidity) or urinary frequency, suprapubic pain, hematuria, urgency, incontinence, or costovertebral pain. The Centers for Disease Control and Prevention (CDC) and the Infectious Disease Society of America both offer specific recommendation on the definition of UTI, including catheter-associated infections. Because a high proportion of nursing home residents have urinary incontinence or chronic symptoms of overactive bladder, significant worsening of these conditions may indicate an infection. In addition to these criteria, the resident should either have fever or delirium, although urinary infection can occur in the absence of both. Acute mental status change or delirium alone or falls with urine bacteruria and pyuria is insufficient to make the diagnosis. Clinical judgment is required to avoid unnecessary antibiotic treatment. The diagnosis

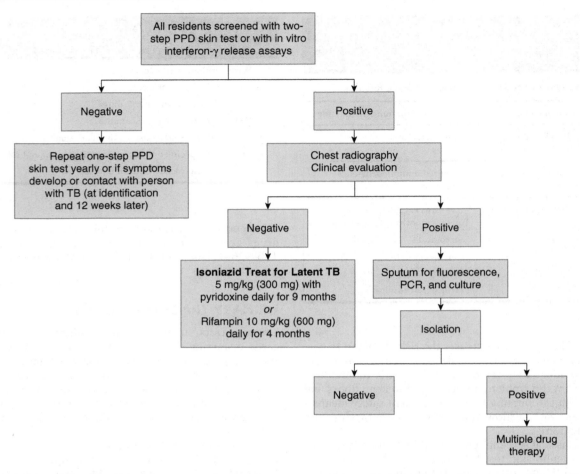

Figure 26–1. Approach to diagnosis and treatment of tuberculosis in nursing homes. PCR, polymerase chain reaction; PPD, purified protein derivative.

is confirmed by the presence of both 100,000 CFU bacteria per high-power field (hpf) or greater and >5 WBCs/hpf in the urine. Specimens cannot be collected from an indwelling catheter because of the biofilm. Thus, the catheter needs to be removed and a clear catheter placed. In women, if a "clean catch" specimen cannot be collected easily, an in-and-out catheterization is often necessary for proper diagnosis. A condom catheter can be used to obtain a specimen in a man. Often UTIs are diagnosed presumptively by on-call clinicians, and an antibiotic is prescribed. In these situations, it is critical to confirm the diagnosis after the culture has been obtained. If the culture result is negative, the antibiotic should be stopped immediately. Elevated interleukin-6 levels in the urine have a high specificity for infection. An elevated or low WBC count and an elevated C-reactive protein may help to confirm the diagnosis. An approach to the diagnosis of a UTI is given in Figure 26–2.

Escherichia coli is the most common infectious organism. *Klebsiella pneumoniae* and *Enterococcus* spp. are other common organism. Other *Enterobacteriaceae* and *Pseudomonas aeruginosa* as well as *Candida* are also seen as causes of infection.

To prevent the development of antimicrobial resistance, antibiotics with the narrowest spectrum should be used. The primary antibiotics to be used should be:

- Trimethoprim–sulfamethoxazole (160/800 mg twice daily) *or*
- Nitrofurantoin monohydrate/macrocrystals 100 mg twice a day if no renal failure

The length of treatment is 5 to 7 days for uncomplicated infections and 10 to 14 days for pyelonephritis. Fluoroquinolones can be used if the resident previously was treated in the past 3 months or if a high rate of resistance to trimethoprim–sulfamethoxazole exists in the nursing home.

In persons with recurrent UTIs, a high intake of cranberry juice may be effective by blocking the adherence of P-fimbriated *E. coli* to uroepithelial cells on the bladder wall. Nursing home residents with recurrent UTIs should be considered for urologic evaluation to exclude a correctable underlying structural abnormality in the urethra, bladder, ureters, or kidneys that may be causing the recurrences.

Table 26–6.   ADVERSE EFFECTS OF CHEMOTHERA-PEUTIC AGENTS FOR TUBERCULOSIS

Drug	Side Effects	Drug Interactions
Isoniazid	Hepatotoxicity	Phenytoin
	Neurotoxicity	Carbamazepine
	Visual disturbances	Aluminum salts
	Anorexia	
	Malaise	
	Fatigue	
	Bruising	
	Jaundice	
Rifampin	Orange urine and contact lenses	Digoxin
		Warfarin
	Hepatotoxicity	β-Blockers
	Thrombocytopenia	Quinidine
Pyrazinamide	Nausea	Insulin
	Hepatoxicity	
	Gout	
	Fever	
	Deep vein thrombosis	
	Hyperglycemia	
Ethambutol	Anorexia	Aluminum salts
	Vomiting	Cephalothin
	Joint pain	
	Altered color perception	
	Gout	
	Dizziness	
	Thrombocytopenia	
Streptomycin	Nephrotoxicity	Loop diuretics
	Ototoxicity	

CELLULITIS

Cellulitis is an infection of dermis and subcutaneous tissues causing a red, warm, swollen, and tender rash. If the borders are raised and there is a clear distinction between infected and uninfected skin, the condition is termed erysipelas and is most likely caused by β-hemolytic streptococci. If the cellulitis has purulent drainage, *S. aureus* is more likely as a diagnosis as is the case if there is an abscess (collection of pus within subcutaneous tissues). MRSA is becoming more common as a causative organism in nursing homes.

The differential diagnosis is outlined in Table 26–7. The recognition of necrotizing soft tissue infection is important because it requires emergent surgery. A normal serum sodium and a WBC count of less than 15.5 cells per mm³

make the diagnosis unlikely. The Laboratory Risk Indicator for Necrotizing Fasciitis (LRINEC) score is given in Table 26–8. Needle aspiration or skin biopsies are not recommended unless the individual fails to respond to antibiotics.

Treatment for nonpurulent cellulitis should be directed at β-hemolytic streptococci with cephalexin, dicloxacillin, or clindamycin. For purulent cellulitis, treatment should include coverage for MRSA with clindamycin, trimethoprim, sulfamethizole, doxycycline, minocycline, or linezolid. Cephalexin can be used if there is a low prevalence of MRSA in the nursing home.

SCABIES

Scabies is a common cause of outbreaks of a severely pruritic skin rash in nursing home residents. Excoriated papules in the web spaces of the fingers together with burrows are the classical presentation. Norwegian scabies is widespread with crusted, papular lesions on the trunk. The diagnosis can be made with skin scrapings.

Residents are treated topically with 5% permethrin cream or 1% lindane lotion from the neck down. These lotions need to remain on the body for 8 hours. A second application may be necessary. Ivermectin (200 μg/kg; two doses 1 week apart) may be necessary to treat Norwegian scabies. All bed linens and clothing need to be washed and heat dried.

Residents should be isolated until treatment is completed and symptoms have improved. Residents sharing a room with the affected resident need to have a single course of topical therapy and their bed linens and clothes washed. Nursing home staff should be screened for symptoms in them and their families because scabies outbreaks can be perpetuated if infections among staff are not recognized and treated.

SHINGLES

Shingles (herpes zoster) is more common in older persons. In nursing homes, it has a frequency of 0.9 occurrences per 10,000 bed days. The disease starts with vesicles on one side of the spine and then spreads in a dermatomal pattern. The vesicles may be preceded by 1 or more days of unilateral pain in the affected area. Shingles can cause severe pain and paresthesias. Treatment consists of oral antiviral therapy begun within 24 hours of the outbreak (Table 26–9). Delirium is a side effect of the antivirals. Occasionally, there is dissemination outside the dermatome or it may involve the eye. Ophthalmologic herpes zoster should be considered an emergency and evaluated and treated rapidly.

Postherpetic neuralgia is when the pain lasts for more than 4 weeks. The pain may be intermittent, disabling, and last for years in some people. Topical lidocaine or a lidocaine patch may help. Other treatments are low-dose tricyclic antidepressants (e.g., desipramine or nortriptyline). More expensive newer therapies include gabapentin and lamotrigine.

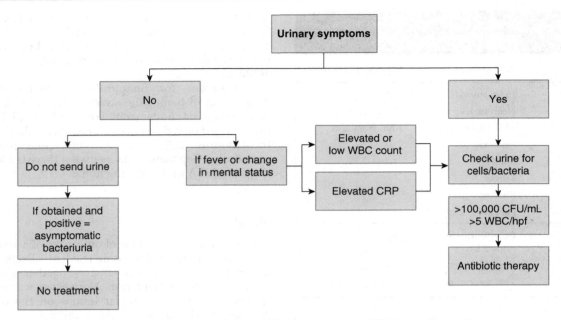

Figure 26–2. Approach to the diagnosis of a urinary tract infection. CRP, C-reactive protein; WBC, white blood cell.

OSTEOMYELITIS

Osteomyelitis occurs secondary to fractures, septicemia, or infected skin ulcers. It is particularly common in persons with diabetes mellitus and peripheral vascular disease. Up to a 25% of individuals who have open fractures develop osteomyelitis, but only 1% to 2% of prosthetic joints become infected.

Clinical features are nonspecific. Normal levels of C-reactive protein and a normal erythrocyte sedimentation rate make osteomyelitis extremely unlikely. Plain radiography may show a periosteal reaction and osteolysis

when the osteomyelitis has been present for some time. As such, radiographs can be helpful in nursing home residents. Magnetic resonance imaging has excellent sensitivity and specificity (about 90%) and is the imaging modality of choice.

Cultures for bacteria obtained directly from bone are needed for the diagnosis. Superficial wound cultures are of little value and should not be obtained. A positive blood culture result may obviate the need for bone biopsy.

Treatment should be driven by bacterial culture with antibiotic susceptibility results. Treatment with antibiotics before biopsy may lead to false-negative bone culture results.

Table 26–7.   DIFFERENTIAL DIAGNOSIS OF CELLULITIS

Condition	Features
Necrotizing fasciitis	Severe pain, blue bullae, crepitus
Erythema migrans	Not painful with tick exposure
Herpetic whitlow	Vesicular on fingers
Gout	Involves joints
Bursitis	Collection of fluid over patella and olecranon
Fixed drug eruption	No pain with recent drug exposure
Hypersensitivity	Pruritus and no pain or fever
Stasis dermatitis	Heme deposition with no fever or pain
Deep vein thrombosis	Pain and swelling but no redness or fever

Table 26–8.   LABORATORY RISK INDICATOR FOR NECROTIZING FASCIITIS SCORE

Test	Points
C-reactive protein >150 mg/L	4
White blood cell count >25 cells/mm³	2
>15 cells/mm³	1
Serum sodium <135 mmol/L	2
Serum creatinine >1.6 mg/dL	2
Serum glucose >180 mg/dL	1
Score Interpretation	
6–7 = 50%–75% possibility of necrotizing infection	
≥8 = >75% possibility of necrotizing infection	

Table 26–9.	TREATMENT FOR SHINGLES
Drug	**Dosage**
Acyclovir	800 mg 5 times a daily for 10 days
Famciclovir	500 mg three times a day for 7 days
Valacyclovir	1G three times a day for 7 days

METHICILLIN-RESISTANT *STAPHYLOCOCCUS AUREUS*

MRSA was first recognized in 1961, and since then, it has become a widespread major cause of bacterial infections. Colonization with *S. aureus* is extremely common in nursing homes with up to 50% of residents being colonized. However, colonization with MRSA varies widely. In a study in 10 nursing homes in Sweden, there was no colonization with MRSA, but 10% of residents were resistant to fluoroquinolones. In other studies in the United States, Belgium, Spain, and the United Kingdom, prevalence varied from 7.8% to 27.5%. Persons with a recent hospitalization are much more likely to be colonized with MRSA. There is evidence that community-acquired MRSA is more virulent than hospital-acquired MRSA. Antibiotics that can be used to treat MRSA are listed in Table 26–10.

MRSA can cause outbreaks in nursing homes involving multiple residents and staff members. This raises the question of the approach to infection control in these residents in a situation where many residents share rooms and others have dementia, making isolation problematic. Screening for nasal colonization and treating with nasal mupirocin (0.7%) is rarely done and places an expense on the nursing home; good practice could argue that hospitals should screen and treat for MRSA carriage before discharge or this should be done on all residents admitted from hospitals. Residents sharing a room with a MRSA-positive resident do not seem to be at high risk for becoming MRSA positive. Regular high-quality hand washing appears to play a major role in prevention of spread. The few studies conducted in nursing homes have shown little benefit of education programs. Isolation should not be overused because residents can quickly become socially isolated and develop symptoms of depression. Isolation is indicated if there is a significant risk of spread from coughing or a wound.

VANCOMYCIN-RESISTANT ENTEROCOCCI

Vancomycin-resistant enterococci (VRE) commonly cause colonization not needing treatment but can cause infections throughout the body, especially in the urinary tract, surgical wounds, and bacteremia. VRE infections have double the mortality of nonresistant enterococci. VRE has a residence time of up to 6 days on furniture. Gloves and gowns should be used for resident care. Hand washing needs to be thorough even if the resident has not been touched. Beds, toilets, and commodes need to be washed with bleach or a hospital-grade disinfectant. Nursing homes may consider doing surveillance cultures in rooms that have been used by residents with VRE.

CANDIDIASIS

Yeast infections can be present in up to 80% of persons in long-term care. Skin lesions classically occur in intertriginous areas. They are fiery red and classically have satellite lesions separated from the edges of the rash. Candidiasis can also involve the mouth, throat, esophagus, areas around dentures (denture stomatitis), paronychia, and cheilitis. In systemic infections, azole-resistant *Candida glabrata* is being more frequently found in older adults. Treatment of candidiasis is with topical antifungals (e.g., nystatin, clotrimazole, and ketoconazole). Severe infections can be treated with fluconazole with caution observed about the many potential drug–drug interactions that can occur with its use.

Table 26–10.	ANTIBIOTICS FOR TREATMENT OF METHICILLIN-RESISTANT *STAPHYLOCOCCUS AUREUS*[a]
Trimethoprim–sulfamethoxazole	
Clindamycin	
Doxycycline	
Minocycline	
Rifampicin plus fusidic acid	
Linezolid	
Vancomycin (IV)	
Tigecycline (IV)	

IV, intravenous.

[a]MRSA can also be resistant to these antibiotics. This is less likely with the newer, more expensive antibiotics and with clotrimazole.

CONJUNCTIVITIS (PINK EYE)

Conjunctivitis occurs at a rate of about 0.5 cases per 1000 resident days and is a classical cause of an epidemic. Infectious conjunctivitis should be distinguished from allergic and traumatic conjunctivitis. The signs of conjunctivitis consist of a purulent exudate or worsening redness in one or both eyes for at least 1 day. Cultures should be obtained whenever possible to establish antibiotic sensitivities. Adenovirus is an important cause of conjunctival epidemics. Common bacterial causes are *S. aureus, Moraxella catarrhalis, Hemophilus* spp. and *S. pyogenes.* When a resident develops conjunctivitis, empirical therapy can be started with antibiotic eye drops, although in some residents, difficulty in administration will make an ointment more practical but limits vision for up to 20 minutes. Most conjunctivitis resolves within 4 days with or without treatment.

HUMAN IMMUNODEFICIENCY VIRUS

HIV is now a treatable disease that remains as a chronic infection. Life expectancy is about 30 years from start of the disease. As such, many older persons are living with the disease, and nursing home admissions with persons with HIV are becoming more common.

In an Australian survey of nursing home personnel in 2009, 55% worried about either catching AIDS or giving it to a family member. Sixty percent were uncomfortable about their ability to look after a patient with HIV. Specialty services for HIV/AIDS are uncommon in nursing homes around the world.

HIV decreases quality of life in older persons by compromising the immune system and causing cognitive decline, depression, and anxiety. HIV residents often face loss of control, and stigma may lead to social withdrawal. If homosexual, a number of sexuality questions may arise, particularly if the resident is younger (see Chapter 15 on sexuality).

HIV patients often have other transmittable infections such as hepatitis B and C. Staff need to be aware that a new onset cough may represent *Pneumocystis carinii* pneumonia or an atypical manifestation of tuberculosis. Diarrhea can be caused by *Campylobacter jejuni*, cytomegalic virus, and a number of parasites. It can also be caused by Kaposi sarcoma of the gut or exocrine pancreatic insufficiency. The HIV treatment regimen itself can also lead to diarrhea.

Nurses need to recognize the importance of maintaining appropriate drug intervals for highly active antiretroviral therapy (HAART) and not missing a dose of medications (Table 26–11). There is a need to recognize which drugs need to be given with or without food and in some cases with a high-fat diet. A pharmacist should review the medication regimen for potential interactions with HAART (Table 26–12).

Prevention of HIV infection in healthcare workers in nursing homes predominantly requires careful hand washing and avoidance of needle sticks. In addition, prevention includes avoidance of blood (e.g., universal precautions) when treating skin lesions and not getting injured if an HIV-positive resident with dementia

Table 26–11.	DRUGS THAT HAVE A CLINICALLY SIGNIFICANT INTERACTION WITH PROTEASE INHIBITORS	
Statins	Alprazolam	St. John's wort
Phenytoin	Triazolam	Bromo-ergocryptine
Carbamazepine	Cisapride	Pimozide
Rifampin	Amiodarone	Quinidine
Proton pump inhibitors	Hydroxyurea	Sildenafil
Warfarin		

becomes aggressive. Wounds should be washed and rinsed immediately. Antiretroviral therapy should be started within 48 to 72 hours. Typical prophylaxis involves an HIV-protease inhibitor (lopinavir plus ritonavir) together with a combination of two nucleoside reverse transcriptase inhibitors (emtricitabine and tenofovir or lamivudine and zidovudine). Unprotected sex should be avoided for 3 months after exposure.

INFECTION CONTROL

Infection control plays a crucial role in nursing homes. Infection control programs help to provide a sanitary environment and to prevent the development and transmission of infection (Table 26–13). The most common infectious epidemics in nursing homes are listed in Table 26–14.

Larger facilities (>100 residents) should have an infection control committee; smaller facilities may wish to handle the infection program as part of their monthly continuous quality improvement program. The infection control committee should be led by an infection control nurse with training and an interest in infection control. Other members should be the director of nursing, the

Table 26–12.	FOOD INTERACTIONS WITH HIGHLY ACTIVE ANTIRETROVIRAL THERAPY			
No Effect	**Take on an Empty Stomach**	**Low-Fat Meal**	**High-Fat Meal**	**Take with Food**
Lamivudine	Zidovudine	Lamivudine–zidovudine	Lopinavir–ritonavir	Tenofovir
Abacavir	Didanosine			Ritonavir
Stavudine	Indinavir			Nelfinavir (high protein)
Zalcitabine	Saquinavir			
Delavirdine				
Efavirenz				
Nevirapine				
Amprenavir				

Table 26–13.	BASIC ELEMENTS OF AN INFECTION PROGRAM

- An infection control committee
- Written protocols and procedures that are updated regularly
- Infection surveillance programs
- Antibiotic resistance surveillance program
- Hand hygiene
- Employee health program
- Education of employees, residents, and visitors
- Rapid intervention for epidemic outbreaks
- Communication of reportable diseases to public health authorities
- Information transfer concerning infections, including culture and antibiotic sensitivities and vaccination status

Table 26–15.	MY FIVE MOMENTS OF HAND HYGIENE

1. Before patient contact
2. Before aseptic task
3. After body fluid exposure risk
4. After patient contact
5. After contact with patient surroundings

administrator, the individual responsible for obtaining admission information from the hospital, and a physician. The committee should be able to access consultation from an infectious disease specialist. Key components of the committee's role are to develop and review policies and procedures and collect and analyze (audit) infections and antibiotic utilization and resistance in the facility. A regular audit should be kept on inappropriate antibiotic usage based on urine cultures and reported infections. Records of the committee meetings together with infection data should be kept for at least 5 years.

Hand hygiene remains the best measure to prevent transmission of infections. Staff needs to be regularly educated about hand hygiene, and regular audits on compliance need to be carried out. It is estimated that in most facilities, hand washing compliance is present between 30%

and 50% of the time. The World Health Organization created the "Clean Care is Safer Care" awareness program in 2005. The basis of this program is "My Five Moments of Hand Hygiene" (Table 26–15). Waterless alcohol-based hand rubs can be used in place of soap and water hand washing. They cause less skin dryness and irritation than soap and water. Alcohol is flammable, and as such, dispensers should only be in resident rooms and not in corridors that are part of fire exit strategy.

All staff should be trained in standard precautions as outlined by the CDC (Table 26–16). These should be used with all residents regardless of the diagnosis. Nursing homes need to regularly audit compliance with these precautions.

Posters in the facility should be available to educate all on cough etiquette. This includes covering mouth when coughing, use of tissue to cover the mouth and nose, appropriate disposal of tissues, and washing hands after exposure to respiratory secretions. Residents displaying respiratory symptoms (cough or running nose) should be kept at least 3 feet (1 m) away from other residents when feasible. Sterile, single-use disposable needles and syringes need to be used facility wide, and appropriate containers for disposal of sharps should be readily available. Residents should have their wounds covered, and their hands should be washed before they are involved in group activities such as dining and recreational activities.

Highly infectious diseases such as tuberculosis (airborne spread), influenza (droplet spread), and *C. difficile* (excretions spread) should have transmission-based

Table 26–14.	MOST COMMON INFECTIOUS EPIDEMICS IN NURSING HOMES	
	Attack Rate	**High Transmission**
Scabies	70[a]	Yes
Chlamydia pneumoniae	46	Yes
Clostridium perfringens	48	No
Noroviruses	45	Yes
Rota viruses	45	No
Adenovirus (epidemic keratoconjunctivitis)	42	No
Respiratory syncytial virus	40[a]	Yes
Influenza virus	33	Yes
Escherichia coli	31	Yes

[a]Fatality rate >20%.

Table 26–16.	ELEMENTS OF "STANDARD PRECAUTIONS" TO BE USED WITH ALL RESIDENTS WHEN THERE IS CONTACT WITH BLOOD, BODY FLUIDS, SECRETIONS, OR EXCRETIONS

Hand hygiene care
Use of gloves
Use of masks
Use of gowns
Use of eye protection
Avoid injuries from sharps
Use of respiratory hygiene and cough etiquette
Safe injection practices

Table 26–17.   MANAGEMENT OF EPIDEMIC OUTBREAKS

- Recognize it early.
- Confirm the diagnosis in the index resident.
- Educate staff on signs and symptoms and rapid reporting.
- Isolate infected residents in one area.
- Inform all physicians and advanced practice nurses of outbreak.
- Work as a team to contain outbreak.
- Initiate treatment as soon as appropriate.
- Plot an epidemic curve showing the development of cases over time.
- Obtain advice from local health department or infectious disease expert when necessary.
- Report epidemic to local health authorities and to any hospitals to which a resident is being transferred.

precautions based on the facilities guidelines for infection control. Use of single rooms is ideal but is rarely available in nursing homes. Cohorting is a reasonable approach to conditions such as influenza. Persons with *C. difficile* infection need to be kept in their rooms if the diarrhea cannot be contained. Toilets need to be thoroughly cleaned after each episode. Persons with active tuberculosis need to be isolated until treatment is started and wear masks until coughing is controlled. Residents with severe immune deficiencies should not be placed in the same room with persons requiring transmission-based precautions.

Infection surveillance requires collection of data of all ongoing infections in the facility. In addition, it is useful to provide maps of the facility delineating where infections occur because this increases the chance of earlier identification of epidemics or of areas where there is poor adherence to universal precautions. Infection rates are reported as infections per 1000 patient days. Patient days can be either actual resident days or more easily based on average resident census multiplied by the days in the month.

Epidemics (infection outbreaks greater than the endemic levels) occur commonly in nursing homes. Table 26–17 outlines an approach to epidemic management.

Tracking antibiotic use and the development of drug resistance in the nursing home is key to improving antibiotic stewardship. Because the number of cases in the nursing home is often insufficient to document antibiotic resistance patterns, it is helpful for the local laboratory to provide information on a number of nursing homes in the area and separately on the patterns from referring hospitals. Recognition and education on inappropriate antibiotic use is an important component of the prevention of the emergence of multidrug resistance.

An employee health program needs to identify and prevent employees with communicable diseases or infected skin lesions from providing direct care to residents or preparing food. Employees who are in the food service section need to be educated that when they develop diarrhea, they need to report it and stop preparing food. Employees should have a medical examination (including

a tuberculosis screen) before starting employment and yearly thereafter. All employee immunizations should be kept current (Table 26–18).

A nurse-led infection prevention program in the United Kingdom successfully improved infection control in care homes in Wolverhampton City. The components of the PREVENT program were:

- **Promotion of best practices by having an infection champion**
- **Regular monitoring of staff**
- **Ensure standards of hand washing**
- **Visible compliance with appropriate clothing**
- **Environmental cleanliness**
- **Never accept poor standards**
- **Take action to protect residents**

VACCINATIONS

Vaccinations are an important component of the infection prevention program in nursing homes. Both residents and healthcare workers, including physicians, need to be vaccinated (Table 26–18). Influenza vaccination represents the most important vaccination program in the nursing home. Influenza vaccination is associated with decreased mortality rates and hospitalizations. The influenza virus has a high mutation rate. This results in a need to produce a new vaccination each year. Efficacy of the vaccine varies from 50% to 70% each year. Because nursing home residents have poor immune systems resulting in poor antibody titers, vaccination should be given as near as possible to the beginning of the influenza season. Some studies have suggested that nursing home residents may benefit from receiving influenza vaccination twice during the winter. At present, there is both a standard trivalent intramuscular vaccine and a higher dose version containing four times as much antigen.

Table 26–18.   VACCINATIONS FOR RESIDENTS AND HEALTHCARE WORKERS IN LONG-TERM CARE

	Residents	Healthcare Workers
Influenza	One dose yearly	One dose yearly
Pneumococcal (polysaccharide)	One dose	One dose every 5 years
Zoster	One dose	No
Tetanus diphtheria	Possibly	Booster every 10 years
Measles, mumps, rubella	No	One dose
Meningococcal	No	Possibly
Hepatitis A	No	Possibly
Hepatitis B	No	Yes

Although the higher dose produces a higher antibody level, there is, at present, no evidence that it reduces attack rates. To reduce attack rates during the influenza season in a nursing home, it is important to obtain "herd immunity." At least 80% of persons in the nursing home, including workers and regular visitors, need to be vaccinated for the program to be successful. During the winter even after successful vaccinations, any resident who develops influenza-like symptoms (fever, cough, headache, body aches, or diarrhea) should be tested with a rapid diagnostic test for influenza. Depending on the test, sensitivity varies from 50% to 70% and specificity from 90% to 95%. Information about the different tests for influenza is available at http://www.cdc.gov/flu/professionals/diagnosis/rapidlab.htm.

Pneumococcal vaccination is 60% to 70% effective in preventing pneumonia. All residents in the nursing home should have received at least one dose within the past 5 years. Immunogenicity wanes more quickly in older sick persons. Although the recommendation is for a single dose of vaccination in those older than 65 years of age, it is possible that nursing home residents may benefit from being vaccinated more frequently.

Vaccination for herpes zoster is recommended in all persons older than 60 years of age. It prevents approximately half of all cases of shingles. It also reduces pain and length of the illness in another half of those who develop shingles. It prevented postherpetic neuralgia in about two thirds of those who develop herpes zoster. Efficacy of the vaccine decreases with age.

Hepatitis A vaccination is an inactivated whole-virus vaccine that has been recommended for healthcare workers. Hepatitis B vaccination has an efficacy of greater than 90%. It is also recommended for healthcare workers.

10. Cellulitis with raised borders and a clear distinction between infected and uninfected skin is caused by B-hemolytic streptococcus.
11. Cellulitis with purulent drainage is caused by *Staphylococcus aureus* and is often methicillin resistant (MRSA).
12. Early recognition of necrotizing soft tissue infection is important for timely surgical intervention.
13. Scabies is a common cause of outbreaks of an itching skin rash. When it is widespread with crusted, papular lesions, it is Norwegian scabies. Staff need to be examined and questioned about their families to prevent recurrent outbreaks.
14. Vesicles in a single dermatome suggest shingles and need to be treated within 24 hours of the outbreak to minimize complications.
15. Hand hygiene represents the primary component for prevention of infectious disease.
16. All staff should be trained in "standard care precautions," and adherence to this program should be audited regularly.
17. Facilities should have a proactive program to recognize possible epidemics and to contain them.
18. Vaccinations are important to reduce morbidity and mortality, and the nursing home should monitor that both residents and healthcare staff have been appropriately vaccinated.
19. Herpes zoster vaccination prevents attacks in half of residents.
20. All staff should have hepatitis B and possibly hepatitis A vaccinations.

KEY POINTS

1. Infections are the most common treatable conditions that occur in nursing homes.
2. All nursing homes need an infectious disease control nurse and an infectious disease committee.
3. The classical triad of cough, dyspnea, and shortness of breath is present in fewer than half of nursing home residents with pneumonia.
4. Not all residents with symptoms or a diagnosis of pneumonia need to be transferred to an acute hospital.
5. All persons in nursing homes should be screened for tuberculosis, and on admission, persons with a negative test result should be retested to exclude the "booster phenomenon."
6. Residents with positive urine cultures or WBCs in the urine should not be treated unless there are symptoms referable to the urinary tract.
7. Nitrofurantoin monohydrate and trimethoprim–sulfamethoxazole are first-line antibiotic treatment for UTIs to prevent antibiotic resistance.
8. Specimens for a urine culture should not be collected from an indwelling catheter before it is changed.
9. Urine dipstick (leukocyte esterase and nitrites) should not be used to diagnose UTIs.

SUGGESTED READINGS

Ariathianto Y. Asymptomatic bacteriuria: prevalence in the elderly population. *Aust Fam Physician.* 2011;40:805-809.

Bentley DW, Bradley S, High K, et al. Practice guideline for evaluation of fever and infection in long-term care facilities. *J Am Geriatr Soc.* 2001;49:210-222.

Beveridge LA, Davey PG, Phillips G, McMurdo MET. Optimal management of urinary tract infections in older people. *Clin Interv Aging.* 2011;6:173-180.

Centers for Disease Control and Prevention. Rapid Diagnostic Testing for Influenza. http://www.cdc.gov/flu.professionals/diagnosis/rapidlab. htm. Access April 29, 2013.

Chien NT, Dundoo G, Horani MH, et al. Seroprevalence of viral hepatitis in an older nursing home population. *J Am Geriatr Soc.* 1999;47:1110-1113.

Cummins D, Trotter G, Murray K, et al. Development of HIV resources for aged care facilities. *Aust Nurs J.* 2010;18:23.

De Schrijver K, Eurosurveillance Editorial Team. Hepatitis B transmission in care homes linked to blood glucose monitoring, Belgium and United States. *Euro Surveill.* 2005;10(3):E050317.1.

DeLeo FR, Otto M, Kreiswirth BN, Chamber HF. Community-associated methicillin-resistant staphylococcus aureus. *Lancet.* 2010;375:1557-1568.

Dreesman JM, Baillot A, Hamschmidt L, et al. Outbreak of hepatitis B in a nursing home associated with capillary blood sampling. *Epidemiol Infect.* 2006;134:1102-1113.

Duffell EF, Milne LM, Seng C, et al. Five hepatitis B outbreaks in care homes in the UK associated with deficiencies in infection control practice in blood glucose monitoring. *Epidemiol Infect.* 2011;139:327-335.

Flanagan E, Chopra T, Mody L. Infection control in alternative healthcare settings. *Infect Dis Clin North Am.* 2011;25:271-283.

Gross L, Barbieri A, Carnevale L. Prevalence of infections in nursing homes in the Vercelli area (Piemonte, Italy). *Ig Sanita Pubbl.* 2012; 68:29-48.

Gunderson CG. Cellulitis: definition, etiology and clinical features. *Am J Med.* 2011;124:1113-1122.

Hatzenbuehler J, Pulling TJ. Diagnosis and management of osteomyelitis. *Am Fam Physician.* 2011;84:1027-1033.

Hauck FR, Neese BH, Panchal AS, El-Amin W. Identification and management of latent tuberculosis infection. *Am Fam Phys.* 2009; 79:879-886.

High KP, Bradley SF, Gravenstein S, et al. Clinical practice guideline for the evaluation of fever and infection in older adult residents of long-term care facilities: 2008 update by the infectious diseases society of America. *J Am Geriatr Soc.* 2009;57:375-394.

Hillson CM, Barash JH, Buchanan EM. Adult vaccination. *Prim Care Clin Office Pract.* 2011;38:611-632.

Hughes C, Smith M, Tunney M, Bradley MC. Infection control strategies for preventing the transmission of methicillin-resistant staphylococcus aureus (MRSA) in nursing homes for older people. *Cochrane Database Syst Rev.* 2011;7(12):CD006354.

INTERACT (Interventions to Reduce Acute Care Transfers). http://interact2.net. Accessed April 15, 2013.

Janssens J-P, Drause K-H. Pneumonia in the very old. *Lancet Infect Dis.* 2004;4:112-124.

Mills K, Nelson AC, Winslow BT, Springer KL. Treatment of nursing home acquired pneumonia. *Am Fam Physician.* 2009;79:976-982.

Nichol KL. Influenza vaccination in the elderly: impact on hospitalisation and mortality. *Drugs Aging.* 2005;22:495-515.

Nicolle LE. Urinary tract infections in the elderly. *Clin Geriatr Med.* 2009;25:423-436.

O'Donnell JA, Hofmann MT. Skin and soft tissues: management of four common infections in the nursing home patient. *Geriatrics.* 2001;56:33-38.

Oh RC, Hustead TR. Causes and evaluation of mildly elevated liver transaminase levels. *Am Fam Physician.* 2011;84:1003-1008.

Olofsson M, Lindgren POE, Ostgren CJ, et al. Colonization with staphylococcus aureus in Swedish nursing homes: a cross-sectional study. *Scand J Infect Dis.* 2012;44:3-8.

Sankar A, Nevedal A, Neufeld S, et al. What do we know about older adults and HIV? A review of social and behavioral literature. *AIDS Care.* 2011;23:1187-1207.

Tjioe M, Vissers WH. Scabies outbreaks in nursing homes for the elderly: recognition, treatment options and control of reinfestation. *Drugs Aging.* 2008;25:299-306.

Utsumi M, Makimoto K, Quroshi N, Ashida N. Types of infectious outbreaks and their impact in elderly care facilities: a review of the literature. *Age Ageing.* 2010;39:299-305.

Vox D, Gotz HM, Richardus JH. Needlestick injury and accidental exposure to blood: the need for improving the hepatitis B vaccination grade among health care workers outside the hospital. *Am J Infect Control.* 2006;34:610-612.

Wilkins T, Malcolm JK, Raina D, Schade RR. Hepatitis C: diagnosis and treatment. *Am Fam Physician.* 2010;81:1351-1357.

Wilkins T, Zimmerman D, Schade RR. Hepatitis B: diagnosis and treatment. *Am Fam Physician.* 2010;81(8):965-972.

Winfield J, Wiley C. tackling infection in care homes. *Nurs Times.* 2012; 108:18-20.

Yoshikawa TT, Norman DC. Approach to fever and infection in the nursing home. *J Am Geriatr Soc.* 1996;44:74-82.

MULTIPLE CHOICE QUESTIONS

26.1   Which of the following makes the diagnosis of pneumonia unlikely in a nursing home resident?

    a. Lack of cough
    b. Leukopenia
    c. Leukocytosis
    d. Normal C-reactive protein
    e. Elevated procalcitonin

26.2   Good quality sputum specimens are obtained in what percentage of nursing home residents?

    a. 5% to 10%
    b. 11% to 15%
    c. 16% to 20%
    d. 25% to 30%
    e. >50%

26.3   Which of the following can produce a false-positive tuberculin skin test result?

    a. BCG vaccination
    b. Immune dysfunction
    c. Protein energy malnutrition
    d. Zinc deficiency
    e. Corticosteroids

26.4   Why does a new admission to the nursing home who has a negative response to tuberculin need a second test 1 to 2 weeks later?

    a. Rule out error in test administration
    b. In case test was improperly read
    c. To test for sarcoidosis
    d. To check for the "booster phenomenon"

26.5   Which vitamin needs to be given with isoniazid?

    a. Vitamin B_1
    b. Pyridoxine
    c. Vitamin B_{12}
    d. Vitamin A
    e. Vitamin E

26.6   Making the diagnosis of UTI requires:

    a. A urine WBC count >20 cells/hpf
    b. ≥100,000 CFU bacteria/hpf in the urine specimen
    c. Dysurea
    d. A positive γ-interferon in vitro test result
    e. A urine WBC count >5 cells/hpf and ≥100,000 CFU bacteria/hpf and symptoms compatible with a UTI

26.7   Which antibiotics are recommended as primary treatment for UTI to limit the development of antibiotic resistance?

    a. Trimethoprim–sulfamethoxazole
    b. Ciprofloxin
    c. Nitrofurantoin
    d. A and B
    e. A and C

26.8   Which of the following make the diagnosis of necrotizing soft tissue infection likely?

    a. Hyponatremia
    b. WBC count >15 cells/mm^3
    c. A normal C-reactive protein
    d. No soft tissue pain

26.9 An 82-year-old woman in the nursing home complains of pain in her back radiating to the left chest wall. On examination, there are a few pustules in a single dermatome on the left side of her back. What is the most likely diagnosis?

a. Scabies
b. Pemphigus
c. Osteomyelitis
d. Shingles
e. Pemphigoid

26.10 Which of the following are cost-effective approaches to limiting the spread of MRSA infection in nursing homes?

a. Regular hand washing
b. Place the resident in a single room and do not allow him or her to wander in the nursing home
c. Screening for nasal colonization and treating with mupirocin
d. All of the above

Chapter 27

ANEMIA

The World Health Organization defines anemia as a hemoglobin level less than 13 g/dL in men and less than 12 g/dL in women. Using this definition, studies in Spain, Israel, and the United States suggest that approximately half of residents in nursing homes have anemia. With this definition, men have more anemia than women. However, it should be recognized that the fall in 1 g/dL in men is attributable to the decline in testosterone, and as such in nursing homes, it is advisable to use levels less than 12 g/dL to diagnose anemia in men. Figure 27–1 sets out the variety of adverse effects anemia has in nursing home residents.

CAUSES OF ANEMIA

The basic causes of anemia are outlined in Figure 27–2. The most common cause of anemia in nursing homes is the anemia of chronic disease. There are two major categories of the anemia of chronic disease, which are (1) anemia caused by chronic inflammation in which iron levels are low and ferritin levels are high and there is a decreased response to erythropoietin, and (2) anemia of kidney failure, which is driven by a reduced production of erythropoietin and a lesser degree of inflammation: The trapping of iron in macrophages resulting in the increase of ferritin is caused by interleukin-6 and other cytokines, causing the release of hepcidin from the liver. Hepcidin then inhibits the ferroportin (iron transporters) in the macrophages.

It has been suggested that there is an idiopathic anemia of old age. However, this can be explained by a number of factors present in the majority of nursing home residents. These include the fall in testosterone in men, a mild increase in inflammation, a decrease in kidney function, protein energy undernutrition, low levels of gastrointestinal (GI) bleeding, and mild forms of myelodysplasia.

The other common anemia in nursing home residents is a microcytic anemia caused by iron deficiency. Iron-deficiency anemia is most commonly caused by bleeding from the GI tract but can also be caused by hemoptysis, recurrent epistaxis, hematuria, or bleeding into tissues after a fall. Nonsteroidal antiinflammatory agents, aspirin, and Coumadin remain the most common causes of GI bleeding. Colonic neoplasms and angiodysplasia also need to be considered. Peptic ulcers are much less common since the recognition that *Helicobacter pylori* represents their major cause and this infection has now been treated in most persons.

Macrocytic anemias are most commonly caused by nutritional disorders such as vitamin B_{12}, folate, or pyridoxine deficiency. Folate deficiency is less common in the United States and other countries where flour is fortified with folate. Hypothyroidism, liver disease, and some drugs can also result in macrocytic anemia.

About 5% of older persons have myelodysplastic anemia. Red blood cells (RBCs) are decreased in 100% of persons with myelodysplasia, white blood cells (WBCs) in 50%, and thrombocytes in 25%. Previously, when only RBC were reduced, this condition was called sideroblastic anemia. Myelodysplasia produces a macrocytic anemia in half of the patients. It also produces hyposegmented nuclei and granular content in WBCs and megakaryocytes. Other causes of bone marrow suppression include drugs, such as amiodarone, and malignancies.

Hemolytic anemia occurs either because of intra-vascular hemolysis or extravascular hemolysis. In older persons, the acquired causes are obviously more common than hereditary. Autoimmune hemolytic anemia is identified by the Coombs' test (direct antiglobulin test). Warm hemolysis is caused by IgG autoimmune antibodies, and cold hemolysis is caused by IgM autoantibodies. Most autoimmune hemolysis is idiopathic but can also be caused by lymphoma, chronic lymphocytic leukemia, infections such as *Mycoplasma pneumoniae* and HIV, and drugs. Microangiopathic hemolytic anemia (fragmentation hemolysis) is caused by RBCs being damaged by injured vascular endothelium. Infections can be directly toxic to RBCs. Of the congenital causes seen in older persons, the most likely are the hemoglobinopathy thalassemia and glucose-6-phosphate dehydrogenase deficiency.

DIAGNOSIS OF ANEMIA

The first test in the diagnosis of anemia is to obtain a corrected reticulocyte count (Figure 27–3). If the count is high, there is an increased unconjugated (indirect) bilirubin, and haptoglobin levels are low, the diagnosis is hemolytic anemia. If the bilirubin is not elevated, hemorrhage is

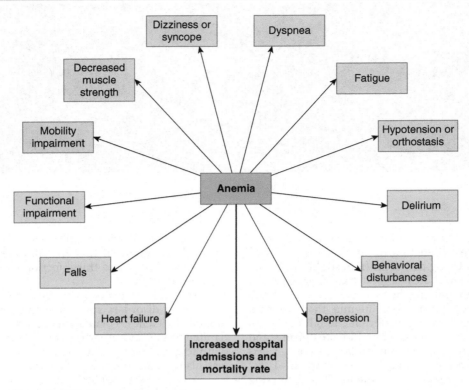

Figure 27–1. Adverse effects of anemia in nursing home residents.

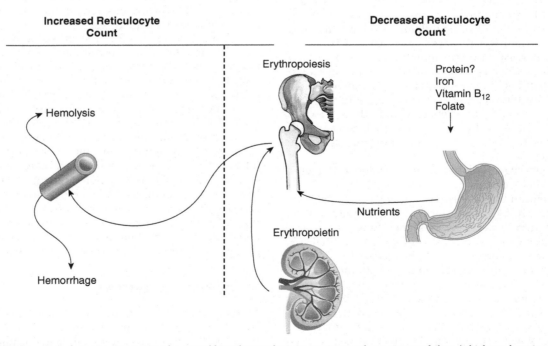

Figure 27–2. Basic causes of anemia. Anemia can be caused by either inadequate nutrients or bone marrow failure (which can be primary or secondary to inadequate erythropoietin stimulus), which is associated with a low reticulocyte count. An increased reticulocyte count occurs in anemia caused by either hemorrhage or hemolysis.

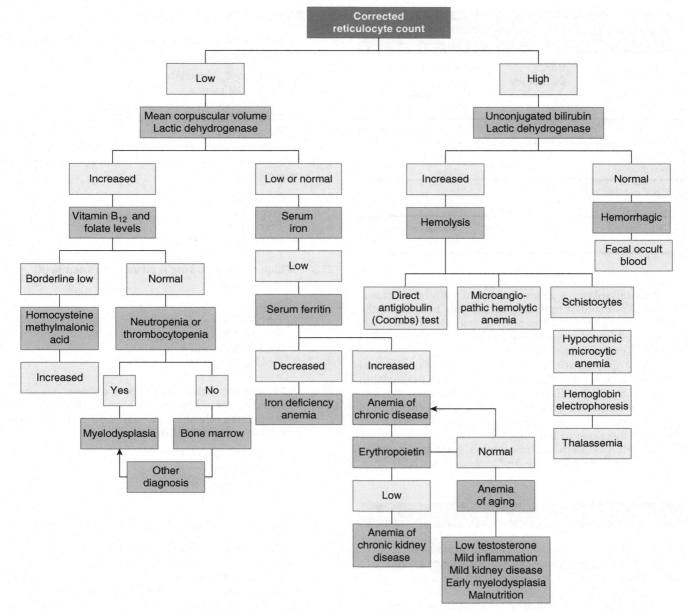

Figure 27–3. Approach to the diagnosis of anemia.

the most likely diagnosis, and a fecal occult blood should be obtained. If the corrected reticulocyte count is low and mean corpuscular volume and lactic dehydrogenase are increased, vitamin B_{12} and folate levels should be obtained. Low levels diagnose deficiency; persons with borderline levels should have a methylmalonic acid (vitamin B_{12} deficiency) or homocysteine (folate and vitamin B_{12} deficiency) measured. If folate and vitamin B_{12} levels are normal, myelodysplasia should be considered. Microcytic or normocytic anemia suggests either iron-deficiency anemia or anemia of chronic disease. These two anemias can be differentiated by carrying out appropriate iron studies (Table 27–1).

MANAGEMENT OF ANEMIA

In most cases, patients with iron-deficiency anemia can be treated with oral iron at a low dose of elemental iron (20 mg) for 6 weeks (325 mg of iron gluconate contains 37 mg of iron, and 300 mg of iron sulfate contains 60 mg of iron). Iron tablets interfere with the absorption other medication and thus cannot be given with other drugs. If there is no increase in the reticulocyte count after 1 week, the possible need for parenteral iron because of malabsorption should be considered.

Vitamin B_{12} deficiency can be treated either with intramuscular, nasal, or high-dose oral vitamin B_{12}.

Table 27–1.   DIFFERENTIAL DIAGNOSIS OF IRON-ASSOCIATED ANEMIAS

	Iron Deficiency	Anemia of Chronic Disease
Iron	Low	Low
Ferritin	Low (<20 ng/mL)	High (>50 ng/mL)
Transferrin receptors	High	Low
Total iron-binding capacity	High	Low
Bone marrow	Absent iron stores	Normal or increased iron stores

Myelodysplasia is generally treated with blood transfusions. Erythroid-stimulating agents can be used if the erythropoietin levels are low and blasts levels are below 5%. Drugs available to treat myelodysplasia are lenalidomide and DNA methyl transferase inhibitors.

Erythropoiesis-stimulating agents (epoetin alfa and darbepoetin alfa) can be used for persons with hemoglobin levels less than 10 g/dL with chronic kidney disease, those on chemotherapy for cancer, persons with rheumatoid arthritis, and those with myelodysplasia. Hemoglobin levels should be increased to 10 g/dL only and at a rate of no more than 1 g/dL per month. These agents cause hypotension, cardiovascular events, stroke, and increased mortality rates.

KEY POINTS

1. The most common causes of anemia are anemia of chronic kidney disease and iron-deficiency anemia.
2. Myelodysplasia occurs in about 5% of nursing home residents.
3. Treatment of iron-deficiency anemia requires only a single tablet of iron gluconate or iron sulfate a day.
4. A corrected reticulocyte count should be the first diagnostic test in a person with anemia.
5. Erythropoietin-stimulating agents should be used in the lowest dose possible, should not increase hemoglobin by more than 1 g/dL per month, and should not be given when the hemoglobin is greater than 10 g/dL.

SUGGESTED READINGS

Bross MH, Soch K, Smith-Knuppel T. Anemia in older persons. *Am Fam Physician*. 2010;82:480-487.

Dhaliwal G, Cornett PA, Tierney LM. Hemolytic anemia. *Am Fam Physician*. 2004;69:2599-2606.

Morley JE. Anemia in the nursing homes: a complex issue. *J Am Med Dir Assoc*. 2012;13:191-194.

MULTIPLE CHOICE QUESTIONS

27.1   What is the most common cause of anemia in nursing homes?

a. Vitamin B_{12} deficiency
b. Folate deficiency
c. Hypothyroidism
d. Myelodysplasia
e. Anemia of chronic disease

27.2   What agent is responsible for trapping iron in the macrophages?

a. Erythropoietin
b. Hepcidin
c. Ferroportin
d. Fibroblast growth factor

27.3   Which of the following is elevated in anemia of chronic disease?

a. Iron
b. Ferritin
c. Transferrin receptors
d. Total iron-binding capacity
e. Red blood cell size

27.4   A 78-year-old male nursing home resident has an elevated corrected reticulocyte count, increased unconjugated bilirubin, and low haptoglobin levels. What is the most likely diagnosis?

a. Hemolytic anemia
b. Hemorrhage
c. Vitamin B_{12} deficiency
d. Iron deficiency

27.5   Which of the following is true of myelodysplasia?

a. Red blood cells are decreased in 25%.
b. Microkaryocytes are common.
c. It is treated with vitamin B_{12}.
d. Lenalidomide can be used to treat some forms of myelodysplasia.
e. Intravenous iron is the treatment of choice.

27.6   Which of the following is true concerning the treatment of anemias?

a. Folate must be given with vitamin B_{12}.
b. Low dose (a single tablet) iron is appropriate to treat most iron-deficiency anemias.
c. Blood transfusions should not be used for myelodysplasia.
d. Iron tablets can be given with other medications.
e. Epoetin alfa should be used at a dose high enough to increase hemoglobin by 2 g/dL per month.

Chapter 28

ENDOCRINE DISORDERS

Endocrine disorders occur commonly in nursing home residents. This is particularly true of autoimmune endocrinopathies (i.e., thyroid disorders, adrenocortical insufficiency, and diabetes mellitus). Persons with these conditions also often have vitamin B_{12} deficiency (pernicious anemia) and celiac disease. Endocrine disorders present subtly in older persons with nonspecific symptoms such as fatigue; cognitive dysfunction; and in the case of diabetes mellitus, polyuria and incontinence. For this reason, regular biochemical screening for endocrine disorders is essential in nursing home residents.

THYROID DISORDERS

In a nursing home in the Canary Islands, the prevalence of hypothyroidism was 7.9%. Euthyroid sick syndrome was present in 14%. In a nursing home in the United States, undiagnosed hypothyroidism was present in just under 1%, subclinical hypothyroidism (thyroid-stimulating hormone [TSH] ≤15 micro IU/mL) in approximately 10%. In the follow-up in these patients, half had their TSH levels return to normal, and only 2% went on to develop hypothyroidism. Both low TSH and elevated free thyroxine (T_4) levels occur in a small percentage of nursing home residents, but these are usually false–positive test results caused by euthyroid sick or psychiatric disturbances. A number of medications also cause low T_4 levels (Table 28–1).

Clinical diagnostic skills are relatively useless in diagnosing hypo- or hyperthyroidism in nursing home residents. Up to 5% of persons with dementia may have hypothyroidism. Other symptoms and signs are nonspecific, including fatigue, depression, constipation, and bradycardia, which are very common in nursing residents. Apathetic hyperthyroidism presents with blepharoptosis instead of exophthalmus, anorexia instead of hyperphagia, depression, weight loss, proximal muscle myopathy, heart failure, and atrial fibrillation.

Based on these considerations, all nursing home residents should have a yearly TSH level checked. If the TSH level is greater than 15 micro IU/mL, the resident should be treated for hypothyroidism. For persons with values between 5 and 15, thyroid peroxidase (TPO) antibodies should be measured, and if elevated, the person has autoimmune thyroid disease, is highly likely to go on to develop overt hypothyroidism, and should be treated. A number

of persons with values between 5 and 10 have abnormal TSH or TSH receptor levels, and these have been associated with longevity and should not be treated. Persons with low TSH levels may have hyperthyroidism or euthyroid sick syndrome (Table 28–2). To make the diagnosis of hyperthyroidism, a free T_4 by dialysis or triiodothyronine (T_3) level needs to be obtained. The direct free T_4 immunoassays provide erroneous results in sick and older persons and should be avoided.

Treatment of hypothyroidism is administration of L-thyroxine with a starting dose of 25 or 50/μg/day and increasing to 75/μg daily. In older persons, there is a decrease in plasma clearance rate, so most older persons' levels are fully replaced in doses between 75 and 100/μg daily. Many residents have received inappropriate thyroid hormone replacement, and in persons given 50/μg or less and having normal TPO levels, thyroid hormone therapy should be withdrawn under careful monitoring. In one study, half of nursing home residents had their thyroid replacement successfully withdrawn. There is no reason not to use generic L-thyroxine. Calcium and iron block the absorption of L-thyroxine and cannot be administered within 2 hours of L-thyroxine. Pocketing L-thyroxine in residents with dementia who then spit out the medication after the nurse has left is another common reason for a resident appearing to require greater L-thyroxine replacement. Thyroid extract should not be used because there is poor standardization from batch to batch.

Older persons with hyperthyroidism are most probably better served by being treated with radioactive iodine. Nevertheless, a number of residents receiving methimazole or propylthiouracil are still seen in nursing homes. In these

Table 28–1.	DRUGS ASSOCIATED WITH LOW THYROXINE LEVELS IN NURSING HOME RESIDENTS
Salicylates	
Phenytoin	
Carbamazepine	
Prednisone	
Furosemide	

Table 28–2.   COMPARISON OF THYROID FUNCTION TESTS IN EUTHYROID SICK, HYPOTHYROIDISM, AND PSYCHIATRIC HYPERTHYRONEMIA

	Euthyroid Sick	Hypothyroid	Psychiatric Hyperthyronemia
Thyroxine	Normal or low	Low	Increased
Triiodothyronine	Very low	Low normal	Normal
Thyrotropin	Normal, increased, or decreased	Increased	Low, normal, or increased
Free thyroxine by dialysis	Normal	Low	Normal or mildly increased

persons, white blood cell counts should be checked regularly to check for agranulocytosis.

All residents should be screened for thyroid nodules. If a solitary thyroid nodule is found, it should be observed for 3 to 6 months. If the nodule is enlarging, a fine-needle aspiration should be performed to exclude anaplastic cancer. If other forms of thyroid cancer (follicular or papillary) are found, management should take into account the life expectancy of the resident, and in most cases, if surgery is appropriate, a hemithyroidectomy should be sufficient.

DIABETES MELLITUS

Diabetes mellitus occurs in about 25% to 30% of all nursing home residents in the United States and Taiwan and about 12% to 20% in Europe. Residents with diabetes mellitus tend to be younger than other residents, more likely to be male, and more disabled, but they often have a longer stay in the nursing home before dying. Residents with diabetes mellitus have a greater comorbidity burden and are more likely to be receiving more medicines and to have recurrent hospitalizations (Table 28–3). Overall high glucose levels (>200 mg/dL or >11.111 mmol/L) produce a number of adverse effects (Table 28–4). Similarly, hypoglycemia needs to be avoided; thus, it is recommended that glucose levels are kept between 100 and 200 mg/dL (5.555–11.111 mmol/L) and an HbA_1C between 7% and 8% (53–106 mmol/mol) in most nursing home residents.

Older persons often have a type of diabetes that is intermediate between type I and II because they produce inadequate insulin as well as having insulin resistance. This means they are often not overweight, but also unlike those with type II diabetes, they can develop ketoacidosis. Other groups of older persons at unique risk of diabetes are those undergoing androgen deprivation therapy and those receiving atypical antipsychotics. These two groups need to be carefully monitored for the development of diabetes.

In persons with diabetes in nursing homes, blood pressure should be maintained between 135 and 150 mm Hg. All residents with diabetes should be checked for orthostasis and postprandial hypotension. If these are present, blood pressure may need to be maintained at a higher level.

α-Lipoic acid has been shown to slow the rate of progression of peripheral neuropathy. There is some evidence that persons with painful peripheral neuropathy may have their nerve damage reversed and pain dramatically reduced with topiramate. Treatment should not be for more than 6 months. Topiramate can cause severe weight loss, which should be monitored for and the drug stopped if it occurs.

Falls occur more commonly in nursing home residents with diabetes than in other nursing home residents. This increase in falls is attributable to poor position and

Table 28–3.   BURDEN OF ILLNESS IN DIABETES MELLITUS: CONDITIONS MORE COMMON IN RESIDENTS WITH DIABETICS THAN OTHERS

Disability
Sensory impairment
Falls or fractures
Incontinence
Dementia
Depression
Amputation
Pressure ulcers

Table 28–4.   REASONS FOR MAINTAINING GLUCOSE LEVELS BELOW 200 MG/DL (11 MMOL/L) IN PERSONS IN NURSING HOMES

Dehydration
Fewer vision disturbances
Decreased pain perception
Decreased urinary tract infections
Decreased recurrence of tuberculosis
Reduced incontinence and nocturia caused by diuretic effect of elevated glucoses
Improved cognitive function
Decreased platelet adhesiveness (reduced chance of stroke or myocardial infarction)
Reduced trace element deficiency
Prevention of secondary complications (retinopathy, nephropathy, and neuropathy)
Prevention of diabetic comas

vibration sense, peripheral neuropathy, poorer vision, and increased renal failure. Falls increase markedly when the HbA_1C is less than 7%. Syncope is also more common in people with diabetes who have autonomic neuropathy caused by orthostasis, postprandial hypotension, and arrhythmias. Although persons with diabetes mellitus often have a higher bone mineral density than others, their bones are more fragile, and they are at an increased risk of hip fracture.

When people with diabetes develop foot ulcers, they are at major risk of losing that leg. As such, they need to be carefully followed by a podiatrist or chiropodist. In nursing homes in England, more than 90% of residents see a chiropodist. Persons with diabetes mellitus also are at increased likelihood of developing pressure ulcers. Zinc deficiency occurs in 10% of older people with diabetes and is more common in those receiving diuretics. As such, in people with diabetes with poorly healing vascular or pressure ulcers, it may be reasonable to provide zinc replacement.

Although statins are commonly given to persons with diabetes mellitus, three major studies (ASPEN, ASCOT-DM, and ALLHAT-LLT) all failed to show an effect of statins on reducing cardiovascular events or mortality.

MANAGEMENT

There is little evidence to support the use of the American Diabetic Association diet in nursing home residents. It has been shown to be ineffective at lowering glucose and weight loss in older people with diabetes and is associated with increased mortality. Residents with diabetes receiving insulin should receive regular meals, and when they eat less than 75% of a meal, this should be reported to the nursing supervisor and a decision made whether to reduce or hold the insulin. All residents with diabetes should have regular physical activity, including resistance exercise, to reduce insulin resistance.

Glucose monitoring is often used excessively in nursing homes. The majority of residents need fasting glucose levels to be monitored by finger sticks once a day or even only once or twice a week. Twice-a-day monitoring should be sufficient for all but those with the most brittle diabetes. The Centers for Disease Control and Prevention has provided guidelines for the use of blood glucose monitoring in long-term care facilities (Table 28–5). Finger sticks need to

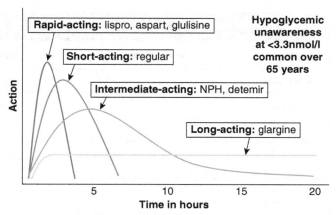

Figure 28–1. Characteristics of available insulin. NPH, neutral protamine Hagedorn.

be done before meals; they should never be done during a meal, which is unfortunately not a rare experience in nursing homes.

The characteristics of the available insulins are given in Figure 28–1. It is important to realize that hypoglycemic unawareness is very common in older persons (Table 28–6). The majority of nursing home residents with hypoglycemia are reported to have had delusions. Variability in the time of meal service, because many residents receive their morning insulin before the night shift leaves and because many residents can decide not to eat a meal makes the use of rapid-acting insulins hazardous in nursing homes. Glargine given once a day in doses of 12 to 20 units will control many residents with minimal hypoglycemia. When possible, the use of sliding scale regular insulin should be avoided. It can result in excessive hypoglycemia and is very time intensive in nursing time.

The different forms of medical management that can be used in nursing home residents are outlined in Table 28–7. With rare exceptions, the use of glucagon-like peptide-1 (GLP-1; exendin) therapies should not be used in nursing home residents because they produce severe anorexia and weight loss in older persons.

Table 28–5.	GLUCOSE MONITORING: CENTERS FOR DISEASE CONTROL AND PREVENTION ADVISORY

Finger stick devices should never be used for more than one person.

Whenever possible, blood glucose meters should not be shared.

If blood glucose meters must be shared, the device must be cleaned and disinfected after every use per the manufacturers' instructions.

If there are no specific instructions for cleaning and disinfecting the device, it should not be shared.

Insulin pens and other medication cartridges and syringes are for single patient use and cannot be shared.

Table 28–6.	POTENTIAL SIGNS OF HYPOGLYCEMIA IN NURSING HOME RESIDENTS

Drowsiness

Lethargy

Confusion

Agitation

Hallucinations

Delusions

Falls

Irritability

Sweating

Seizures

Strokes

Table 28–7.   ORAL MEDICATIONS FOR DIABETES MELLITUS THAT CAN BE USED IN NURSING HOME RESIDENTS

Class	Medications	Cost	Comments
Sensitizers			
Biguanides	Metformin	Inexpensive	Less effective in older persons; not to be used in renal failure or uncontrolled heart failure because of risk of lactic acidosis
Thiazolidonediones	Rosiglitazone, pioglitazone	Expensive	Cause edema and osteoporosis and are associated with cardiac disease and bladder cancer
Secretagogues			
Sulfonylureas	Tolbutamide, glipizide, glybunde (glibenelamide), glimepiride	Inexpensive	Increased risk of hypoglycemia
Meglitinides	Repaglinide, nateglide	Expensive	Increased risk of hypoglycemia
α-Glucosidase Inhibitors			
	Miglitol, acarbose, voglibose	Intermediate	Gut side effects Treat postprandial hypotension
Dipeptidyl Peptidase-4 Inhibitors			
	Vildagliptin, sitagliptin, saxagliptin, linagliptin	Very expensive	Minimal hypoglycemia Cause skin rash and Angioedema Can occur with ACE inhibitors

ACE, angiotensin-converting enzyme.

Metformin was shown in the United Kingdom Prospective Diabetes Study to decrease mortality rate, myocardial infarction, and microvascular disease. Although it is less effective in older persons, it is the first-line treatment for people with diabetes. It should not be used in persons older than 70 years of age with creatinine above 1.2 mg/dL. It is contraindicated in uncontrolled type IV heart failure and needs to be stopped before using radioiodinated contrast material. Its major side effects are gastrointestinal (GI) distress, diarrhea, and anorexia. Thus, excess weight loss should be monitored in all persons receiving metformin.

Two sets of agents increase endogenous GLP-1. These are the α_1-glucosidase inhibitors (acarbose, miglitol, and voglibose) and the gliptins (sitagliptin, vildagiptin, saxagliptin, and linagliptin). The α_1-glucosidase inhibitors need to be taken before each meal and cause relatively severe GI distress, making them less usable in nursing homes. However, they are the drugs of choice in persons with postprandial hypotension. The gliptins tend not to produce hypoglycemia and have fewer GI side effects. They can produce severe skin rashes and should be stopped in any persons with a new skin rash. They can interact with angiotensin-converting enzyme inhibitors to rarely produce angioedema. Their doses need to be reduced in persons with renal failure.

The sulfonylureas (glipizide, glyburide, glimepiride) produce hypoglycemia. Chlorpropramide has a long half-life and should not be used in older persons. Studies suggest that the sulfonylureas do not decrease mortality rate and may even increase mortality rate and cardiovascular

disease. If they need to be used, they should be used in low doses. Although glipizide is believed to produce less hypoglycemia than glyburide, this is not true with the long-acting glipizide formulation and appears to be more attributable to glyburide's being more effective at lowering blood glucose.

Thiazolidinediones (rosiglitazone and proglitazone) rarely produce hypoglycemia. They do increase edema, and rosiglitazone may increase heart failure and myocardial infarction. Pioglitazone has been associated with an increase in bladder cancer. Both drugs decrease bone mineral formation and have a higher risk of fracture, making them less than ideal for use in nursing home residents use in nursing home residents." "Canagliflozin is a sodium-glucose co-transporter-2 (SGLT2) inhibitor that lowers blood glucose by increasing its excretion in the urine. It is associated with genital infections and possibly increasing cardiovascular disease and osteoporosis. The FDA approved its use in March 2013. At present, it most probably should not be used in older persons."

Three recent studies have shown little advantage of lowering HbA$_1$C below 7% in community-dwelling middle-aged and young old persons (Table 28–8). A community study in the United Kingdom suggested that addition of a second hypoglycemic drug increased the mortality rate up to an HbA$_1$C of 7.5%. Thus, it seems reasonable to aim at an HbA$_1$C greater than 7% (53 mmol/mol) in nursing home residents. An HbA$_1$C between 8% and 9% (106–159 mmol/mol) may be reasonable for some very frail nursing home residents.

Table 28–8.   OUTCOMES OF INTENSIVE DIABETES TRIALS

	Patients (*n*)	Years	Intensive A$_1$C (%)	Std A$_1$C (%)	Outcome
ACCORD	10,521	3.5	6.4	7.5	Includes CVD mortality; 3 deaths/1000/yr
ADVANCE	11,140	4.5	6.5	7.3	No effect on CVD
VADT	1791	6.3	6.9	8.4	No effect on CVD

CVD, cardiovascular disease.

In summary, the approach to the management of diabetes in nursing home residents has undergone radical change in the past decade. The principles are now:

- Do not use therapeutic diets.
- Use metformin, gliptins, and α-glucosidase inhibitors as monotherapy before considering sulfonylureas.
- Do not add a second drug until the HbA$_1$C is above 7.5%.
- Do not add insulin until the HbA$_1$C is above 8%.
- In most residents, check fasting accuchecks one or two times a week and in those on insulin twice a day.
- Many nursing home residents can have their diabetes medication withdrawn completely if their HbA$_1$C is less than 7%.
- When possible, sliding scale insulin should be avoided (in the United States, half of residents on insulin are on a sliding scale). If it is used, it should be limited to treating very high glucose levels (>300 mg/dL; 16.6 mmol/L) and should only be a twice-daily scale.
- Errors in diabetic medication use are most often associated with insulin use.

All nursing homes should develop protocols for the management of diabetes mellitus. They should stress what should be done when a resident does not eat. They should move away from four times a day accuchecks. An approach to hypoglycemia should be included with limitation of the use of glucagon to only true hypoglycemic emergencies. They should include a plan for regular eye and foot examinations and measurement of HbA$_1$C and renal function at least every 6 months.

HYPONATREMIA

Hyponatremic episodes are common in nursing home residents. In Taiwan, 31% of nursing home residents had a hyponatremic episode and in the United States, the prevalence was 53% over a year. The incidence of hyponatremia in the nursing home is approximately double that seen in community dwelling older persons. There are numerous causes of hyponatremia in the nursing home (Table 28–9). Pseudohyponatremia occurs in the presence of hyperglycemia or hypertriglyceridemia.

The major clinical effects of hyponatremia are balance problems; falls; delirium; and in severe cases, convulsions and death. Water restriction remains the treatment of choice in most persons with hyponatremia. This is difficult in persons with dementia. The development of arginine vasopressin antagonists known as "vaptans" (e.g., tolvaptan, conivaptan) provide an expensive alternative therapy. At present, no clear long-term advantages have been demonstrated for "vaptan" treatment in the syndrome of inappropriate antidiuretic hormone secretion or edematous states. These drugs are justified when the serum sodium is less than 120 mEq/L and water restriction is not feasible.

ADDISON'S DISEASE (HYPOADRENALISM)

Addison's disease is not rare in nursing home residents. Clinical features include fatigue, abdominal pain, constipation or diarrhea, and cognitive dysfunction. Nursing home residents with high or borderline high potassium level, low or borderline low sodium level, and eosinophilia should have the diagnosis of Addison's disease ruled out. This is done by administering 250 μg of cosyntropin and obtaining cortisol levels at 0, 30, and 60 minutes. Failure of cortisol levels to increase by at least 8 μg/dL (210 nmol/L)

Table 28–9.   CAUSES OF HYPONATREMIA

Congestive heart failure

Liver disease

Hypothyroidism

Adrenocortical insufficiency

Diuretic induced hyponatremia especially thiazides

SIADH

- Ectopic hormone production (outcell cancer of lung)
- Lung disease
- Lung ventilation
- Brain diseases (e.g., tumors, multiple sclerosis)
- Neurosurgery
- Drugs (e.g., amiodarone, NSAIDs, SSRIs, TCAs, antineoplastic drugs, phenothiazines, carbamazepine)

Polydipsia (e.g., as seen with lithium or thioridazine)

Tube feeding with inadequate salt

NSAID, nonsteroidal antiinflammatory drug; SIADH, syndrome of inappropriate antidiuretic hormone secretion; SSRI, selective serotonin reuptake inhibitor; TCA, tricyclic antidepressant.

or for the level of cortisol not to be greater than 25 µg/dL (690 nmol/L) makes the diagnosis. Replacement therapy is 25 mg of hydrocortisone in the morning and 12.5 mg at lunchtime. When steroids are given in the evening, they may interfere with sleep. Doses of corticosteroids should be doubled when the resident has an infection. Similarly, residents on chronic steroids should receive stress doses of corticosteroids when they become ill.

KEY POINTS

1. Hypothyroidism is common in nursing homes.
2. The diagnosis of thyroid disease requires regular screening (TSH) because thyroid diseases present insidiously and atypically.
3. Calcium and iron block the absorption of L-thyroxine and as such should not be given with thyroid hormone replacement.
4. Diabetic therapeutic diets should not be used in nursing home residents.
5. The appropriate HbA$_1$C for people with diabetes in nursing homes is between 7% and 8%.
6. Most medication errors occur when insulin is used. Do not add insulin until HbA$_1$C is greater than 8%.
7. Avoid using sliding scale insulin if possible.
8. Withdrawal of diabetic medication is often possible in nursing home residents.
9. Falls are more common in residents with diabetes, especially if the HbA$_1$C is greater than 7%.
10. Hyponatremia is a common cause of falls and delirium in nursing home residents.
11. Use of selective serotonin reuptake inhibitors is a common cause of hyponatremia.
12. Addison's disease (hypoadrenalism) is often missed in nursing home residents.

SUGGESTED READINGS

Afshinnia F, Sheth N, Perlman R. Syndrome of inappropriate antidiuretic hormone in association with amiodarone therapy: a case report and review of literature. *Ren Fail.* 2011;33:456-458.

Amberson J, Drinka PJ. Medication and low serum thyroxine values in nursing home residents. *South Med J.* 1998;91:437-440.

Anía Lafuente BJ, Suàrez Almenara JL, Fernàndez-Burriel Tercero M, et al. Thyroid function in the aged admitted to a nursing home [Spanish]. *An Med Interna.* 2000;17:5-8.

Bouillet B, Vaillant G, Petit JM, et al. Are elderly patients being overtreated in French long-term care homes? *Diabetes Metab.* 2010;36:272-277.

Chen LK, Lin MH, Hwang SJ, Chen TW. Hyponatremia among the institutionalized elderly in 2 long-term care facilities in Taipei. *J Chin Med Assoc.* 2006;69:115-119.

Chen L-K, Lin M-H, Lai H-Y, et al. Care of patients with diabetes mellitus in long-term care facilities in Taiwan: diagnosis, glycemic control, hypoglycemia, and functional status. *J Am Geriatr Soc.* 2008;56:1975-1976.

Coll PP, Abourizk NN. Successful withdrawal of thyroid hormone therapy in nursing home patients. *J Am Board Fam Pract.* 2000;13:403-407.

Currie CJ, Peters JR, Rynan A, et al. Survival as a function of HbA(1C) in people with type 2 diabetes: a retrospective cohort study. *Lancet.* 2010;375:481-489.

Drinka PJ, Amberson J, Voeks SK, et al. Low TSH levels in nursing home residents not taking thyroid hormone. *J Am Geriatr Soc.* 1996;44:573-577.

Drinka PJ, Nolten WE. Prevalence of previously undiagnosed hypothyroidism in residents of a midwestern nursing home. *South Med J.* 1990;83:1259-1261.

Drinka PJ, Nolten WE, Voeks S, et al. Misleading elevation of the free thyroxine index in nursing home residents. *Arch Pathol Lab Med.* 1991;115:1208-1211.

Drinka PJ, Nolten WE, Voeks SK, Langer EH. Follow-up of mild hypothyroidism in a nursing home. *J Am Geriatr Soc.* 1991;39:264-266.

Dybicz SB, Thompson S, Molotsky S, Stuart B. Prevalence of diabetes and the burden of comorbid conditions among elderly nursing home residents. *Am J Geriatr Pharmacother.* 2011;9:212-223.

Feldman SM, Rosen R, DeStasio J. Status of diabetes management in the nursing home setting in 2008: a retrospective chart review and epidemiology study of diabetic nursing home residents and nursing home initiatives in diabetes management. *J Am Med Dir Assoc.* 2009;10:354-360.

Gadsby R, Barker P, Sinclair A. People living with diabetes resident in nursing homes—assessing levels of disability and nursing needs. *Diabet Med.* 2011;28:778-780.

Gassanov N, Semmo N, Semmo M, et al. Arginine vasopressin (AVP) and treatment with arginine vasopressin receptor antagonists (vaptans) in congestive heart failure, liver cirrhosis and syndrome of inappropriate antidiuretic hormone secretion (SIADH). *Eur J Clin Pharmacol.* 2011;67:333-346.

Hix JK, SIlver S, Sterns RH. Diuretic-associated hyponatremia. *Semin Nephrol.* 2011;31:553-566.

Holt RM, Schwartz FL, Shubrook JH. Diabetes care in extended care facilities: appropriate intensity of care? *Diabetes Care.* 2007;30: 1454-1458.

Joseph J, Koka M, Aronow WS. Prevalence of a hemoglobin A1C less than 7.0%, of a blood pressure less than 130/80 mm Hg, and of a serum low-density lipoprotein cholesterol less than 100 mg/dL in older patients with diabetes mellitus in an academic nursing home. *J Am Med Dir Assoc.* 2008;9:51-54.

Meyers RM, Broton JC, Woo-Rippe KW, et al. Variability in glycosylated hemoglobin values in diabetic patients living in long-term care facilities. *J Am Med Dir Assoc.* 2007;8:511-514.

Miller M, Morley JE, Rubenstein LZ. Hyponatremia in a nursing home population. *J Am Geriatr Soc.* 1995;43:1410-1413.

Milligan FJ, Krentz AJ, Sinclair AJ. Diabetes medication patient safety incident reports to the National Reporting and Learning Service: the care home setting. *Diabet Med.* 2011;38:1537-1540.

Pandya N, Thompson S, Sambamoorthi U. The prevalence and persistence of sliding scale insulin use among newly admitted elderly nursing home residents with diabetes mellitus. *J Am Med Dir Assoc.* 2008;9:663-669.

Resnick HE, Heineman J, Stone R, Shorr RI. Diabetes in U.S. nursing homes, 2004. *Diabetes Care.* 2008;31:287-8.

Sinclair A, Morley JE, Rodriguez-Manas L, et al. Diabetes mellitus in older people: position statement on behalf of the International Association of Gerontology and Geriatrics (IAGG), the European Diabetes Working Party for Older people (EDWPOP), and the International Task Force of Experts in Diabetes. *J Am Med Dir Assoc.* 2012;13:497-502.

Sjöblom P, AndersTengblad, Löfgren UB, et al. Can diabetes medication be reduced in elderly patients? An observational study of diabetes drug withdrawal in nursing home patients with tight glycaemic control. *Diabetes Res Clin Pract.* 2008;82:197-202.

Turner SA. Update on blood glucose monitoring in long-term care facilities. *Geriatr Nurs.* 2010;31:446-447.

Wedick NM, Barrett-Connor E, Knok JE, Wingard DL. The relationship between all-cause mortality in older men and women with and without diabetes mellitus: the Rancho Bernardo study. *J Am Geriatr Soc.* 2002;50:1810-1815.

Yarnall AJ, Hayes L, Hawthorne GC, et al. Diabetes in care homes: current care standards and residents' experience. *Diabet Med.* 2012;29: 132-135.

Zhang X, Decker FH, Luo H, et al. Trends in the prevalence and comorbidities of diabetes mellitus in nursing home residents in the United States: 1995-2004. *J Am Geriatr Soc.* 2010;58(4): 724-7730.

MULTIPLE CHOICE QUESTIONS

28.1   A 87-year-old woman has fatigue, depression, and weight loss. On examination, she has blepharoptosis, atrial fibrillation, and proximal muscle myopathy. What is the most likely diagnosis?

    a. Inclusion body myositis
    b. Dermatomyositis
    c. Polymyalgia rheumatica
    d. Apathetic hyperthyroidism
    e. Polymyositis

28.2   A 95-year-old resident is receiving 0.150 mg of L-thyroxine daily. His TSH is 35 micro IU/mL. What is the most likely cause of his requiring such large doses of L-thyroxine?

    a. Thyroid receptor abnormality
    b. Abnormal TSH level
    c. Taking calcium carbonate
    d. Diarrhea
    e. Primary malabsorption of L-thyroxine

28.3   The HbA$_1$C for nursing home residents who are receiving oral medications or insulin should be:

    a. 5% to 6%
    b. 6% to 7%
    c. 7% to 8%
    d. 9% to 10%
    e. greater than 10%

28.4   Evidence supports the use of the American Diabetic Association's diet for residents with diabetes in nursing homes.

    a. True
    b. False

28.5   Which of the following is not a cause of hyponatremia?

    a. Liver disease
    b. Paroxetine
    c. Digoxin
    d. Hypothyroidism
    e. NSAIDs

28.6   A 72-year-old man with diarrhea and weight loss is admitted to a nursing home. His blood pressure is 90/50 mm Hg. He has hyponatremia and a high normal potassium level. He has eosinophilia. What is the diagnosis?

    a. SIADH
    b. Hypothyroidism
    c. Hyperthyroidism
    d. Diabetes mellitus
    e. Addison's disease

Chapter 29

GASTROINTESTINAL DISORDERS

GASTROINTESTINAL DISEASES

Approximately 20% of residents in nursing homes have gastroesophageal reflux disease (GERD). Rates of gastrointestinal (GI) bleeding requiring hospital admission are approximately 2.5% for men younger than age 85 years and 3% in older male residents. Female residents have a lower rate between 1.5% and 2%. These rates are about five times higher than that of community-living older persons. Use of nonsteroidal antiinflammatory drugs (NSAIDs) more than doubled the admission from nursing homes for GI bleeding. The operative mortality rate for nursing home residents for abdominal surgery is about double that seen in community-dwelling elders. For cholecystectomy and appendectomy, the death rate is about 11%. For colonectomy, the death rate is 31%, and the death rate for surgery for bleeding ulcers is 41%. Even these higher rates do not suggest that surgery should be avoided in nursing home residents, but less invasive therapies may be appropriate for a subset of residents (Table 29–1).

GASTROESOPHAGEAL REFLUX DISEASE

Indigestion is only present in half of older persons with GERD. GERD can present with water brash, anorexia, weight loss, hoarseness, chronic cough, asthmatic symptoms, and dysphagia. Erosive gastritis is present in 20% of older persons. Older persons are more likely to develop Barrett esophagus and esophageal cancer. Hiatal hernia is common in older persons and increases the likelihood of GERD. Numerous medications can aggravate GERD (Table 29–2).

Proton pump inhibitors (PPIs) are the treatment of choice for severe GERD. They have a number of long-term side effects, making it important to try to wean residents off PPIs when possible and not to continue PPIs started in hospital or for dyspepsia. Drugs used for the treatment of GERD are summarized in Table 29–3. All persons with GERD should be tested for *Helicobacter pylori* with serologic (IgA or IgM), stool antigen, or urea breath tests and treated when the results are positive.

GASTROINTESTINAL BLEEDING

Bleeding can be caused by either upper of lower intestinal bleeding. Peptic ulcer disease is the most common cause of upper intestinal bleeding. It is usually associated with the ingestion of aspirin or NSAIDs or it caused by *Helicobacter pylori* infection. Esophageal varies is associated with liver disease. Repeated vomiting or retching can lead to a Mallory-Weiss tear. Residents with gastric cancer can have cachexia, supraclavicular adenopathy, and an abdominal mass or pain.

In older persons, painless lower intestinal bleeding is often caused by diverticular disease or arteriovenous malformations. Colonic neoplasms can present with painless bleeding. Other causes of lower intestinal bleeding include radiation colitis; colonic tuberculosis; and in persons with aortic aneurysm repair, aortoduodenal fistula. Persons with inflammatory bowel disease (Crohn [regional ileitis] or ulcerative colitis) usually have an onset between 20 and 50 years of age.

Diagnosis usually requires endoscopy. Capsule endoscopy is becoming useful for diagnosing small bowel disease, especially angiodysplasia. Technetium-99m–tagged red blood cell scanning can be used to identify where the bleeding is occurring in the intestinal tract.

It is important to recognize that the half of nursing home residents who have coffee ground emesis or occult GI bleeding may have serious infections or respiratory failure leading to gastritis. These residents need treatment of the underlying disorder, should receive temporary treatment with PPIs, and do not require endoscopy.

ABDOMINAL PAIN

In an older person with mild to moderate abdominal pain and stable vital signs, one should consider urinary tract infection or diverticulitis if they have a fever or delirium and constipation or irritable bowel syndrome if no other symptoms. If the abdominal pain is severe, the abdomen is distended, and the resident is constipated, sigmoid volvulus should enter the differential diagnosis. At the other end of the spectrum, a resident with unstable vital signs, ischemic bowel disease (acidotic), septicemia, and perforated viscus are possibilities.

The differential diagnosis of abdominal pain is driven by the site of the pain (Table 29–4).

ELEVATED TRANSAMINASE LEVELS AND HEPATITIS

Elevated transaminases (alanine transaminase [ALT] and aspartate transaminase [AST]) are present in 9% of the general population. Whereas ALT comes mostly from the

Table 29–1.	LESS INVASIVE SURGERIES TO BE CONSIDERED FOR NURSING HOME RESIDENTS
Disease	**Procedure**
Cholecystitis	Percutaneous aspiration or cholecystostomy
Appendicitis	Antibiotics
Bleeding	Endoscopic embolization for bleeding duodenal ulcers
Large bowel obstruction	Endoluminal stents

Table 29–3.	DRUGS USED TO TREAT GASTROESOPHAGEAL REFLUX DISEASE
Drug	**Effects**
Antacids	Limited effectiveness
	Salt overload, constipation, and diarrhea
	Interfere with drug absorption
Histamine-2 receptor antagonists	Poorly effective when esophageal
	Mucosal injury
	Mental status changes
	Especially in persons with renal or liver dysfunction
	Drug interaction with warfarin, theophylline, and phenytoin
Proton pump inhibitors	Twice as effective as H2RAs for erosive esophagitis
	Drug interaction with warfarin, clopidogrel, phenytoin and some benzodiazepines
	Interstitial nephritis
	Bone fracture (osteoporosis)
	Pneumonia
	Decreased vitamin B_{12} levels
	Increased *Clostridium difficile*
	Possible increased cardiovascular disease

liver, AST comes from the muscles and red blood cells as well as the liver. Table 29–5 provides the causes of elevated transaminases. In general, in a nursing home, the workup consists of discontinuing possible hepatoxic medications, and if the elevated transaminases persist after 4 weeks, the practitioner should check hepatitis C virus antibodies and hepatitis B surface antigen, iron, and ferritin levels and if the patient has anemia, rule out hemolysis. If the patient is obese ultrasonography of the liver should be considered to rule out nonalcoholic fatty liver disease.

Hepatitis B is a common disorder that can lead to cirrhosis, liver failure, and hepatocellular cancer. Although the prevalence of hepatitis B in the United States is less than 0.4%, 90% of the world's population reside in areas where the prevalence is greater than 2%. Hepatitis B outbreaks have been commonly described in nursing home residents, usually related to blood glucose testing but also from resident-to-resident transmission. Nursing assistants develop hepatitis from needle sticks, mostly from insulin

Table 29–2.	MEDICATIONS THAT AGGRAVATE GASTROESOPHAGEAL REFLUX DISEASE
Medications That Alter Esophageal Function and Gastric Emptying	**Medications That Injure the Mucosa**
Calcium channel blockers	Aspirin
Anticholinergics	NSAIDS
Narcotics	Ferrous sulfate
Nitrates	Vitamin C
Benzodiazepines	Potassium chloride
	Bisphosphonates
	Trimethoprim–sulfamethoxazole corticosteroids

NSAID, nonsteroidal antiinflammatory drug.

needles or pens. Diagnosis of hepatitis B infection requires measurement of hepatitis antibodies. Persons who are hepatitis B surface antibody positive are immune; those who are hepatitis B core antibody positive are most probably infected if the surface antibody result is negative. The presence of the hepatitis B antigen indicates that the person is infected. In a United States nursing home, hepatitis B core antibody was positive in 24% and surface antibody in 19%.

Hepatitis C infects about 3% of the world's population. Hepatitis C infection occurs on exposure to blood products. Most persons who have hepatitis C infection are asymptomatic or have nonspecific symptoms. About 10% go on to develop cirrhosis. They have a marked increase in the propensity to develop hepatocellular carcinoma if they develop cirrhosis. Screening for hepatitis C is done with an enzyme immunoassay for antibodies. If the result is positive, it is necessary to do a recombinant immunoblot assay and a hepatitis C RNA polymerase reaction. The prevalence of antihepatitis C antibodies was 4.8% in the United States and 11.1% in Italy.

Hepatitis E is the most common form of viral hepatitis and jaundice around the world but is rare in developed countries. It occurs mostly in older persons. Besides hepatitis, the acute form of the disease can also manifest with anemia, arthritis, pancreatitis, and a variety of neurologic conditions. Chronic infection is usually limited to persons who are immune compromised.

Table 29–4.	DIAGNOSIS OF ABDOMINAL PAIN IN NURSING HOME RESIDENTS	
Site of Pain	**Causes**	**Diagnostic Test**
Right upper quadrant	Pulmonary embolus	Chest radiography
	Pneumonia	D-Dimer
	Cholecystitis	Urinalysis
	Pyelonephritis	Ultrasonography
	Nephrolithiasis	
Epigastric	Cholecystitis	Ultrasonography
	Pancreatitis	Computed tomography
	Myocardial infarction	
	Gastritis	Lactic acid
	Ischemic bowel disease	Troponin
	Aortic dissection	
Left upper quadrant	Myocardial disease	Troponin
	Pancreatic mass	Computed tomography
	Gastric cancer or gastritis	
		Urinalysis
	Nephrolithiasis	Endoscopy
	Pyelonephritis	
Right lower quadrant	Peritonitis	Urinalysis
	Appendicitis	Computed tomography
	Urinary tract infection	
Left lower quadrant	Diverticulitis	Urinalysis
	Urinary tract infection	Computed tomography
	Gynecologic	
		Colonoscopy
Suprapubic	Cystitis	Urinalysis
	Gynecologic	Ultrasonography

Table 29–5.	CAUSES OF ELEVATED TRANSAMINASES
Liver	**Medications**
Alcohol	Isoniazid
Cirrhosis	Statins
Fatty liver	Rifampin
Hepatitis B	Acetaminophen (paracetamol)
Hepatitis C	Valproic acid
Hemochromatosis	NSAIDs
Non-liver	Methotrexate
Muscle disorders	
Hyperthyroidism	
Hemolysis	
Celiac disease	

NSAID, nonsteroidal antiinflammatory drug.

KEY POINTS

1. GERD occurs in one in five older persons and is associated with erosive gastritis, which is ideally treated with PPIs.
2. Medications such as calcium channel antagonists, anticholinergics, narcotics, NSAIDs, aspirin, iron sulfate, and vitamin C aggravate GERD.
3. In older persons, small amounts of coffee ground emesis are most commonly caused by serious infections or respiratory failure.
4. Diverticular disease and arteriovenous malformations commonly cause painless GI bleeding.
5. Urinary tract infection is the most common cause of abdominal pain in persons with fever.
6. The diagnosis and diagnostic tests for abdominal pain depend on the site of the pain.
7. Abdominal pain with severe acidosis suggests ischemic bowel disease.
8. Elevated transaminase levels are common in nursing home residents and are mostly caused by medications.
9. Hepatitis B and C are common conditions, and in persons with elevated transaminases, appropriate testing to rule out active infection is necessary.
10. Needle sticks and inappropriate use of glucose testing materials are a common reason for hepatitis transmission to staff in the nursing home.
11. Hepatitis E is the most common hepatitis worldwide but rare in developed countries. It most commonly occurs in older men.

SUGGESTED READINGS

Baldo V, Floreani A, Menegon T, et al. Prevalence of antibodies against hepatitis C virus in the elderly: a seroepidemiological study in a nursing home and in an open population. The Collaborative Group. *Gerontology.* 2000;46:194-198.

Cartwright SL, Knudson MP. Evaluation of acute abdominal pain in adults. *Am Fam Physician.* 2008;77:971-978.

Finlayson E, Wang L, Landefeld S, Dudley RA. Major abdominal surgery in nursing home residents: a national study. *Ann Surg.* 2011; 254:921-926.

Hoofnagle JH, Nelson KE, Purcell RH. Hepatitis E. *N Engl J Med.* 2012; 367:1237-1244.

Manning-Dimmitt LL, Dimmitt SG, Wilson GR. Diagnosis of gastrointestinal bleeding in adults. *Am Fam Physician.* 2005;71:1339-1346.

Suatengco R, Posner GL, March F. The significance and work-up of minor gastrointestinal bleeding in hospitalized nursing home patients. *J Natl Med Assoc.* 1995;87:749-750.

MULTIPLE CHOICE QUESTIONS

29.1 Which of the following is *not* a side effect of PPIs?

    a. Increased *Clostridium difficile* diarrhea
    b. Pneumonia
    c. Bone fracture
    d. Mental status changes
    e. Decreased vitamin B_{12} levels

29.2   Which of these commonly leads to coffee ground emesis in nursing home residents?

   a. Pneumonia
   b. Regional ileitis
   c. Diverticulitis
   d. Meckel's diverticulum
   e. Angiodysplasia

29.3   What is the most common cause of moderate abdominal pain and fever or delirium in nursing home residents?

   a. Urinary tract infection
   b. Crohn disease
   c. Diverticulitis
   d. Colonic polyp
   e. A and C

29.4   What has been a cause of hepatitis B outbreaks in nursing homes?

   a. Chickens
   b. Birds
   c. Dogs
   d. Blood glucose testing

29.5   Which of the following is true about hepatitis C?

   a. About 1% will develop cirrhosis.
   b. Hepatitis C is usually symptomatic in nursing home residents.
   c. Hepatocellular carcinoma is not associated with hepatitis C.
   d. The diagnosis of hepatitis C requires a recombinant immunoblot assay and an RNA polymerase reaction test.

Chapter 30

PULMONARY DISORDERS

This chapter focuses on chronic obstructive pulmonary disease (COPD) and pulmonary embolism (PE).

CHRONIC OBSTRUCTIVE PULMONARY DISEASE

Chronic obstructive pulmonary disease was present in 20% of men and 14% of women in nursing homes in the United States. Over 2 years, 90% of residents with COPD had at least one emergency department visit or hospital admission. Persons with comorbid asthma were more likely to go to the emergency department.

Screening for COPD on admission to a nursing home should involve three questions:

1. Does the resident have greater than or equal to a 19 pack-year smoking history?
2. Does the resident have shortness of breath at rest or on exertion?
3. Does the resident have a diagnosis of asthma?

Chronic obstructive pulmonary disease is a disease in which limitations of air flow to and from the lungs results in dyspnea. Dyspnea is a subjective feeling of being short of breath and is different from tachypnea, which is measurable. A normal respiratory rate in a nursing home resident is 14 to 18 breaths/min. Breathing rates above 28 breaths/min represent severe respiratory distress caused by emphysema or chronic bronchitis. An approach to dyspnea management is given in Table 30–1. Besides dyspnea, residents have a chronic cough with sputum production (Table 30–2), breathing out taking longer than breathing in, active use of accessory muscles for breathing, and cyanosis and wheezing or crackles in the lung. Weight loss is common and is an independent prognosticator of poor outcome. Pulmonary hypertension is commonly associated with COPD, leading to increased jugular venous pressure and edema. Respiratory failure results in drowsiness, asterixis (flapping tremor), and delirium. Chest radiography shows hyperinflation of the lungs with a flattened diaphragm and bullae. The diagnosis is made by spirometry demonstrating a ratio of forced expiratory volume in 1 second (FEV_1) to forced vital capacity (FVC) of less than 10%. Severe COPD is present when the FEV_1 ratio is less than 50%. Pulse oximetry at rest, during exertion, and while asleep can be done to determine the need for oxygen.

The key components to management are to stop smoking and to receive supplemental oxygen. These are the only two approaches that have been demonstrated to reduce the mortality rate. In persons who are CO_2 retainers ("blue bloaters"), care must be taken to give the minimal amount of oxygen necessary because their respiratory drive is dependent on hypoxia. Bronchodilators reduce dyspnea, wheezing, and exercise limitation. There are two types: β_2-agonists (short-acting terbutaline and salbutamol and long-acting salmeterol and formoterol) and anticholinergics (short-acting ipratropium and long-acting tiotropium). β-Agonists can be given to persons with coronary artery disease receiving β-blockers. Cholinesterase inhibitors should be avoided in persons with COPD. Corticosteroids decrease exacerbations in persons with moderate to severe COPD. They increase pneumonia and do not decrease mortality. Theophylline (dimethylxanthine) is a bronchodilator with a very narrow therapeutic window, making its use difficult and requiring regular monitoring. It has multiple drug interactions, including erythromycin, fluoroquinolones, and phenytoin.

Antibiotics should be used in persons who develop purulent sputum or have an increase or decrease in white blood cell count. Postnasal drip (sinus drainage) can aggravate COPD and produce acute exacerbations of asthma. When residents with COPD have sinus disease, they need to be given antihistamines and possibly nasal steroids. Antihistamines that cross the blood–brain barrier poorly (e.g., fexofenadine, loratadine) cause less drowsiness and so are preferred to first-generation histamine-receptor antagonists. It is important to recognize that men with lower urinary tract symptomatology may have it aggravated by antihistamines and may even have acute urinary retention. In these residents, antihistamine nasal sprays (e.g., azelastine and olopatadine) may produce relief without causing urinary obstruction. Table 30–3 lists the side effects of drugs used to treat COPD. All residents with COPD should be immunized for influenza and pneumonia.

Pulmonary rehabilitation, with the addition of a high-protein supplementation or multiple small meals, decreases dyspnea and fatigue and has a borderline effect on 6-minute walking distance. It improves quality of life. Thus, rehabilitation with a regular maintenance program plays a key role in the care of residents with COPD.

Table 30–1.	APPROACH TO DYSPNEA MANAGEMENT IN PERSONS WITH CHRONIC OBSTRUCTIVE PULMONARY DISEASE IN A NURSING HOME

- The level of dyspnea should be recorded at each shift using a visual analog scale where the resident can answer the questions or nursing observation. This should be compared with previous levels and categorized as stable or unstable. If unstable, pulse oximetry should be obtained.
- Recognize danger signs (i.e., chest pain, severe dyspnea at rest, high fever, agitation, delirium, drowsiness).
- If the resident has acute respiratory distress, a nurse should remain with the resident and the physician or emergency medical services contacted immediately.
- To clear secretions, teach the resident to do deep breathe and blow out through pursed lips, cough after a deep breath with the mouth closed, and make a sound like "ha" or "huff" to increase air movement out (huffing).
- Chest percussion may loosen secretions.
- Energy conservation techniques include pacing one's self, eliminating unnecessary tasks, use equipment such as long-handled equipment to avoid reaching or bending, control breathing using pursed lips, and diaphragmatic breathing.
- Elevate head of bed to at least 30 degrees at all times.
- If the resident cannot finish meals because of breathlessness, give multiple small meals or supplements between meals.
- Teach relaxation techniques.
- Recognize oral thrush caused by improper use of a corticosteroid inhaler by providing good dental hygiene, rinsing the mouth after use of corticosteroid inhaler, and using a holding chamber.
- Train the resident in the appropriate use of metered-dose inhalers, dry powder inhalers, and nebulizers. Know when to use holding chamber spacer. Understand which inhaler is more appropriate for the resident.
- Consider referral to pulmonary rehabilitation.
- Understand the medications available and what can be used if symptoms worsen.
- Check oximetry and recognize the appropriate use of oxygen and the limits to increasing oxygen in persons with hypercapnia.
- Make sure all residents with COPD have had influenza and pneumococcal vaccinations.
- Develop end-of-life planning and recognize when it is time to refer the resident to hospice.
- The nursing home needs access to an education specialist in pulmonary care.

COPD, chronic obstructive pulmonary disease.

PULMONARY EMBOLISM

Venous thromboembolic events occur in between 1.3 and 1.5 per 100 residents every year. In two autopsy studies in nursing homes, PE was found to cause death in 8% and 12.8%. Seventy-one percent of the deaths caused by PE were not attributed to PE. The major risk factors for venous thromboembolism (VTE) are immobility

Table 30–2.	MANAGEMENT OF COUGH IN CHRONIC OBSTRUCTIVE PULMONARY DISEASE

- If caused by nasal or sinus drainage, consider antihistamine or nasal steroids.
- If it occurs at night or first thing in morning, consider gastric acid reflux and treat appropriately.
- Exclude that cough is caused by a medication, especially ACE inhibitors.
- Recognize that cough could be caused by an infection, particularly if there is a change in sputum color.
- Cough can be a sign of an acute asthmatic attack in COPD.
- Eosinophilic bronchitis causes a cough with eosinophils in the sputum and is treatable with steroids.
- Consider that the person has developed left-sided heart failure, especially if the cough is dry.
- Teach the resident to control cough by relaxing, taking two deep breaths, and then coughing while leaning forward and pushing on the abdomen.
- Teach the resident the "huffing" technique for coughing.
- Consider using a mucolytic (e.g., acetylcysteine [Mucomyst]).
- The resident can use an expectorant (e.g., guaifenesin), but effectiveness has not been shown.
- Cough suppressants (e.g., dextromethorphan and codeine) are ineffective in COPD and should not be used.

ACE, angiotensin converting enzyme; COPD, chronic obstructive pulmonary disease.

(Table 30–4), receiving rehabilitation, and having a pressure ulcer. Atypical antipsychotic use in nursing homes is also associated with increased thromboembolism. Newer residents are more likely than long-term residents to have thromboembolism. In skilled nursing facilities, 85% of residents have indications for VTE prophylaxis with half having contraindications, including quality of life and resident or caregiver wishes. In a study in the United States, about

Table 30–3.	SIDE EFFECTS OF DRUGS USED TO TREAT CHRONIC OBSTRUCTIVE PULMONARY DISEASE

Drug	Side Effects
Anticholinergics	Dry mouth, urinary retention, orthostasis, tremor
β-Agonists	Headache, tremor, angina, palpitations, tachycardia, vomiting
Corticosteroids	Myopathy, psychosis, delirium, indigestion, increased glucose, gut bleeding, infections
Theophylline	Nausea, diarrhea, hypertension, tachyarrhythmias, dizziness, insomnia, seizures, headaches

Table 30–4.	FACTORS INCREASING IMMOBILITY THAT ARE ASSOCIATED WITH VENOUS THROMBOEMBOLISM IN NURSING HOMES

- Bedfast
- Wheelchair use
- Assistance with grooming or transferring
- Inability to walk 10 feet
- Lower limb cast
- Recent lower limb orthopedic surgery
- Recent acute infection

Table 30–5.	ALTERNATIVE DIAGNOSES TO DEEP VEIN THROMBOSIS

- Muscle rupture
- Ruptured Baker's cyst
- Chronic venous insufficiency
- Cellulitis
- Superficial venous thrombosis
- Unilateral edema caused by other causes of edema

two thirds of those who were eligible for receiving skilled care received prophylaxis.

The primary approach to the prevention of PE is the early recognition and treatment of deep vein thrombosis (DVT). Half of DVT's have minimal symptoms and may present with mildly increased edema in one leg and an increase in calf circumference. Others present with a sore, swollen, red, warm leg. DVTs are more common in the veins of the left leg. Table 30–5 provides alternative diagnoses to DVT. Criteria that should lead to further evaluation for DVT are given in Table 30–6.

If probability is low, a D-dimer (cross-linked fibrin degradation product) can be obtained. Elevated levels require further investigation but do not make the diagnosis. The diagnosis is made by duplex ultrasonography, which has high sensitivity, specificity, and reproducibility.

Low-molecular-weight heparin (LMWH) may be slightly superior to unfractionated heparin in the prevention of DVT (Table 30–7). Thrombocytopenia occurs in 1.2% of those receiving unfractionated heparin and 0.6% of those receiving LMWH. The doses of fondaparinux and enoxaparin should be reduced if the creatinine clearance is less than 30 mL/min. When the resident's weight is less than 50 kg, the dose of LMWH and fondaparinux should be reduced. DVT treatment should be carried out in the

nursing home if appropriate diagnostic tools are available. Available studies suggest that a person with a DVT should receive at least 1 year's therapy with warfarin, with an international normalized ratio maintained between 2 and 3. If this is not feasible, aspirin can be used in the place of warfarin after 3 months. Long-term treatment with LMWH may be preferable to warfarin. The newer anticoagulants (factor Xa inhibitors [fondaparinux, rivaroxaban] and thrombin inhibitors [dabigatran]) are easier to use but are problematic in persons with poor renal clearance, and no direct antagonists to reverse bleeding exist. The latest

Table 30–6.	CRITERIA TO CONSIDER FURTHER EVALUATION FOR DEEP VEIN THROMBOSIS

- Calf swelling >3 cm compared with the other calf
- Unilateral edema of new onset
- Calf tenderness
- Acute onset
- Recent hospitalization or immobility
- Cancer or exacerbation of heart failure
- Pressure ulcer
- Previous DVT or family history of DVT

DVT, deep vein thrombosis.

Table 30–7.	LOW-MOLECULAR-WEIGHT HEPARIN COMPARED WITH UNFRACTIONATED HEPARIN	
	Low-Molecular-Weight Heparin	**Unfractionated Heparin**
Once- or twice-daily administration	Yes	No
Safer to administer in nursing homes	Yes	No
No laboratory monitoring	Yes	No
More efficacious	Yes	No
Risk of bleeding	Lower	Higher
Incidence of thrombocytopenia	Lower	Higher
Incidence of heparin-induced osteoporosis	Lower	Higher

Table 30–8.	WELLS SCALE TO DETERMINE THE NEED TO TRANSFER TO A HOSPITAL

- Clinically suspected DVT: 3 points
- Tachycardia (>100 beats/min): 1.5 points
- Immobilization or surgery in past 4 weeks: 1.5 points
- Previous history of DVT or PE: 1.5 points
- Hemoptysis: 1.0 point
- Malignancy with treatment in last 6 months: 1.0 points

Score >4: Highly likely to have PE: Transfer
Score ≤4: PE unlikely; consider D-dimer

DVT, deep vein thrombosis; PE, pulmonary embolism.

Beers list includes dabigatran, but this is most probably not supported by the literature as long as the dose is reduced in persons with poor creatinine clearance. In nursing homes, aspirin should be avoided in combination with any of the anticoagulants. Compression stockings reduce the post-thrombotic syndrome. There is minimal evidence to support the use of vena caval filters.

Symptoms of PE include an acute onset of dyspnea, chest pain on breathing in, and palpitations. In some residents, this produces acute anxiety. Signs include tachycardia, respiratory rate greater than 28 breaths/min, and low blood oxygen saturation. Persons with a multiple small PEs may develop basal crepitations. With a small PE, all symptoms and signs may dissipate within 30 minutes. The Wells prediction rule can be used to decide if the resident needs transfer to a hospital (Table 30–8).

KEY POINTS

1. All nursing home residents should be screened for COPD with three simple questions.
2. Persons with COPD and comorbid asthma are more likely to go to the emergency department; patients with new asthmatic symptoms should be promptly treated with corticosteroids to decrease nursing home admissions.
3. The key components of COPD management are to stop smoking and supplemental oxygen when appropriate.
4. Pulmonary rehabilitation with exercise and a high-protein supplement improves quality of life.
5. PE accounts for nearly 10% of nursing home deaths.
6. DVT should be treated aggressively in immobile residents and new admissions from the hospital.
7. New anticoagulants may improve the ability to treat DVTs but are very expensive.
8. New-onset shortness of breath, chest pain, or unexplained anxiety may indicate a PE in a nursing home resident.

SUGGESTED READINGS

Dharmarajan TS, Nanda A, Agarwal B, et al. Prevention of venous thromboembolism: practice patterns in 17 geographically diverse long term care facilities in the United States: part 1 of 2 (an AMDA Foundation project). *J Am Med Assoc.* 2012;13:298-302.

Evensen AE. Management of COPD Exacerbations. *Am Fam Physician.* 2010;81:607-613.

Gomes JP, Shaheen WH, Truong SV, et al. Incidence of venous thromboembolic events among nursing home residents. *J Gen Intern Med.* 2003;18:934-936.

Gross JS, Neufeld RR, Libow LS, et al. Autopsy study of the elderly institutionalized patient. Review of 234 autopsies. *Arch Intern Med.* 1988;148:173-176.

Lacasse Y, Brosseau L, Milne S, et al. Pulmonary rehabilitation for chronic obstructive pulmonary disease. *Cochrane Database Syst Rev.* 2002;(3):CD003793.

Leibson CL, Petterson TM, Bailey KR, et al. Risk factors for venous thromboembolism in nursing home residents. *Mayo Clin Proc.* 2008;83:151-157.

Liperoti R, Pedone C, Lapane KL, et al. Venous thromboembolism among elderly patients treated with atypical and conventional antipsychotic agents. *Arch Intern Med.* 2005;165:2677-2682.

Segal JB, Streiff MB, Hofmann LV, et al. Management of venous thromboembolism: a systematic review for a practice guideline. *Ann Intern Med.* 2007;146:211-222.

Simoni-Wastila L, Blanchette CM, Qian J, et al. Burden of chronic obstructive pulmonary disease in Medicare beneficiaries residing in long-term care facilities. *Am J Geriatr Pharmacother.* 2009;7: 262-270.

Stephens MB, Yew KS. Diagnosis of chronic obstructive pulmonary disease. *Am Fam Physician.* 2008;78:87-92.

Taubman LB, Silverstone FA. Autopsy proven pulmonary embolism among the institutionalized elderly. *J Am Geriatr Soc.* 1986;34: 752-756.

Zarowitz BJ, Tangalos E, Lefkovitz A, et al. Thrombotic risk and immobility in residents of long-term care facilities. *J Am Med Dir Assoc.* 2010;11:211-221.

Zarowitz BJ, O'Shea T, Lefkovitz A, Peterson EL. Development and validation of a screening tool for chronic obstructive pulmonary disease in nursing home residents. *J Am Med Dir Assoc.* 2011;12: 668-674.

MULTIPLE CHOICE QUESTIONS

30.1   A 75-year-old man with benign prostate hypertrophy has a COPD exacerbation associated with increased sinus drainage. After treatment is started, he develops acute urinary retention. Which drug is most likely to have caused this?

a. Corticosteroids
b. Terbutaline
c. Antihistamine
d. Formoterol
e. Salbutamol

30.2   Which of the following is improved by an exercise program together with a high-protein supplement?

a. Quality of life
b. Mortality
c. Dyspnea
d. Hospitalization
e. A and C

30.3   More than two thirds of deaths from PE in nursing homes are attributed to other causes.

   a. True
   b. False

30.4   Which of the following is *not* a criteria to further investigate a person with a swollen leg in the nursing home?

   a. New onset
   b. Diagnosis of cancer
   c. Previous DVT
   d. Calf tenderness
   e. Calf swelling <3 cm compared with the other calf

30.5   An 85-year-old woman complains of anxiety and was noted to have had a brief episode of shortness of breath. Her pulse rate is 112 beats/min. She has bibasilar crepitations. She has a left leg that is swollen. She has recently been treated for ovarian cancer. Her Wells score to determine need to transfer to a hospital or acute treatment and evaluation for a pulmonary embolus is:

   a. 1.5
   b. 2.5
   c. 3.5
   d. 4.5
   e. 5.5

Chapter 31

ONCOLOGY

Cancer is three times more common in persons older than age 75 years and is the second most common cause of death in persons older than 80 years of age. Lung cancer is the most common cancer in persons older than 60 years of age. The other major causes of cancer in men are colorectal, prostate, and pancreatic cancer and non-Hodgkin's lymphoma. In women, the other major causes are breast, colorectal, pancreatic, and ovarian cancer.

About 10% of nursing home residents have cancer. The most common cancer diagnoses in nursing homes are breast cancer in women and prostate cancer in men. Residents in nursing homes with cancer are more likely to have pain, a poorer health-related quality of life, and worse general health than other nursing home residents. They also have more dyspnea, constipation, anemia, and weight loss than residents with dementia. Persons with cancer in nursing homes receive less physical, psychological, occupational, and speech therapies. They receive more ostomy care and intravenous medications. Of nursing home residents, 4% are receiving chemotherapy, and 14% are having radiation therapy. Approximately half of nursing home residents with cancer die within 1 year of admission. There has been an increase in cancer patients dying in nursing homes with nearly 20% now dying there.

A quarter of residents in nursing homes with cancer are diagnosed within 1 month of death. Early diagnosis of residents with cancer is less likely if the person is older or has dementia. Of interest is residents in nursing homes with lower nursing staffing were most likely to be diagnosed with cancer. This conundrum has no obvious explanation.

Residents with colon cancer commonly undergo surgery. In these residents, both mortality rates and functional decline are greater than expected.

In residents with breast cancer, one third were not referred for treatment. The residents who were not referred had end-stage dementia, resident or family preference, and limited life expectancy. In about 15% of residents, hormonal treatment is started without a cancer diagnosis. For many residents whose life span is less than 5 years, a simple lumpectomy will prevent ulceration and improve their quality of life.

Screening for cancer in nursing home residents has minimal value (see recommendations of the United States Preventive Service Task Force in Table 31-1). For most residents, screening should be guided by observing the basic CAUTION mnemonic (Table 31-2) and considering cancer when treatable causes of weight loss are not found. The majority of oral cancers occur in older persons. They are present on the tongue and floor of the mouth. Screening for oral cancer is poorly done even by dentists in nursing homes.

It is important to recognize the harms of standard types of cancer therapy that are magnified in nursing home residents with poor functional status (Table 31-3). Early withdrawal of therapy that is unlikely to produce a cure can prolong life and improve function.

Oncologists use two functional status scales for cancer patients. They are the Karnofsky index (0 = dead; 100 = normal function) and the Eastern Cooperative Oncology Group (ECOG) scale (0 = normal; 5 = dead). Persons with an ECOG score greater than 3 or a Kanofsky index less than 40% have a cancer survival period of about 3 months.

Most cancer patients develop cachexia. Cachexia is characterized by loss of muscle and fat and is predominantly caused by excess circulating cytokines. The features of cachexia are listed in Table 31-4. High-quality nutritional support (protein and caloric supplementation) can slow the progression of cachexia. Megestrol acetate (600–800 mg) can increase appetite and produce weight gain, predominantly in increasing fat gain. There is no evidence that megestrol increases life expectancy, but it may improve quality of life. Dronabinol produces a small increase in appetite and weight gain. It also enhances taste of food, relaxes the person, and is an antiemetic. Many persons find smoking cannabis (marijuana) more effective than taking dronabinol, but this is illegal in many parts of the world.

CHRONIC LYMPHOCYTIC LEUKEMIA

Chronic lymphocytic leukemia (CLL) is a disease of older persons characterized by a progressive increase of afunctional lymphocytes. Early in the disease, there are minimal symptoms, and the diagnosis is usually made when a blood count is obtained for other purposes. The majority of persons with CLL live between 5 to 10 years. The clinical features of CLL are given in Table 31-5.

Table 31–1.	UNITED STATES PREVENTIVE SERVICES TASK FORCE RECOMMENDATIONS FOR SCREENING

Cancer	Recommendation
Colorectalg	No screening in adults older than 75 years of age
Lung	No screening in asymptomatic individuals
Ovarian	No routine screening
Prostate	No screening in men older than 75 years of age
Cervical	No screening in women with hysterectomy or older than 65 years of age with normal Pap smear results
Breast	No screening older than 75 years of age

Table 31–2.   SIGNS OF POSSIBLE CANCER
Change in bowel or bladder habits
A sore that does not heal
Unusual bleeding or discharge
Thickening or lump in breast or elsewhere
Indigestion or difficulty in swallowing
Obvious change in wart or mole
Nagging cough or hoarseness

Table 31–3.	SIDE EFFECTS OF CANCER THERAPY

Therapy	Side Effects
Chemotherapy	Nausea, vomiting, fatigue, diarrhea, hair loss, anorexia, weight loss, infections
Radiation	Fatigue, anorexia, skin irritation, radiation enteritis
Surgery	Pain, muscle atrophy, bleeding, fatigue, loss of mobility, loss of limbs, pulmonary embolus
Hormone therapy	Mood changes, insomnia, osteoporosis, fluid retention, diabetes mellitus, coronary artery disease, fatigue

Table 31–4.   THE FEATURES OF CACHEXIA
• Weight loss
• Muscle loss
• Fat loss
• Inflammation
• Anemia
• Hypoalbuminemia
• Anorexia
• Fatigue
• Insulin resistance
• Slowed gastric emptying

Table 31–5.	CLINICAL FEATURES OF CHRONIC LYMPHOCYTIC LEUKEMIA
• Fatigue	
• Weight loss	
• Lymphadenopathy	
• Predilection to infections (e.g., pneumonia, herpes zoster, herpes labialis)	
• Early satiation (anorexia)	
• Fever or night sweats	
• Anemia	
• Thrombocytopenia (petechial or mucocutaneous bleeding)	
• Splenomegaly	
• Hepatomegaly	
• Markedly elevated lymphocyte count	
• Muscle wasting	

The diagnosis of CLL includes an elevated lymphocyte count and peripheral blood flow cytometry to demonstrate more than 5000 β-lymphocytes/μL. The differential diagnosis is acute lymphoblastic and hairy cell leukemia as well as a variety of lymphomas.

Most persons with CLL should receive no treatment and just have periodic measurement of their blood count. If the residents becomes severely symptomatic or there is a doubling of lymphocytes in 6 months, therapy can be considered.

Chlorambucil (an alkylating agent) is cheap and has the same progression-free survival time as the more expensive fludarabine (a purine nucleoside analog). Other drugs do not appear to be more effective. Early therapy has no benefit and increases side effects and mortality rate.

KEY POINTS

1. Residents with cancer have more pain, worse health-related quality of life, and more weight loss than residents with dementia.
2. Residents with cancer receive less physical, occupational, psychological, and speech therapies than other residents.
3. Residents in nursing homes often have new cancer diagnoses late, and one third are not referred for treatment.
4. The CAUTION mnemonic should be used to screen for cancer in nursing home residents.
5. Routine screenings for cancer are not recommended in the majority of nursing home residents.
6. CLL is a common condition in the nursing home and should only be treated when the resident is symptomatic.

SUGGESTED READINGS

Clement JP, Bradley CJ, Lin C. Organizational characteristics and cancer care for nursing home residents. *Health Serv Res.* 2009;44: 1983-2003.

Drageset J, Eide GE, Ranhoff AH. Cancer in nursing homes: characteristics and health-related quality of life among cognitively intact residents with and without cancer. *Cancer Nurs.* 2011;35(4):295-301.

Fennell ML. Nursing homes and cancer care. *Health Serv Res.* 2009; 44:1927-1932.

Finlayson E, Zhao S, Boscardin WJ, et al. Functional status after colon cancer surgery in elderly nursing home residents. *J Am Geriatr Soc.* 2012;60(5):967-973.

Hamaker ME, Hamelinck VC, van Munster BC, et al. Nonreferral of nursing home patients with suspected breast cancer. *J Am Med Dir Assoc.* 2012;13:464-469.

Korc-Grodzicki B, Wallace JA, Rodin MB, Bernacki RE. Cancer in long-term care. *Clin Geriatr Med.* 2011;27:301-327.

Mahalaha SA, Cheruva VK, Smyth KA. Oral cancer screening: practices, knowledge, and opinions of dentists working in Ohio nursing homes. *Spec Care Dentis.* 2009;29:237-243.

MULTIPLE CHOICE QUESTIONS

31.1 Which of the following is *not* true of residents in a nursing home?

a. They have worse health-related quality of life.
b. They get more ostomy care.
c. They are more likely to have pain.
d. They have more anemia.
e. They get more physical therapy.

31.2 What percentage of residents who develop cancer are diagnosed within 1 month of their death?

a. 5%
b. 10%
c. 25%
d. 30%
e. 40%

31.3 Which of the following is a sign of cancer in nursing home residents, as delineated by the CAUTION mnemonic?

a. Edema
b. Dyspnea
c. Angina
d. A sore that does not heal
e. Delirium

31.4 Which of the following is *not* true concerning residents with cachexia?

a. Cachexia is associated with insulin resistance.
b. Megestrol acetate does not produce weight gain in persons with cancer.
c. Most cachectic residents are anemic.
d. Cytokine increase leads to hypoalbuminemia.

31.5 Which of the following is true concerning CLL?

a. Early use of fludarabine decreases mortality rate.
b. Flow cytometry needs to demonstrate a count greater than 1000 β-lymphocyte per μL.
c. Persons with CLL live for less than 2 years on average.
d. Chlorambucil is a cheap, effective treatment for CLL.

Appendix

MULTIPLE CHOICE QUESTIONS ANSWERS

PART 1. INTRODUCTION TO NURSING HOME LIFE AND ALTERNATIVES

Chapter 1

Question 1.1   Answer **e**
Although nursing visits and other visits by healthcare professionals are essential for successful aging in place, physician visits are not necessary because either transport can be provided to the physician office or, in the future, telemedicine may be an alternative.

Question 1.2   Answer **d**
This is based on a Swedish study using the Safe Medication Assessment tool.

Question 1.3   Answer **a**
Hong Kong has approximately one in 10 older persons institutionalized. Sweden has approximately a 7% institutionalization rate. The United States and United Kingdom each have institutionalization rates below 5%. South Korea has one of the lowest institutionalization rates in the world.

Question 1.4   Answer **a**
A variety of electronic monitoring methods are being developed in demonstration "smart homes" to allow older persons to safely live at home.

Question 1.5   Answer **b**
Persons in the PACE program are twice as likely to die at home. Persons in the PACE program also have better health, better functional status, and better quality of life.

Question 1.6   Answer **c**
The key driver was the known variations in the quality of nursing home practice around the world and imperative to protect vulnerable older people from unacceptable healthcare inequalities.

Chapter 2

Question 2.1   Answer **b**
Helena, the wife of the Emperor Constantine, was credited with developing the first nursing homes in Constantinople (Istanbul). The first hospice was established in Rhodes by the Knights Hospitals of St. John.

Question 2.2   Answer **c**
OBRA is a yearly act passed by the United States Congress called the Office of Budget Reconciliation Act. In 1987, a number of nursing home regulations were attached to this bill.

Question 2.3   Answer **e**
The United States has only half of its nursing residents having dementia. This is because much more rehabilitation with the intention of returning people to their homes is done in skilled nursing facilities in the United States compared with other countries.

Question 2.4   Answer **a**
Polypharmacy is far more common in the United States than in Europe. This is partly because nursing homes in the United States treat many people undergoing rehabilitation. All the others are more common in Europe, presumably related to the higher prevalence of dementia in European nursing homes.

Question 2.5   Answer **c**
Windows should be at a lower level to allow persons in wheelchairs to be able to easily look outside.

Chapter 3

Question 3.1   Answer **b**
The medical model has an active role for physicians not only in medical care but also in administration. This is the classical model in the United States.

Question 3.2   Answer **d**
Although knowledge of the history of the time a person has lived through can be very useful, it is not considered a component of personalized care. Personalized care is focused on the person.

Question 3.3   Answer **a**
Surprisingly, many older persons are grateful that their admission to a nursing home has improved life for their spouse. Overwhelmingly in most cases, admission to a nursing home is at least as stressful for the spouse staying at home as the spouse being admitted to the nursing home.

Question 3.4   Answer c
All of the other conditions are associated with "rust out." "Burnout" occurs because of either quantitative or qualitative overload.

Question 3.5   Answer b
Lack of language fluency leads to an inability to communicate with residents and boredom. All the other conditions cause "burnout."

Chapter 4

Question 4.1   Answer d
In the Pioneer Network, voices of residents and caregivers are given equal import. The Pioneer Network advocates person-centered care to bring about culture change.

Question 4.2   Answer e
Allowing staff to make their own decisions and to change things to improve the residents or their quality of life is a key for culture change to occur. An overfocus on health needs tends to lead to an underfocus on social needs. A top-down management structure is inhibitory to providing a home-like structure.

Question 4.3   Answer b
Terminology and forms of address that may be appropriate in one country may be considered highly inappropriate in another country. In some areas, residents prefer to be addressed by their first names. Obviously, all residents should be asked how they wish to be addressed.

Question 4.4   Answer d
The primary caregiver (usually a nurse's aide) and resident are at the center of care. All other staff and family need to focus on improving the quality of life for this dyad. All of the other answers listed are important components of cultural change.

Question 4.5   Answer d
Making staff feel good about themselves and central to cultural change is the single component most important to creating successful culture change. Organizational culture is a major determinant of values. In negative cultures, staff are often unaware of the differences in each of their understandings of their tasks. Involving family members is a key component of culture change.

PART 2. FUNDAMENTALS OF NURSING HOME PRACTICE

Chapter 5

Question 5.1   Answer c
Participation, the right to remain integrated in society, to serve as volunteers, and to form movements or associations of older persons, is the missing principle. Although freedom from illness is a laudable aim, it is not a realistic principle.

Question 5.2   Answer d
Lack of truth telling leads to a culture in which persons are uncertain what to believe. Family members are often unaware of what the person wants or needs to hear. Truth telling is essential for self-realization and autonomy. There are marked cultural differences in the acceptability of "truth telling."

Question 5.3   Answer d
Intentional neglect requires the failure to knowingly provide help to a resident. An inappropriately trained staff member is not performing intentional neglect. When a staff member is legitimately busy with another resident, this is not neglect. Failing to provide care because of inappropriate knowledge is a form of passive neglect. An act of violence is a form of physical abuse.

Question 5.4   Answer a
The addition of a sixth drug has an equal change of causing benefit or harm. This is independent of the type of the drug. For this reason, increasing drugs above five requires a very clear rationale for the addition of another drug.

Question 5.5   Answer a
Restraints have led to strangulation of residents and pulmonary emboli. Physical restraints as opposed to posturing devices or mobility-enhancing devices (e.g., walkers) are generally considered abusive and increase injurious falls.

Chapter 6

Question 6.1   Answer d
Although medical needs are important, social and psychological needs need a greater focus. The individual needs to be able to choose to reject medical therapies.

Question 6.2   Answer a
The STOP AND WATCH tool is a simple tool to allow nursing assistants to have early recognition of changes in the resident condition. Although the other three approaches are potentially important in reducing transitions, they are not part of INTERACT II.

Question 6.3   Answer a
Acute renal failure, although occasionally avoidable (e.g., drug toxicity), is not a common cause of potentially avoidable hospital admissions. The other four and chronic obstructive pulmonary disease are all on the list of five.

Question 6.4   Answer d
Urinary incontinence occurs much earlier in persons with dementia.

Question 6.5   Answer c
Although acceptance is common, death is rarely associated with happiness. Bargaining is the other of the stages of dying.

Chapter 7

Question 7.1   Answer a, b, and d
Teamwork involves working together, and this requires a shared and explicit value base. To achieve resident-centered care, all team members must believe this is appropriate and understand what this means in terms of their discipline and individual contributions in the context of the wider team. Staff need clarity about their own roles and

those of other team members to enable the development of mutual respect and reciprocity. A dedicated development budget is also desirable because this investment helps forge teamwork and succession planning.

Question 7.2   Answer b
This is false. The largest staff group is nursing aides and care assistants, who are ideally supervised by registered nurses. The ratio of registered nurses to nursing aides will depend on the category of home and regulatory guidance.

Question 7.3   Answer d
The medical director is an important member of the multiprofessional team with a major administrative role. The medical director plays a role as an educator of other physicians and monitors their performance.

Question 7.4   Answer e
Rapid cycles are teams that try to solve a newly recognized problem as rapidly as possible. They usually meet as necessary. They are usually fairly small. Although they do collect data, they also need to fix the problem.

Question 7.5   Answer b
Loners tend to hold the team's functioning back even if they are performing their own jobs at a high level. All of the others are important members of functioning teams.

Chapter 8

Question 8.1   Answer b
Leaders create and drive change, leading to reform, and managers manage the present, creating stability through rationality and control.

Question 8.2   Answer a, b, and c
All three answers are correct but should be used selectively for particular situations.

Question 8.3   Answer b
Medical leadership may or may not be useful or indeed available and depends on the change project. When a medical director is available, his or her support is essential, but the medical director is not necessarily the most effective leader for all projects. Potentially, all nursing home practitioners make leadership contributions, and the most appropriate person irrespective of discipline or rank should be identified to lead particular projects.

Question 8.4   Answer d
Persons are empowered to do their own corrections. Control is not a component of the cycle.

Question 8.5   Answer c
In most nursing homes, the pharmacist and possibly the medical director supervise physician prescribing practices.

Chapter 9

Question 9.1   Answer c
Institutions tend to promote conformity, leading to apathy and submissiveness. All of the other behaviors are common after admission to a nursing home but are not considered "social breakdown behaviors."

Question 9.2   Answer b
Family caregivers who have poor self-reported health have problems adjusting to their family member being in a nursing home.

Question 9.3   Answer a
The MDS 3.0 covers extensive medical and social details but does not ask question directed to whether or not the resident can afford the care.

Question 9.4   Answer d
The geronte is a wonderful simple communication tool.

Question 9.5   Answer d
Fatigue is one of the components together with climbing a flight of stairs, walking a block, more than five illnesses, and weight loss.

Chapter 10

Question 10.1   Answer d
Most nursing home research has focused on geriatric syndromes.

Question 10.2   Answer b
For a variety of reasons, the majority of research-based best care practices have not been implemented in nursing homes.

Question 10.3   Answer b
Trials in nursing homes tend to be of short duration and are often underpowered. Trials of new drugs are rare in nursing homes. There is a paucity of randomized controlled trials. There are inadequate quality data to perform meta-analyses in most areas of nursing home care.

Question 10.4   Answer c
COP models require continued learning at a distance, including sharing information between the students. It requires a sophisticated infrastructure. It is evidence based and emphasizes culture change.

Question 10.5   Answer b
In the United States, it was found that 38% of medical students felt uneasy caring for nursing home residents. Worldwide there is limited training for medical students in nursing homes.

PART 3. MANAGING AGE-RELATED SYNDROMES AND CHANGES

Chapter 11

Question 11.1   Answer b
NSAIDs account for a quarter of hospitalizations for drug side effects in older persons. All drugs have side effects, and drug–drug interactions are a particularly important cause of side effects.

Question 11.2   Answer d
Constipation is the most common side effect. In most cases, it can be treated with osmotic laxatives. Methylnaltrexone and lubiprostone may be effective in severe cases.

Question 11.3   Answer a
Tramadol is eleptogenic. The others either have no effect or are antiseizure medications.

Question 11.4   Answer d
Spinal stenosis is classically relieved by sitting or bending forward. Herniated discs lead to sciatic pain. Cancer, compression fracture, and spinal infection are associated with localized tenderness.

Question 11.5   Answer a
Acetaminophen (paracetamol) increases the INR in persons taking warfarin. NSAIDs reduce the effect of warfarin. The others have no effect.

Question 11.6   Answer b
Interpersonal relationships play a major role in the effectiveness of pain programs.

Question 11.7   Answer e
Acupuncture has not been shown to be highly effective in nursing home residents. All of the other approaches have been studied and shown to decrease pain in nursing home residents.

Chapter 12

Question 12.1   Answer d
Privacy and maintaining a locus of control are key factors in allowing a person to adjust to the nursing home. Although family attitude can be helpful, it can also hinder adjustment. Having a roommate decreases but, though for some persons, a compatible roommate can be helpful. The need for conformity is a negative factor in adjustment to nursing homes. Buildings need to be designed to allow maximum privacy.

Question 12.2   Answer a
The PHQ-9 is now becoming the screening test of choice for depression. There is no test called the PDQ-9. The other three have all been used in nursing home residents and are valid. The PHQ-9 performs better than the Geriatric Depression Scale. The Cornell Depression Scale is used for persons with depression. The PHQ-9 in the MDS 3.0 has a version that has been adapted for persons with dementia and is valid.

Question 12.3   Answer e
All four approaches have been shown to perform better than placebo. The combination of drug therapy with cognitive behavioral therapy has the best outcomes.

Question 12.4   Answer d
Dysphoria (unhappiness) is a symptom of depression. All of the other symptoms are part of the generalized anxiety disorder.

Question 12.5   Answer d
SSRIs pull calcium off bone, leading to osteoporosis and hip fracture. All of the others are side effects of tricyclic antidepressants.

Question 12.6   Answer b
Disorganized sleep is a negative symptom. All of the others are positive symptoms. Only positive symptoms respond well to antipsychotics.

Chapter 13

Question 13.1   Answer b
Delirious residents have a decline in function. All of the other statements are true of delirious residents in nursing homes.

Question 13.2   Answer a
The MMSE differentiates MCI poorly. The other three tests have reasonable sensitivity and specificity to screen for MCI.

Question 13.3   Answer c
Normal-pressure hydrocephalus is considered the wacky, wobbly, and wet syndrome. All forms of dementia can be associated with incontinence. Falls caused by executive dysfunction lead to poor ability to dual task. Lewy body dementia usually presents with behavioral disturbances early. Fragile X syndrome has an essential tremor. People with Pick's disease and hypothyroidism tend to present with apathy.

Question 13.4   Answer c
Memantine is an NMDA antagonist and as such can reduce chronic pain. This can lead to a decrease in agitation. Both nightmares and hypotension are side effects of memantine.

Question 13.5   Answer a
Cognitive stimulation therapy is at least as effective as treatment with cholinesterase inhibitors for persons with dementia. It is associated with fewer side effects.

Question 13.6   Answer a
Antipsychotics increase mortality rates. They have a variety of adverse effects and have not been demonstrated to decrease nonpsychotic behaviors.

Chapter 14

Question 14.1   Answer c
Studies have demonstrated that it takes approximately 45 minutes.

Question 14.2   Answer c
Between 1 and 1.5 g/kg protein/day is recommended. The recommended daily allowance is 0.8 g/kg/day, which is believed to be too low for individuals actively building protein. Greater than 1.5 g/kg/day may be toxic to the kidneys and lead to acidosis.

Question 14.3   Answer b
Megestrol acetate is a powerful orexigenic. Therapeutic diets need to be avoided in nursing home residents. Buffet dining stimulates food intake as does the involvement of families. Caloric supplements should be given between meals.

Question 14.4   Answer c
Hypodermoclysis rarely causes bruising.

Question 14.5   Answer d
Colchicine proton pump inhibitors and mineral oil are associated with vitamin B_{12} deficiency.

Question 14.6   Answer e
1,25(OH) vitamin D has great variability in the serum and is a poor measure of vitamin D status. If a level of vitamin D status is required, 25(OH) vitamin D should be measured.

Chapter 15

Question 15.1   Answer d
All of the other factors are ones that can legitimately lead to a decrease in a person's sexual intimacy. Homosexuality should not prevent an intimate relationship in the nursing home.

Question 15.2   Answer a
Persons who are cognitively impaired can still have relationships as long as a series of rules are used to approach the consent process. If the relationship makes the person happy, this is positive. Depression is not. There are approaches allowing proxy consent. A single individual or a group of individuals should not have veto power over a relationship.

Question 15.3   Answer c
Testosterone increases hematocrit. If the hematocrit is greater than 55, testosterone needs to be stopped because of the risk of stroke.

Question 15.4   Answer d
Residents must always be told if their behavior is inappropriate. Antipsychotics do not work. Medroxyprogesterone has an unacceptably high rate of thrombosis. Staff members need to openly discuss the behavior and potential approaches to curbing it among themselves. Staff members need to be careful not to have behaviors that may be inappropriately interpreted by residents.

Question 15.5   Answer a
Studies have shown that residents in nursing homes often view themselves as unattractive. Staff members need to work with residents to help make them feel more attractive and enhance their self-esteem.

Chapter 16

Question 16.1   Answer d
Urination occurs when the parasympathetic nervous system stimulates the detrusor muscle together with inhibition of the sympathetic nervous system, leading to relaxation of the internal urethral sphincter.

Question 16.2   Answer b
Increasing abdominal pressure by sneezing or coughing leads to stress incontinence.

Question 16.3   Answer d
Lower urinary tract symptomatology is often related to a large prostate and has a high postvoid residual.

Question 16.4   Answer c
Soap and water increases the propensity to develop incontinence-associated dermatitis. All others are protective.

Question 16.5   Answer d
Indwelling catheters increase infection and should be avoided whenever possible.

Chapter 17

Question 17.1   Answer b
Lactulose, sorbitol, and polyethylene glycol are all osmotic laxatives. On the whole, these are more effective than stimulant laxatives such as senna and bisacodyl. Stool softeners, such as dioctyl sodium, are ineffective. Lubiprostone, which activates chloride-2 channels, is highly effective.

Question 17.2   Answer d
Both Almivopan and methylnatrexone are specific drugs that inhibit the peripheral constipating effects of opiates.

Question 17.3   Answer a
Although all can cause fecal incontinence, overflow incontinence from constipation is the most common.

Question 17.4   Answer e
All of the others are correct. Diarrhea in persons receiving antibiotics is caused by infection with *Clostridium difficile.*

Question 17.5   Answer a
The presence of cytotoxin A or B makes the diagnosis. Culture of *Clostridium difficile* often finds commensal *C. difficile* organisms that do not produce diarrhea-inducing cytotoxins.

Chapter 18

Question 18.1   Answer b
The outside of the heel strikes the ground first with the forefoot being used to push off. The feet are 2 to 4 inches apart, and the knees are flexed.

Question 18.2   Answer e
This is a classical gait of spinal stenosis. Retropulsion is leaning backward while walking. Antalgic is a limp caused by pain. Claudication is a slow gait with increased pain while walking. A sensory gait is broad based with short steps.

Question 18.3   Answer c
It is generally believed that 1.7 falls per bed per year is the average, but both higher and lower numbers of falls are seen in individual nursing homes.

Question 18.4   Answer b
Delirium, SSRIs, and dopamine agonists all cause falls. Extrinsic causes are common causes of falls in nursing homes.

Question 18.5   Answer c
Calcitonin reduces vertebral but not hip fractures. Resistance exercises have been shown to reduce recurrent hip fractures in the year after a fracture. In persons with multiple falls, hip pads reduce hip fractures. Calcium together with vitamin D and bisphosphonates reduce hip fractures.

Chapter 19

Question 19.1   Answer b
Noise and switching on light by staff are the major causes of sleep disruption. Patients with severe Alzheimer's disease sleep longer. Although all of the other three disrupt sleep, none are as common as the problems created by excessive staff surveillance.

Question 19.2   Answer a
Beta antagonists do not cause insomnia. All of the other drugs have been implicated as causes of insomnia.

Question 19.3   Answer e
Coffee interferes with sleep.

Question 19.4   Answer d
AVP decrease and ANH increase are implicated in nocturia. Diuretics in the evening increase nocturia. Diabetes mellitus causes an osmotic diuresis and nocturia.

Question 19.5   Answer d
All except for nightmares are symptoms of possible sleep apnea.

Question 19.6   Answer c
Low levels of CPAP work and are less disruptive for older persons CPAP breathing is noisy. Cognitive function improves in residents with Alzheimer's disease who are treated for sleep apnea.

Chapter 20

Question 20.1   Answer d
Cherry angiomas are round, red, nonblanching papules. Pemphigus and pemphigoid present with blisters. Tinea versicolor consists of dark or light scaly lesions.

Question 20.2   Answer a
Other treatments for actinic keratosis include imiquimod, ingenol mebutate, and cryosurgery. Isotretinoin is used topically for keratoacanthomas and systemically for sebaceous hyperplasia. Coal tar paste is used for psoriasis. Selenium sulfide shampoo is used for tinea versicolor.

Question 20.3   Answer e
Beans increase flatus. Garlic, asparagus, and onions increase ostomy odor.

Question 20.4   Answer a
Lack of skin (epidermal) flap is a hallmark of category III in both classifications. Category IIA is less than 225% epidermal flap loss. No tissue loss is category IA. For stage IIB, skin needs to be able to be realigned.

Question 20.5   Answer c
Stage III is full-thickness tissue loss without exposure of bone, muscle, or tendons. Tunneling can be present.

Question 20.6   Answer c
Hydrocolloids are the only dressings with all of these characteristics. All of the other dressings are water permeable. Wet saline, gauze, and polymers may macerate skin and damage epithelial cells. Only hydrocolloids are bacterial resistant.

Question 20.7   Answer d
Pearly translucency is characteristic of basal cell cancer.

Chapter 21

Question 21.1   Answer d
This is the classical definition of erythema migrans or geographic tongue. Erythroplakia is a fiery red patch or a bright red velvety plaque. Lichen planus is either white lines or a painful redness. *Candida* infection is either white or red scaling lesions that can be removed. Canker sores are painful ulcers covered by a white or yellow membrane.

Question 21.2   Answer c
Erythema migrans is an inflammatory condition. All of the others are thought to be premalignant.

Question 21.3   Answer c
The tongue is the most common site for oral cancer. Most oral cancers are squamous. The 5-year survival is about 50%. Oral cancers are responsible for 2% to 3% of cancers. Surgical excision is the treatment of choice for oral cancer, but radiation and chemotherapy are used as adjunctive therapies.

Question 21.4   Answer c
Teeth grinding is not an age-related activity, although it is common in older persons who are agitated.

Question 21.5   Answer a
Oral pathology increases risk of aspiration of infectious material and saliva, leading to respiratory infection, which can be life threatening in vulnerable patients. Systematic reviews have shown that one in 10 deaths from pneumonia in long-term facilities for elderly adults are preventable through appropriate mouth care.

Question 21.6   Answer d
All types of dentures should be cleaned after meals to remove debris. Although overnight soaking is recommended, the choice solution will depend if the denture is made entirely of plastic materials or has metal parts; chlorhexidine can be used for dentures with metal parts. For all plastic sets, dilute sodium hypochlorite should be used.

Question 21.7   Answer d
Caries in older people can advance considerably before the person recognizes or reports a painful tooth. This is caused by secondary dentine increasing the distance from the outer surface of the tooth to the pulp; large holes can develop within teeth before they are felt.

Chapter 22

Question 22.1   Answer b
Screening questions are not reliable compared with a visual acuity tests or ophthalmologic examination; they are not accurate for identifying residents with vision impairments.

Question 22.2   Answer a
The prevalence of age-related hearing loss rises exponentially with increasing age. Studies of long-term care populations suggest prevalence rates higher than general population studies.

Question 22.3   Answer b
Acute-onset closed-angle glaucoma is an ophthalmologic emergency.

Question 22.4   Answer e
Water-based agents are preferred for softening ear wax.

Question 22.5   Answer c
Cognitive behavioral therapy improves quality of life and decreases dysphoria associated with tinnitus. It does not change the loudness or the quality of the sound.

PART 4. DISEASE MANAGEMENT

Chapter 23

Question 23.1   Answer d
The HYVET study and the Cochrane meta-analysis showed that treating fairly healthy people older than 80 years of age when the systolic blood pressure was greater than 160 mm Hg decreased subsequent heart failure. The data on decreasing mortality rates in this group are controversial.

Question 23.2   Answer c
Postprandial hypotension occurs in more than 25% of nursing home residents. It leads to falls, syncope, myocardial infarction, stroke, and increased mortality rates. Measurements by nurses are often spuriously high as shown by ambulatory blood pressure measurements.

Question 23.3   Answer b
Weight loss leads to a reduction in blood pressure, and failure to recognize this and discontinue antihypertensives is a common reason for hypotension and inappropriate medication use in nursing homes.

Question 23.4   Answer d
Sitting all day leads to pooling of fluid in the legs. Basal crepitations can be a normal finding in up to 10% of normal older persons. The absence of jugular venous distension excludes heart failure.

Question 23.5   Answer a
The blood urea nitrogen criteria for hospice referral for congestive heart failure is above 30 mg/dL (mmol/L).

Question 23.6   Answer b
Her $CHADS_2VAS_c$ score is 3, and anyone with a score of 2 or more should receive oral anticoagulation.

Question 23.7   Answer c
Blood transportation on a hot day alters INR values as do a variety of green vegetables, beef liver, and influenza vaccination.

Chapter 24

Question 24.1   Answer b
The unaffected limb performs the task in front of the mirror while the affected arm is not in view. This increases activation of the affected brain hemisphere.

Question 24.2   Answer c
Ten percent of residents in nursing homes have Parkinson's disease. Persons with Parkinson's disease cost four times more to treat. Parkinson's disease is characterized by akinesia.

Question 24.3   Answer a
Antipsychotics are antagonists of dopamine and worsen Parkinson's disease.

Question 24.4   Answer e
Botulinum toxin can stop drooling. Modafinil is used for excessive daytime somnolence. Amantadine may help fatigue. Propantheline helps excessive sweating. Midodrine is used to treat orthostasis.

Chapter 25

Question 25.1   Answer d
Paracetamol (acetaminophen) up to 4 g/day should be the initial treatment for pain caused by osteoarthritis. NSAIDs and celecoxib have more side effects than acetaminophen. Capsaicin cream can be used as an adjunctive therapy. Opioids are used when paracetamol is ineffective.

Question 25.2   Answer a
EORA is more aggressive and disabling than classical rheumatoid arthritis. Rheumatoid arthritis occurs in 2% of persons older than 60 years of age. EORA involves mainly large joints. Both diagnostic tests are present in about 80% of persons with rheumatoid arthritis.

Question 25.3   Answer c
Only Botox injections have been shown to improve range of motion and decrease caregiver burden.

Question 25.4   Answer d
Both allopurinol and colchicine need to have their doses reduced in kidney disease.

Question 25.5   Answer c
Giant cell arteritis is suggested by headaches and intermittent jaw claudication. Magnetic resonance imaging is only positive for vasculitis in one third of cases. The diagnosis is made with a temporal artery biopsy. The other findings are classical of polymyalgia rheumatica. Inclusion body myositis occurs in persons older than age 50 years and may mimic polymyalgia rheumatica. There is no synovitis or pitting edema, and pseudogout is a disorder of joints.

Question 25.6   Answer b
This is a classic description of elderly-onset rheumatoid arthritis with acute-onset large joint involvement and rapid functional decline. It is often rheumatoid factor negative. The large joint involvement and rapidity of progression suggest that this is not classical rheumatoid arthritis. Polymyalgia rheumatica mainly involves muscle. There are no skin lesions to suggest psoriasis.

Chapter 26

Question 26.1   Answer d
C-reactive protein is a sign of inflammation and is elevated in people with pneumonia. Older persons with pneumonia can have either leukopenia or leukocytosis. Although procalcitonin is not useful in older persons, an elevated level is compatible with pneumonia. Cough is often not present in persons with pneumonia.

Question 26.2   Answer c
Good-quality sputum specimens in the nursing home are obtained in about one in five residents.

Question 26.3   Answer a
BCG produces a false–positive result. All of the other possibilities produce a false-negative result.

Question 26.4   Answer d
Persons with a small previous exposure to tuberculosis or one a long time in the past may need a second injection to produce a positive test result; this is called "the booster phenomenon."

Question 26.5   Answer b
Isoniazid depletes body stores of vitamin B_6 (pyridoxine).

Question 26.6   Answer e
Making the diagnosis of urinary tract infection requires all three criteria in an older person. Elevated interleukin-γ levels in the urine may be useful. The γ-interferon in vitro test is used to diagnose tuberculosis.

Question 26.7   Answer d
Fluoroquinolones are only recommended if the resident was previously treated in the previous 3 months or if there is a high rate of resistance to the other two antibiotics.

Question 26.8   Answer a
Hyponatremia and a white blood cell count above 15 cells/mm³ are usually present when the patient has a necrotizing soft tissue infection.

Question 26.9   Answer d
Shingles is classically limited to a single dermatome. Often it starts with only a few blisters next to the spinal cord.

Question 26.10   Answer a
Although all of the answers have some merit, only regular hand washing has been shown to be cost effective in nursing homes.

Chapter 27

Question 27.1   Answer e
Anemia of chronic disease, including anemia caused by renal failure, is the most common anemia in nursing homes.

Question 27.2   Answer b
Interleukin-6 releases hepcidin from the liver that inhibits ferroportin-trapping iron in the macrophages.

Question 27.3   Answer b
All but ferritin are either normal or decreased.

Question 27.4   Answer a
These are the classic findings of hemolytic anemia.

Question 27.5   Answer d
Lenalidomide can be used to treat some forms of myelodysplasia. Red blood cells are decreased in 100% of patients. Megakaryocytes are diagnostic. Neither iron nor vitamin B_{12} is used as treatment.

Question 27.6   Answer b
Low-dose iron corrects most iron deficiency unless there is an iron absorption defect. Vitamin B_{12} can be given alone. Blood transfusions remain the primary treatment for myelodysplasia. Iron tablets inhibit absorption of other medicines and must be given alone. Epoetin alfa should not increase hemoglobin by more than 1 g/dL per month to decrease the risk of thrombosis.

Chapter 28

Question 28.1   Answer d
Blepharoptosis and atrial fibrillation strongly suggest that this is apathetic hyperthyroidism. Polymyalgia rheumatica

is associated with painful muscles. Dermatomyositis has a heliotrope rash around the eyes.

Question 28.2   Answer c
Calcium inhibits the absorption of L-thyroxine. Thyroid-hormone receptor abnormalities and primary malabsorption of L-thyroxine are extremely rare. Abnormal thyroid-stimulating hormone rarely reaches such high levels. Chronic diarrhea rarely causes loss of L-thyroxine. The other common cause is the resident not taking the L-thyroxine.

Question 28.3   Answer c
Most experts suggest an HbA_1C between 7% and 8% is less likely to produce hypoglycemia and at the same time produce minimal negative effects from the hyperglycemia.

Question 28.4   Answer b
Studies have failed to show any effect of diet in nursing home residents.

Question 28.5   Answer c
Only digoxin does not cause hyponatremia.

Question 28.6   Answer e
This person has the classical presentation of Addison's disease.

Chapter 29

Question 29.1   Answer d
Histamine-2 receptor antagonists cause mental status changes.

Question 29.2   Answer a
More than half of residents in nursing homes have pneumonia-causing gastritis as the cause of their coffee ground emesis.

Question 29.3   Answer e
Both urinary tract infections and diverticulitis should be the first diagnostic choices.

Question 29.4   Answer d
Blood glucose testing has been reported multiple times as a cause of institutional hepatitis B outbreaks.

Question 29.5   Answer d
About 10% develop cirrhosis. Hepatitis C is rarely symptomatic. Hepatocellular carcinoma incidence is increased in persons who have cirrhosis secondary to hepatitis C.

Chapter 30

Question 30.1   Answer c
Antihistamines used to reduce sinus drainage can interfere with bladder muscle function and cause acute urinary retention. β-Agonists tend not to interfere with urination. The inhaled anticholinergics, not given as an option in this question, can also decrease detrusor muscle function.

Question 30.2   Answer e
Pulmonary rehabilitation decreases fatigue and dyspnea and improves quality of life. It does not decrease hospitalization or mortality rates in nursing home residents.

Question 30.3   Answer **a**
Pulmonary embolism is greatly underdiagnosed in nursing homes.

Question 30.4   Answer **e**
Calf swelling greater than 3 cm compared with the other leg is an indication for further investigation for deep vein thrombosis in a nursing home resident.

Question 30.5   Answer **e**
Her unilateral leg swelling suggests a DVT (3 points). She has tachycardia (>100 mm; 1.5 points). She has had cancer treatment recently (1.0 points). She needs acute investigation for pulmonary embolism. Crepitations are present in persons who have had a number of small pulmonary emboli.

Chapter 31

Question 31.1   Answer **e**
Cancer residents in nursing homes get less physical, occupational, psychological, and speech therapy than other residents.

Question 31.2   Answer **d**
Cancer diagnoses are often missed and made late in the nursing home.

Question 31.3   Answer **d**
Poorly healing sores should be considered as possibly being caused by cancer.

Question 31.4   Answer **b**
Megestrol increases weight gain in cancer patients. Low albumin in persons with cancer is caused by proinflammatory cytokine excess. Insulin resistance and anemia are commonly seen in residents with cachexia.

Question 31.5   Answer **d**
Chlorambucil is a cheap drug that produces the same progression-free survival time as other drugs. Early treatment increases side effects and does not decrease mortality. Persons with CLL live from 5 to 10 years from diagnosis. The flow cytometry diagnosis of CLL requires 5000 β-lymphocytes/μL.

INDEX

Page numbers followed by *f* or *t* indicate figures or tables, respectively.